Ménière's Disease

Helmut Schaaf

Ménière's Disease

Vertigo - Hearing Loss - Tinnitus: A Psychosomatically Oriented Presentation

Springer

Helmut Schaaf
Tinnitus-Klinik
Bad Arolsen, Germany

The translation was done with the help of artificial intelligence (machine translation by the service DeepL.com). A subsequent human revision was done primarily in terms of content.

ISBN 978-3-662-63609-1 ISBN 978-3-662-63610-7 (eBook)
https://doi.org/10.1007/978-3-662-63610-7

This Springer imprint is published by the registered company Springer-Verlag GmbH, DE part of Springer Nature.
The registered company address is: Heidelberger Platz 3, 14197 Berlin, Germany

Preface to the 1st English edition

Menière's disease with its mostly unpredictable attacks of vertigo can confound people's bodies as well as their souls. Those who lose their balance, which they previously regarded as being secure and stable, very often also lose their overall assurance and confidence in other fundamental pillars of daily life which they had taken "for granted" until then.

When I began my study on Meniere's disease in 1987 due to my own desperation as a patient, I was looking for helpful information and research that would give me some reliable orientation. What I found were numerous, scholarly articles and some abstracts from symposiums. They presented the state of current, approximate knowledge in diverse and often speculative ways. What was missing was a reliable orientation for dealing with the disease and taking care of those suffering from Meniere's disease.

After a few tolerable years, in 1993, "Meniere's disease and its accompanying symptoms" threw me off track. I then had no choice but to deal intensively with the illness myself. In this way, the disease had found an author rather than an author finding a disease to study and write about.

This had its effect on my – somewhat personal – approach and style of presentation.

Therefore, this book is written for patients with Meniere's disease in the hopes of giving them an understanding of the essentials of the disease and its consequences, but also of the available possibilities and chances for compensating for these consequences.

At the same time, I have made it a point to support the medical aspects with reference to important and current scholarly publications in such a way that colleagues in the fields of medicine and psychotherapy can also find a coherent and comprehensive presentation.

Altogether, the neurotological and psychosomatic foundations should show clearly what is known, what can be implemented, and what needs to be questioned critically. I have incorporated the experience of dealing with my own suffering from Meniere's disease and decades of experience with Meniere's patients in a specialty hospital in Germany, which offered neurological as well as psychosomatic-based treatment, into this book.

The better we understand the disease and the better we can reduce the uncertainty, the more possibilities of dealing with vertigo will become apparent. Then the subsequent problems become smaller. This is especially true for the phenomena of reactive psychogenic dizziness and of the escalation of anxiety components.

This means that Meniere's disease is not a "terminal diagnosis" and not a (central) disease of the brain, as Prosper Meniere already suspected more than 160 years ago. Even if the disease itself cannot be cured, many of the effects of M. Menière can be largely compensated for or at least influenced favorably. Medical science can lay the foundation for such a therapy in this individually complex and interwoven puzzle of an illness with its various physical and psychological components.

These foundations include:
1. Diagnosis, which has been improved by the possibilities of mobile recording of nystagmus and hearing test in acute cases. The range of vestibular diagnostics has also been expanded considerably including visualization of endolymphatic hydrops in MRI-findings.
2. Education and counseling.
3. Effective mitigation of acute attacks.
4. Medical therapy between attacks, including intratympanic cortisone injections.
5. Vestibular training for rehabilitation and compensation.
6. Providing technical aids to compensate hearing loss ranging from hearing aids to cochlear implants.
7. Reduction or elimination of the function from the affected vestibular organ as a final option to stop vertigo spells.

It should be noted that false or "inadequately substantiated" promises may increase the confidence of those seeking help in the short term, but the resulting disappointment represents a serious side effect. For this purpose, the book includes a lengthy chapter on Betahistine, which is still prescribed too often as a kind of reflex action, even though it has been shown in a well-structured research by Betahistine advocates(!) that this substance is no more effective than a placebo, whether with low or high dosage.

At the same time, many questions remain unanswered, including what triggers Meniere's disease. What seems most significant to me when we look at the progression of the disease – in the absence of effective invasive intervention – is the effect of time and duration. The longer the damage to the vestibular organ progresses with the duration of the disease, the less frequent and less severe the vertigo attacks usually become. This also explains why therapeutic measures can appear more "effective" the later they are administered.

I am grateful to Springer for making it possible for me to update this book with current knowledge in Germany at foreseeable intervals and to align it with long-standing practical approaches.

I have always been able to profit from the meetings and discussions with my colleagues in Germany:
- in Arolsen, Prof. Dr. Gerhard Hesse, Dr. Georgis Kastellis, and Dagmar Beyrau;
- in Mainz, Prof. Dr. Kai Helling; in Königstein/Sulzbach, Prof. Dr. Leif Walther; and in Berlin, Prof. Dr. Thomas Lempert.

Once again, I would like to thank the staff at Springer, Monika Radecki (planning), Hiltrud Wilbertz (project management/production), and Stephanie Kaiser-Dauer (external editing) and the team of Snehal Surwade, namely Anamika Kumari and Akshay Supalkar.

Helmut Schaaf
Bad Arolsen, Germany
2021

Contents

1	**Ménière's Disease – The Clinical Picture**	1
1.1	**Vertigo, Hearing Loss, Tinnitus**	2
1.2	**An Exemplary Case – The Classical Case**	4
1.3	**Forms of Appearance**	6
1.4	**Uncertainty and (Reactive) Psychogenic Dizziness**	8
1.5	**Insecurity in the Partnership**	10
1.6	**Swindle in the Therapeutic Relationship**	10
1.7	**Suddenly One Is Affected Oneself**	11
1.8	**Is Ménière's Disease a Psychosomatic Disease?**	12
1.9	**Perspective**	14
	Literature	14
2	**Physiological and Anatomical Basics**	17
2.1	**The Vestibular Organ**	21
2.1.1	Orientation Via Gravity	21
2.1.2	Otolith Organs – Utricule and Saccule	22
2.1.3	Semicircular Canals	24
2.1.4	The Saccus Endolymphaticus and the Sinus Endolymphaticus	27
2.2	**Auditory Part**	28
2.2.1	From Sound to Nerve Impulse	28
2.2.2	From the Otolithic Organs to the Cochlea	31
2.2.3	Organ of Corti	33
2.3	**Vestibular Nerve**	34
2.4	**Vestibulo-Ocular Reflex (VOR)**	34
2.4.1	Suppression of the VOR – a Central Achievement	36
2.5	**Oculomotor System**	36
2.6	**Nystagmus**	37
2.7	**Who Is Able to Do What!**	38
2.8	**Other Conditions for Equilibrium**	39
2.8.1	Information from the Skin, Hands and Feet	39
2.8.2	The "Belly Feeling"	40
2.8.3	Heart, Lungs, Food and Drink	40
2.8.4	Implementation in Motion	40
2.9	**Interface Points in the Brain**	41
2.9.1	Advantages and Disadvantages	41
2.10	**Balance of the Soul**	42
	Literature	44
3	**Pathophysiology of Ménière's Disease**	47
3.1	**Vertigo from the Inner Ear**	49
3.1.1	Stadium Classification According to Jahnke (1994)	54
3.2	**Eye Tremor (Nystagmus) During an Acute Attack**	54
3.3	**Impaired Balance After Vertigo Attacks**	55
3.4	**Hearing Loss**	57

3.5 **Dysacusis (Distorted Hearing)** 57
3.6 **Lack of Loudness Compensation and Noise Sensitivity (Hyperacusis)** 58
3.7 **Hearing Impressions Without External Sound Source – Tinnitus** 59
3.7.1 Forms of Tinnitus 59
3.7.2 Psychological Conflicts 61
3.7.3 Tinnitus in Endolymphatic Diseases Such as Ménière's Disease 61
3.8 **Feeling of Pressure in and Behind the Ear** 62
3.9 **Sensory Sensations (Paresthesia)** 63
3.10 **Lack of Compensation and Double Inhibition** 63
3.11 **Reactive, Psychogenic Vertigo** 67
3.11.1 How Can Organic Vertigo Become Psychogenic Dizziness in Ménière's Disease? 68
3.11.2 Maintenance of Vertigo in Cases of Previous Mental Illness 74
3.11.3 Can Fear and Panic Cause Ménière's Attacks? 79
Literature 81

4 **Special Forms of Meniere's Disease** 85
4.1 **Lermoyez Syndrome** 86
4.2 **Tumarkin Drop** 86
4.3 **Cochlear Form** 87
Literature 87

5 **Differentiation from Other Clinical Pictures** 89
5.1 **A Misdiagnosis and its Treatment** 93
5.1.1 From Body to Soul and Back Again 93
5.2 **Fluctuating Hearing with Low Tone Tinnitus Without Vertigo** 96
5.2.1 Diagnosis 100
5.2.2 Therapy 100
5.3 **Migrainous Vertigo (Basilar Migraine)** 101
5.3.1 Symptomatology 102
5.3.2 Pathophysiology 103
5.3.3 Diagnostics 103
5.3.4 Treatment 103
5.4 **Benign Paroxysmal Positional Vertigo (BPPV)** 105
5.4.1 Diagnostics and Therapy 105
5.5 **Vestibular Neuritis – Acute Unilateral (Idiopathic) Vestibulopathy** 107
5.5.1 Possible Causes 107
5.5.2 Diagnostics: Complete or Partial Failure? 108
5.5.3 Therapy 109
5.5.4 Balance Training 110
5.5.5 Lack of Compensation 111
5.5.6 Possible Functional Reduction for Too Fast Movements 111
5.5.7 Hearing Impairment and Ringing in the Ears 112
5.5.8 A Subsequent Paroxysmal Positional Vertigo 112
5.5.9 Confusion in Experience 112
5.6 **Perilymph Fistula** 113
5.6.1 Diagnostics 115
5.6.2 Therapy 115

5.6.3 Excursus: Influences of Air Pressure on the Ear (Tullio Phenomenon) 116
5.6.4 Tube Ventilation Disorder 116
5.7 **Vestibular Paroxysmia** 116
5.8 **Isolated Otolith Dysfunction** 117
5.9 **Psychogenic Dizziness** 118
5.9.1 Dizziness Instead of Unpleasant Feelings 118
5.9.2 The Problem of Understanding 120
5.9.3 Where Does the Psychogenic Dizziness Take Place? 121
5.9.4 From the "Phobic Postural Vertigo" (PPV) to "Persistent Perceptual and Postural Dizziness" (3P-D) 121
5.9.5 Dizziness in Sociophobia (Social Phobia) 128
5.10 **Multiple Sclerosis** 129
5.11 **Central Vestibular Vertigo Syndrome** 130
5.11.1 Diagnostics 130
5.11.2 Prevention 131
5.12 **Blood Pressure Fluctuations** 131
5.13 **Acoustic Neuroma** 132
5.13.1 Diagnostics 132
5.14 **Bilateral Loss of Vestibular Function** 132
5.15 **Head-Extension Vertigo: Cervicogenic?** 133
5.15.1 Diagnostics 134
5.15.2 Therapy 134
5.16 **Drug-Induced Dizziness** 135
5.16.1 Gentamycin for the Elimination of Ménière's Disease 136
Literature 137

6 **Diagnostics and Examination Methods** 141
6.1 **Medical History** 144
6.2 **Balance Examination (Vestibular Examination)** 147
6.2.1 Standing and Walking Examination 147
6.3 **Examination of Eye Movement** 149
6.3.1 Suppression of the VOR 150
6.3.2 Head Impulse Test – Testing von the Vestibulo-Ocular-Reflex (VOR) 151
6.3.3 Positioning Maneuvers 152
6.3.4 Overall Evaluation of the Investigation 152
6.4 **Apparative Examination of the Semicircular Canals** 153
6.4.1 Caloric (Thermal) Test 153
6.4.2 Rotational Testing: Examination in a Swivel Chair 154
6.5 **Examination of the Otolith Organs** 155
6.5.1 Examination of the Sacculus 155
6.5.2 Examination of the Utricle 158
6.6 **Hearing Tests** 162
6.6.1 Pure Tone Audiogram 162
6.6.2 Speech Audiogram 165
6.7 **Tinnitus Determination** 165
6.8 **Otoacoustic Emission and Distortion Products** 166
6.9 **Electrocochleography** 166
6.10 **Brain-Evoked-Response Audiometry (BERA)** 167

6.11	**Glycerol Load Test (Klockhoff Test)**	167
6.12	**Manual Examination of the Vertebral Segments**	168
6.13	**Imaging Techniques**	168
6.14	**Psychological-Psychosomatic Diagnostics**	169
6.15	**Psychological Questionnaires/Test Diagnostics**	172
6.15.1	Dizziness Handicap Inventory (DHI)	172
6.15.2	Hospitality Anxiety and Depression Score (HADS)	173
6.15.3	Patient Health Questionnaire (PHQ-D)	173
6.15.4	University Research	174
6.16	**The Most Important Thing at the End: Evaluating and Assigning**	175
	Literature	177
7	**Therapy of Ménière's Disease**	179
7.1	**Enlightenment and Counselling**	182
7.1.1	Attention: Interactions Between Patient and Doctor – The Doctor–Patient Relationship	183
7.2	**Acute Therapy**	187
7.2.1	Emergency Medical Assistance: First and Second Vertigo Attack	187
7.2.2	Own Emergency Preparation	189
7.3	**Therapy Between Vertigo Attacks**	192
7.3.1	How Can Therapeutic Success Be Determined?	192
7.3.2	Proven Therapies	195
7.3.3	Non-proven Conservative Therapies	213
7.3.4	Surgical Interventions – without Proven Effect	221
7.4	**Basic Outline of Psychosomatic Treatment**	226
7.4.1	Relaxation Techniques	226
7.4.2	Psychotherapy	227
7.4.3	Psychodynamic Psychotherapy	228
7.4.4	Behavioral Therapy Approaches	229
7.4.5	Systematic Desensitization	229
7.4.6	Psychotropic Drugs	238
7.4.7	Inpatient Psychosomatic Treatment	240
7.5	**Alternatives/Outsiders: Opportunities and Threats**	242
7.5.1	Homeopathy	243
7.5.2	Acupuncture	243
	Literature	244
8	**Bilateral Disease**	249
8.1	**Consequences**	250
8.1.1	For Therapy	250
8.1.2	In Case of Bilateral Vestibular Loss	251
8.2	**Perspectives**	252
	Literature	253
9	**What Might Make a Good Therapist?**	255
9.1	**Careful Diagnostics**	257
9.2	**Comprehensible Enlightenment**	257
9.3	**Therapeutic Measures**	258

9.4 **Support and Therapy Between Vertigo Attacks** 259
9.5 **Psychological Measures** 259
9.6 **What Might Make a Good Patient?** 260
9.6.1 Factors that Can Be Influenced 260
9.6.2 Compensable Factors 260
9.6.3 And myself? 261
Literature 262

10 **Short Answers to Frequently Asked Questions** 263
10.1 **What Is Ménière's Disease?** 265
10.2 **What Causes Ménière's Disease?** 265
10.3 **How Common Is Ménière's Disease** 265
10.4 **Are Hearing Fluctuations in the Low-Frequency Range with Low Tone Tinnitus a Sign of Ménière's Disease?** 265
10.5 **Can Ménière's Disease Be Bilateral?** 266
10.6 **Is There a Cure for Ménière's Disease?** 266
10.7 **When Can Therapy Be Helpful for Ménière's Disease?** 266
10.8 **Is There a Connection Between Migraine and Ménière's Disease?** 267
10.9 **Are Ménière's Sufferers Allowed to Drive?** 267
10.10 **Are Ménière's Sufferers Allowed to Travel (Fly)?** 268
10.11 **Are Ménière's Patients Allowed to Swim and What Do they Need to Be Aware of?** 268
10.12 **Are Ménière's Sufferers Allowed to Dive?** 269
10.13 **Is Ménière's Disease Hereditary?** 269
10.14 **Does Ménière's Disease Affect Pregnancy?** 269
10.15 **Do Hearing Aids Help with Ménière's Disease?** 269
10.16 **Can Anesthesia Influence Ménière's Symptoms?** 270
10.17 **And What Other Use Is There?** 270
Literature 270

Supplementary Information
Self-help Groups 272
Glossary 273
Literature 279
Index 295

About the Author

Helmut Schaaf, MD

worked as a specialist in anesthesia in Cologne before he himself became ill with Ménière's disease. He therefore had to give up his original occupation.

He has been a senior physician in Bad Arolsen since 1994 and has been working at the Balance Institute and the Tinnitus Clinic Dr. Hesse since 2008.

He has written several books on balance, vertigo, tinnitus, and hyperacusis – in the attempt to write understandably for those concerned – as well as published numerous scientific articles.

For publications see: ► http://www.drhschaaf.de/hslit.html

Dr. med. Helmut Schaaf
Senior physician at Tinnitus Clinic Dr. Hesse, Bad Arolsen Hospital,
Große Allee 50, D-34454 Bad Arolsen Hessen, Germany
hschaaf@tinnitus-klinik.net; ► www.drhschaaf.de

Ménière's Disease – The Clinical Picture

How It Can Start – And How It May Go On

Contents

1.1 Vertigo, Hearing Loss, Tinnitus – 2

1.2 An Exemplary Case – The Classical Case – 4

1.3 Forms of Appearance – 6

1.4 Uncertainty and (Reactive) Psychogenic Dizziness – 8

1.5 Insecurity in the Partnership – 10

1.6 Swindle in the Therapeutic Relationship – 10

1.7 Suddenly One Is Affected Oneself – 11

1.8 Is Ménière's Disease a Psychosomatic Disease? – 12

1.9 Perspective – 14

Literature – 14

H. Schaaf, *Ménière's Disease*, https://doi.org/10.1007/978-3-662-63610-7_1

1.1 Vertigo, Hearing Loss, Tinnitus

Vertigo attacks, hearing loss and tinnitus are the clinical of hallmarks Meniere's disease. The incidence of Ménière's disease in industrialised countries is estimated at approximately 1:1000 (0.1%). It is also estimated that 3200–9000 new cases occur per year (Wladislavosky-Wasserman et al. 1984).

In the majority of cases, it is a disease of adulthood. Increasingly, people over the age of 60 can also be affected for the first time (Shojaku et al. 2009). Occasionally, the disease can already occur in childhood, although the diagnosis was often only confirmed during the course of the disease (Choung et al. 2006).

The vertigo usually varies from attacks lasting at least 20 minutes to severe spinning attacks lasting for hours with severe vomiting. Shorter and longer attacks probably have other causes.

▪ Benign and peripheral

In contrast to malignant tumor diseases Menière's disease is "benign" and – in distinction from diseases of the central nervous system it is a peripheral disease of the vestibular and hearing organ. In the favorable case this can take a mild course. Then the attacks of vertigo remain manageable, the hearing loss is small and one-sided, and the patient is able to cope with the ringing in the ears.

In the worst case, however, Ménière's disease can also lead to:

- serve hearing loss,
- a suffering from tinnitus,
- prolonged insecurity, helplessness, development of anxiety and panic as a result of the vertigo spells, as well as
- depressive courses.

▪ Reactive psychogenic expansion

Vertigo attacks in many cases are experienced as existentially threatening. When they occur more often, the fear of the vertigo can become so great that it is itself experienced as insecurity and dizziness and becomes an illness component in its own right. Then often a "constant" feeling of vertigo, a "psychogenic dizziness", can establish itself. These mostly gradual transitions between organically caused and (reactive) psychogenic vertigo make Ménière's disease one of the most multifaceted vertigo phenomena. It therefore requires special attention both in terms of diagnosis and therapy.

■ When is a Ménière's disease a Ménière's disease?

In 2015, five experts association agreed on two categories for classifying Ménière's disease (Lopez-Escamez et al. 2015):

- the Bárány Society, which represents an international community of basic scientists, neurootologists and other experts on equilibrium research. It was named after Robert Bárány, who received the Nobel Prize in 1914 for his work on the physiology and pathology of the vestibular organ;
- the Japan Society for Equilibrium Research;
- the European Academy of Otology and Neurotology (EAONO);
- The Equilibrium Committee of the American Academy of Otolaryngology-Head and Neck Surgery (AAO-HNS);
- the Korean Balance Society.

■ The current consensus on diagnosis: definite versus probable

The diagnosis of definite Ménière's disease is based on clinical criteria and requires the observation of an episodic vertigo syndrome associated with low- to medium-frequency sensorineural hearing loss (more than 30 dB between 250 and 2000 Hz) and fluctuating aural symptoms (hearing, tinnitus and/or fullness) in the affected ear. Duration of vertigo episodes is limited to a period between 20 minutes and 12 hours. (Lopez-Escamez et al. 2015).

Probable Ménière's disease is a broader concept defined by episodic vestibular symptoms (vertigo or dizziness) associated with fluctuating aural symptoms occurring in a period from 20 minutes to 24 hours. (Lopez-Escamez et al. 2015).

The category "possible Ménière's disease" was abandoned, probably also because in practice it had resulted in more ambiguity than certainty. It seems that this definition becomes accepted in scientific studies and publications, so it will replace the previous (older) definition of the American "Committee on Hearing and Equilibrium" from 1995. Hearing loss in the mid-frequency ranges would thus also be given more importance, albeit with higher threshold values.

In parallel, a new Ménière's classification – "hydropic inner ear disease" – is already being discussed, which would also like to take into account variants of Ménière's disease and the secondary Ménière's syndromes (Gürkov et al. 2016).

Neither the old nor the new classification names findings in the balance part. This is certainly unsatisfactory in a disease that also subjectively predominantly affects the sense of balance. But in fact, there exists not the "*one* marker" that could assure Ménière's disease alone.

Thus, further overlaps with the – frequent – vestibular migraine as well as with the rare perilymph fistulae and vestibular paroxysmia are possible (► Chap. 5), if one refers only to the criteria of the classification. Therefore, half of the diagnoses could be wrong. If one also has to estimate how many psychogenic vertigo symptoms are not identified, this leaves a very uncertain starting position for determining the diagnosis – appropriate to the disease.

Nevertheless, in the course of the disease, a puzzle of hearing and balance findings usually come together, which at least allows a more reliable assessment – and thus also more reliable therapy recommendations.

> Table 1.1 compares the diagnostic criteria defined in 2015 with the older of the "Committee on Hearing and Equilibrium" from 1995.

1.2 An Exemplary Case – The Classical Case

▪ Things buzzing around the room

The following impressive description was written in 1861 by the Prosper Menière himself.

"A Young healthy man experience, for no apparent reason, vertigo, nausea, and vomiting; an inexpressible state takes all his strength away; his pale face bathed with sweat announces a near fainting. Often the patient after feeling unsteady, falls dazed to the ground without being able to get up again. Lying on his back, he is then unable to open his eyes without seeing surrounding objects spinning around him. The slightest movement of his head increases vertigo and nausea; vomiting recurs as soon as the sick person attempts to change his position.

The patient can neither lift his head nor turn to the right or left without losing his balance; his gait becomes unsteady, he leans to one side without intending it, often he is even forced to lean against a wall. The ground seems uneven to him, he bumps against the smallest obstacles, the two legs are no longer equally skillful in going up a flight of stairs. In other words, the standing and walking muscles no longer work with their usual regularity. Every somewhat violent movement causes functional disturbances of the same kind. If, while lying down, the patient suddenly lets himself fall into a horizontal position, the bed, together with all the surrounding things, begins to move violently in a circular motion; he believes himself to be on the bridge of a ship on high sea, rocked by a mighty lurch, and immediately nausea sets in, just as in the beginning of seasickness.

Table 1.1 Comparison of international diagnostic criteria

	Diagnostic criteria of the Bárány Society and other four expert association 2015	Committee on Hearing and Equilibrium 1995
Certain Ménière's disease	–	Clinic with additional histological confirmation of endolymph hydrops
Definite Ménière's disease/	Two or more spontaneous episodes of vertigo, each lasting 20 minutes to 12 hours. Audiometrically documented low- to medium-frequency sensorineural hearing loss in one ear, defining the affected ear on at least one occasion before, during or after one of the episodes of vertigo. Fluctuating aural symptoms (hearing, tinnitus or fullness) in the affected ear. Not better accounted for by another vestibular diagnosis	Two or more episodes of vertigo of at least 20 minutes Audiometrically documented hearing loss on at least one occasion Tinnitus or aural fullness Other causes excluded
Probable Ménière's disease	Two or more episodes of vertigo or dizziness, each lasting 20 minutes to 24 hours. Fluctuating aural symptoms (hearing, tinnitus or fullness) in the affected ear. Not better accounted for by another vestibular diagnosis.	One definite episode of vertigo attack Audiometrically documented hearing loss on at least one occasion Tinnitus or aural fullness Other causes excluded
Possible Ménière's disease	–	Episodic vertigo without documented sensorineural hearing loss, fluctuating or fixed, with disequilibrium, but without definitive episodes Other causes excluded

If, on the other hand, the patient suddenly assumes a vertical posture when he gets up, the same phenomena occur, and if he wants to start moving, he turns around himself and immediately falls over. As one can then observe, his face is pale, there is a threat of fainting, his body is covered with cold sweat, and everything points to a deep fear. But it is not long before the attentive patient reports that certain phenomena have occurred, such as often strong, persistent noises in the ears, and then the hearing is wont to become perceptibly weaker on one, sometimes on both sides."

▪ Typical rotational vertigo

The rotational vertigo described here, typical of the disease, usually occurs in attacks and repeatedly. This can happen at any time of day, even at night from deep sleep. Sometimes the ringing in the ears is amplified beforehand, the hearing performance is reduced and there may be a feeling of pressure in the ear.

My own major attacks usually started in the morning. Soaking wet with sweat, waking up from bad dreams, the whole room around me turned to the right, I felt sick, I had to vomit and would have loved to jump out of one of the many windows that were turning around me, if only I could have gotten there the few meters from the bed and then still known which of the turning windows was the right one. Often enough I wished I had passed out. But the typical thing about a Ménière's attack is that there is no unconsciousness. This makes Ménière's disease very different from many other forms of shock or attacks, such as epileptic attacks. My luck was that I was usually not alone in the apartment and my fellow men could often help me.

In a major dizzy spell, nausea and vomiting predominate. The affected person is pale, cold sweaty and looks so "shocked" that during the first attack even experienced emergency doctors can misinterpret this as a circulatory collapse or possible heart attack. In the case of further attacks, the patient, if he knows about the disease, will be able to tell very precisely what is present and independently initiate the first measures with a suppository that dampens the nausea.

1.3 Forms of Appearance

And then? – After the attack, most sufferers feel insecure, weak and shattered for a long time. Afterwards, everything seems to be the same as before. What may remain are noises in the ears (tinnitus), hearing loss and the hope that this was a one-time event.

▪ First vertigo is difficult to assess

Thereafter it is important to distinguish the clinical picture from other diseases. This is not easy and so Ménière's disease, especially in its early stages, is often a diagnosis of exclusion, i.e. what remains after weighing all other possible causes.

These include first the “benign positional vertigo” and the vestibular neuritis, a “one-time loss of balance”. In the case of repeated attacks of vertigo without permanent hearing loss, one must think above all of “vestibular migraine” (▶ Chap. 5).

In Ménière’s disease, the interval until the next vertigo attack can vary greatly – sometime years. Unfortunately, much shorter intervals between attacks are also possible. These can be months, weeks or even just days.

In most cases, the severity and length of organically induced vertigo decrease over time. In the absence of surgery or treatment with gentamycin (▶ Chap. 7), long studies suggest that Ménière’s disease seems to reach a plateau where the number of vertigo attacks decreases and their intensity weakens or even disappears in more than 75% of patients. This appears to be somewhere between the first onset and the 9-year mark (Stahle et al. & Kitahara in: Huang 1991). This may be due to the fact that the vestibular organ loses more and more of its function with time and especially with each attack. In addition, however, it is possible that if one has good processing abilities and capacities, one can still find ways to cope with the disease (Tyrrell et al. 2015). Nevertheless, even this is not certain, at least not in the experience of patients.

What is “certain” is that the character of the vertigo changes over time. More often than in people without M. Menière’s disease, a so-called “benign paroxysmal positional vertigo” can occur. This is then – too often – misjudged as part of Meniere’s disease. If it is not recognized, it is not treated properly.

Even more often, a psychogenic event “overlays” Meniere’s disease – which can also lead to unfavorable additional fears (van Esch et al. 2016).

▪ "Tumarkin events": rarely in the late stage

Not quite as often, a so-called “Tumarkin” can occur in the late stages.

More often, in the course of life, the rare Menière disease is joined by other, more common diseases with effects on the vestibular system. This can be misjudged with Ménière’s disease, which is already known in this patient, and therefore may not be treated appropriately.

▪ Fluctuating hearing loss

In addition to vertigo, two other important symptoms of Ménière’s disease are a fluctuating hearing loss, typically in the low-frequency range, and a predominantly low-frequency roaring or rushing in the ears. Both symptoms can be a lasting reminder of a violent event in the attack-free interval.

Often the hearing loss fluctuates and makes hearing difficult, but still possible. Hearing then benefit from proper hearing aids. However, hearing loss may extend from the low-frequency range to the higher frequencies. This mostly stops in hearing loss around 60 dB. This can lead to a restriction of directional hearing, which is only possible with both ears. So usually residual hearing is preserved (Morgenstern 1985; Savastano et al. 2006), which can be used for hearing aid fitting.

▪ Distorted hearing

Speed and severity of the progression vary greatly from individual to individual. The hearing impairment is perceived as unpleasant, especially in the area of speech. Sounds can be distorted and music heard dissonantly (dysacusis).

▪ Low-frequency tinnitus

The roaring, rushing and ringing in the ears (medical term: tinnitus) is typically perceived in the low-frequency area. In the further course, however, whistling and hissing may develop, especially in the case of failures in the high-frequency range. Character and intensity can change – this is also typical for Ménière's disease.

Usually the suffering from vertigo is dominates. Something unpleasant is displaced by something worse. Nevertheless, tinnitus can be disturbing during the attack-free period – often even more then the hearing loss.

▪ Feeling of pressure and fullness in the ear (aural fullness)

Many Ménière's sufferers experience a feeling of pressure or fullness in the affected ear or in the area of the mastoid, that can be felt directly behind the earlobe. This feels like a middle ear infection, sometimes even associated with a stinging sensation that can radiate to the affected side of the face.

▪ Hypersensitivity to noise

Despite hearing loss, the hearing may temporarily – seemingly paradoxically – become particularly sensitive to loud noises. This is especially true for the low-frequency range, which is also affected by the hearing loss.

1.4 Uncertainty and (Reactive) Psychogenic Dizziness

The consequences for normal life can hardly be described if the vertigo occurs in attacks, unpredictably and above all frequently. So Ménière's disease can then lead to considerable impairment of life.

Even if patients do not experience any organically caused vertigo further, they often feel no longer sure of themselves. Whereas it used to be a matter of course to be able to rely on one's balance, remains now uncertainty as to how the day, the week, the month could turn out.

Without the reliability of one's senses, there is a risk of being thrown off track. This has consequences for living with a partner, for friends and acquaintances, and for many everyday activities that are otherwise taken for granted – from brushing teeth to shopping. In addition, there is a loss of driving and often also of job security. In the meantime, the affected person appears to most acquaintances to be too healthy for the severity of the burden to be taken seriously. During an attack, on the other hand, the others often believe they are looking at a drunkard rather than a serious emergency, so that help is rarely expected here either.

■ Fearful observation

Frequent consequences are anxious observations, sometimes panic, when another attack threatens to announce itself. This can lead to depressive processing with social withdrawal and isolation, which can be intensified by the lack of understanding of the environment. If the vertigo, experienced as existentially threatening, occurs more often, the fear of recurrence understandably also grows. If the fear persists, it can also inhibit the processing of balance impulses (Balaban et al. 2011, Staab 2012). Thus, fear also delays the recovery of the vestibular system.

■ "Constant" dizziness

At the same time, fear can become so dominant that it itself is experienced as uncertainty and dizziness up to a feeling of spinning vertigo. In this way it becomes an additional component. Beyond the pure attacks, a "constant" feeling of dizziness can become noticeable. Medically and psychologically, this is called "psychogenic dizziness". If Ménière's disease occurs first and then the psychogenic dizziness, this is called " reactive psychogenic dizziness".

Affected persons often describe it like this: they are unsteady, wobbly, twitchy, confused in the head, have a droning feeling and fear, often a lot of fear. Whole days are now "Meniere days". In certain situations, this feeling, combined with fear and panic, can be experienced like an inner ear evoked Ménière's attack.

If the job is in danger or lost, relationships break up or wear down, the question of the meaning of one's own existence often arises.

"Already this morning, as soon as I put my foot on the floor in front of the bed, I realized it was going to be another one of those days. The first thought that comes to mind is escape," describes a Ménière's patient impressively. "I feel like a stork in a salad. With spindly, wooden legs I push myself to the bathroom ... All the mundane things of morning personal hygiene become torture – today I can't look out the window because the steps to the window are too difficult. I don't like to think about being sick. I don't feel sick either. My world has just become different. And then there are days that cruelly remind me of my new life first thing in the morning. Then the thought is also there again, how beautiful it was, all that I once could do. How nice it was to be an acquaintance in family, friends and neighbors. One who was no different from them." (Kraft 1992).

1.5 Insecurity in the Partnership

Ménière's disease not only affects the sufferer, but usually also the persons who live with the sufferer. Often it is the social and family environment that decides whether the disease can be coped and whether and how the affected person can be supported.

In the case of a joint depressive processing of the illness, the partner withdraws like the ill relative. In this course of the illness, social contacts are increasingly reduced; the circle of friends shrinks. As a result, important opportunities for regeneration and social support are lost.

More favorable is, if the partner is both enlightened and supportive, can help with attacks and pushes the sufferer when he avoids more than is necessary. The prerequisite is that the sufferer shows a lot of personal responsibility and takes the burden that the partner shares seriously. Both should not fail to explore coping options in order to be able to address changes in the course of the disease (Praetorius 1995).

1.6 Swindle in the Therapeutic Relationship

Even "simpler" vertigo disorders can trigger many different, often contradictory (ambivalent) feelings, not only in those affected, but also in therapists. These range from insecurity and helplessness to feelings of protectiveness and anger. This is especially the case if causes for a dizziness goes beyond the organic and are not clearly recognizable. In such cases, doctors in particular are seldom sure: sometimes they can even feel "swindled". At the same time, they feel the patients' expectations and pressure to do something helpful in any case.

▪ Contradictory feelings

Sometimes it happens that they – although they have found nothing in their field of expertise – nevertheless try to help with their means in order to leave nothing undone. Then, in the best effort (!), something unfavorable is done in the "mutual" distress (patient and doctor), for example, an ear is operated, although this was only the expression, but not the cause of the vertigo. After that, one also has – really – an organic problem in addition to the mental one. Occasionally there is also an angry and ultimately "dismissive" reaction – born of helplessness: "I have found nothing" – instead of – more correctly: "I have found nothing in my field", which can be allowed.

Then patients are "sent away" to the "specialized" colleagues of neurology, otorhinolaryngology, orthopedics and internal medicine, but also psychiatry. Until there is no one left to "refer", patients with vertigo often go through a true odyssey from doctor to doctor or "healers".

▪ The puzzle must be put together

Often someone is missing who can put together the variety of the "nothing" in the physical realm and the "so different" mental realm into a picture which then again enables steps of action. Also, a psychotherapist needs a clear, secure, firm idea of what lies ahead. Otherwise he is in danger of becoming dizzy together with the patient However, such a therapist must also be sought by the patient. However, this can often only become possible when the patients face the challenge of rearranging their own "coordinate system" and, if necessary, changing the direction of their lives. This could be the most important step on the way to an improved equilibrium.

1.7 Suddenly One Is Affected Oneself

I myself lost my job as an anesthetist with my Ménière's disease. After two violent attacks within half a year, I initially believed that the usual tablets and relaxation procedures would be enough to deal with the misery. Seven years later I was shaken so often and violently that I couldn't manage my normal workload. Months later, when then – as I know (only) today (!) – an increasingly psychogenic dizziness and a depressive exhaustion were added, nothing worked at all.

After half a year of inability to work, my employer gave me notice. I thought I no longer had any place in this world. It took me a year of intensive therapeutic support to get back on my feet. At the end gentamycin stopped the organically vertigo attacks. It took me years to see for myself that all this ultimately also initiated a positive turnaround for me, even if I would have wished for less dizzying drama.

▪ Self-help groups

A circle of friends, which can now prove to be sustainable or become very small, is immensely supportive. Self-help groups are also beneficial.

However, the step into the self-help groups seems to be even more difficult than with "pure" tinnitus diseases. This is certainly also due to the nature of the disease: in dizziness distress, one does not get out of the door, and when one is well, the tendency to just want to be left alone is great. As a result, the insecurity caused by the disease can also be perpetuated in missing interpersonal and organizational contacts.

▪ A prominent victim

A prominent victim of this disease was Martin Luther. In 1530, Martin Luther saw the work of Satan in his Ménière's disease, which had not yet been recognized and named in this way: "I thought it had been the black shaggy companion from hell, who probably does not like me in his kingdom on earth ...". ... "No one believes me how much torment the dizziness, the ringing and buzzing of the ears causes me. I do not dare to read for an hour without interruption, nor to think or contemplate anything clearly, for immediately the ringing is there, and I sink down the length of it." (Feldmann et al. 1998).

1.8 Is Ménière's Disease a Psychosomatic Disease?

If, with Lamparter (2002), psychosomatic vertigo is taken to mean phenomena in which the symptom of vertigo is directly "organically" caused, but in which psychological factors play a significant role in the maintenance, aggravation and possibly even the development of the underlying clinical picture, then Ménière's disease is a psychosomatic vertigo.

▪ Disturbed inner ear processes, different ways of coping

Ménière's disease is clearly explained by disturbed processes in the inner ear. Obviously, however, the extent and nature of the disease experience and suffering depend not only on the number and duration of Ménière's attacks, but also to a significant extent on the coping abilities of the affected person.

Thus, there are:
- Ménière's sufferers who are quickly back on their feet after the attack and a relatively short period of rest and tick off the attack
- Ménière's disease sufferers who are distressed for a long time afterwards and relive the event depressively
- Ménière's sufferers who are anxiously awaiting the next attack, so that the anxiety and psychogenic dizziness component becomes the decisive part of Ménière's disease

The compensable consequences include:
- Hearing loss
- Experience of the disease
- Social impact
- Interpersonal intrusions and challenges

Factors that can be influenced include:
- Extension of the vertigo coming from the inner ear to psychogenic vertigo with its – possible – repercussions on the inner ear events
- Psychologically treatable constellations that lead to vertigo and – perhaps also via a tension that does not dissipate – to alterations in the inner ear.
- Mixing with other forms of vertigo (positional vertigo, migraine, anxiety disorders, blood pressure fluctuations, visual defects, etc.)

It is important for each individual Ménière's disease patient to understand as many parts as possible of his complex "Ménière's disease", in order to tackle, what can be changed or at least compensated and improved and to accept, what cannot be changed, even if it is often very painful and difficult. Then the necessary help can be requested and accepted and perhaps some detours can be avoided.

■ Possibilities for improvement exist

Often – until proven otherwise – there is still a chance for improvement. This may include balance training, improvement of the hearing situation and for all of which it may also make sense to seek professional help.

Thus, whoever has read this book is – unfortunately – not cured, but he at least knows what he is ill with, and this knowledge could be helpful in order not to additionally intensify fear and despair, as justified and understandable as they may be.

1.9 Perspective

Tyrrell and his co-authors (Tyrrell et al. 2015) were able to analyze health data from the English "UK Biobank" of 1376 individuals assessed as having Ménière's disease and compare them with data from 500,000 other individuals. The UK Biobank is supported by the English National Health Service as a not-for-profit institution with the aim of prevention. Between 2000 and 2010, it was able to motivate 500,000 people in England between the ages of 40 and 69 to take part in a screening. Participants were interviewed by a trained nurse using a questionnaire, and laboratory data were collected. A "Ménière's disease group" was formed on the basis of the data on dizziness, hearing disorders and tinnitus.

As expected, the Ménière's disease group had a significantly higher incidence and longer duration of depression, fatigue, tension and dejection than the control group. They visited a doctor more often for depression or anxiety disorders and took antidepressants more frequently. Health satisfaction was also experienced as reduced in the Ménière's disease group.

> In other aspects of life, *however,* such as general cheerfulness, work, family, friends and financial aspects, the Ménière's patients did *not* differ from the control group.

The evidence on mental health and well-being showed a clear correlation with the duration of the disease. For example, patients with longer-standing Ménière's disease symptoms performed significantly better than those with a more recent problem. This indicates in the longitudinal correlation that there may be adaptation strategies that help long-term sufferers to cope better with the disease and significantly reduce the highly understandable psychological impairments. The authors suggest that increased social support and social interaction may contribute to a satisfying way of coping with life despite the symptomatology (Tyrrell et al. 2015).

Accordingly, the support of the social environment is seen as very important, and it is logically advised that relatives should also be involved in counselling.

Literature

Balaban CD, Jacob RG, Furman JM (2011) Neurologic bases for comorbidity of balance disorders, anxiety disorders and migraine: neurotherapeutic implications. Expert Rev Neurother 11(3):379–394. https://doi.org/10.1586/ern.11.19

Choung YH, Park K, Kim CH, Kim HJ, Kim K (2006) Rare cases of Menière's disease in children. J Laryngol Otol 120(4):343–352

Committee on Hearing and Equilibrium (1995) Guidelines for the diagnosis and evaluation of therapy in Menière's disease. Otolaryngol Head Neck Surg 113:181–185

Feldmann H, Lennarz H, von Wedel H (1998) Tinnitus, 2. Aufl. Thieme, Stuttgart

Gürkov R, Pyyko I, Zou J, Kentala E (2016) What is Menière's disease? A contemporary re-evaluation of endolymphatic hydrops. J Neurol 263(Suppl 1):71–81

Huang TS (ed) (1991) Menière's disease: recent advances in basic and clinical aspects. Acta Otolaryngol Suppl 485:7–154

Kraft R (1992) Das Schleifchen. Tinnitus Forum 4:89

Lamparter U (2002) Schwindel. In: Ahrens S, Schneider W (Hrsg) Lehrbuch der Psychotherapie und psychosomatischen Medizin, 2. Aufl. Schattauer, Stuttgart, S. 354–361

Lopez-Escamez JA, Carey J, Chung WH, Goebel JA, Magnusson M, Mandalà M, Newman-Toker DE, Strupp M, Suzuki M, Trabalzini F, Bisdorff A (2015) Diagnostic criteria for Menière's disease. J Vestib Res 25(1):1–7. https://doi.org/10.3233/VES-150549

Morgenstern C (1985) Pathophysiologie, Klinik und konservative Therapie der Menièreschen Erkrankung. Arch Otorhinolaryngol 1:1–66

Praetorius C (1995) Krankheitserleben und Bewältigungsformen bei Morbus Menière-Patienten. Neuthor, Michelstadt

Savastano M, Guerrieri V, Marioni G (2006) Evolution of audiometric pattern in Menière's disease: long-term survey of 380 cases evaluated according to the 1995 guidelines of the American Academy of Otolaryngology-Head and Neck Surgery. J Otolaryngol 35(1):26–29

Shojaku H, Watanabe Y, Yagi T, Takahashi M, Takeda T, Ikezono T, Ito J, Kubo T, Suzuki M, Takumida M, Takeda N, Furuya N, Yamashita H (2009) Changes in the characteristics of definite Menière's disease over time in Japan: a long-term survey by the peripheral vestibular disorder research Committee of Japan, formerly the Menière's disease research Committee of Japan. Acta Otolaryngol 129(2):155–160

Staab J (2012) Chronic subjective dizziness. Continuum 18(5):1118–1141

Tyrrell J, White MP, Barrett G, Ronan N, Phoenix C, Whinney DJ, Osborne NJ (2015) Mental health and subjective well-being of individuals with Ménière's: cross-sectional analysis in the UK Biobank. Otol Neurotol 36(5):854–861. https://doi.org/10.1097/MAO.0000000000000732

van Esch BF, van Benthem PPG, van der Zaag-Loonen HJ, Bruintjes TD (2016) Two common second causes of dizziness in patients with Menière's disease. Otol Neurotol

Wladislavosky-Wasserman P, Facer GW, Mokri B (1984) Menière's disease: a 30–year epidemiologic and clinical study in Rochester, Mn, 1951–1980. Laryngoscope 94:1098–1102

Physiological and Anatomical Basics

What Happens in the Vestibular and in the Auditory System?

Contents

2.1 The Vestibular Organ – 21
2.1.1 Orientation Via Gravity – 21
2.1.2 Otolith Organs – Utricule and Saccule – 22
2.1.3 Semicircular Canals – 24
2.1.4 The Saccus Endolymphaticus and the Sinus Endolymphaticus – 27

2.2 Auditory Part – 28
2.2.1 From Sound to Nerve Impulse – 28
2.2.2 From the Otolithic Organs to the Cochlea – 31
2.2.3 Organ of Corti – 33

2.3 Vestibular Nerve – 34

2.4 Vestibulo-Ocular Reflex (VOR) – 34
2.4.1 Suppression of the VOR – a Central Achievement – 36

2.5 Oculomotor System – 36

2.6 Nystagmus – 37

2.7 Who Is Able to Do What! – 38

2.8 Other Conditions for Equilibrium – 39
2.8.1 Information from the Skin, Hands and Feet – 39
2.8.2 The "Belly Feeling" – 40
2.8.3 Heart, Lungs, Food and Drink – 40
2.8.4 Implementation in Motion – 40

H. Schaaf, *Ménière's Disease*, https://doi.org/10.1007/978-3-662-63610-7_2

2.9 Interface Points in the Brain – 41
2.9.1 Advantages and Disadvantages – 41

2.10 Balance of the Soul – 42

Literature – 44

■ **Endolymphatic Hydrops**

In Ménière's patients, there is an increase in the pressure of the (endolymphatic) fluid in the auditory and vestibular ducts in the inner ear. Medically, this fluid congestion – is called "endolymphatic hydrops" (◘ Fig. 2.1a, b).

This is presumably the result of an imbalance between the production and removal of fluid in the inner ear ducts. A reduced performance of the endolymphatic sac (saccus endolymphaticus), which is responsible for the removal of the fluid, seems to be responsible for this. As a result, the finely tuned system of sensory perception can be disturbed, leading to a veritable chaos in the vestibular organ as well as to disturbances and failures in the organ of hearing. This manifest themselves in typically unpredictable, vertigo attacks, in hearing loss and in ringing or roaring in the ears, as well as aural fullness and a sensation of pressure in or behind the ear. This can have effects on the whole person in the experience of vertigo, hearing loss, suffering from tinnitus and may induce a development of anxiety with insecurity and depressive processing.

> The vestibular system comprises much more than the two organs of balance in the inner ear, which are mirror images of each other.

Important players of the balance system are (◘ Fig. 2.2):

- Two eyes capable of receiving an image of space, self and external motion, and acceleration
- Skin and touch organs, which can register an immediate impression of the environment

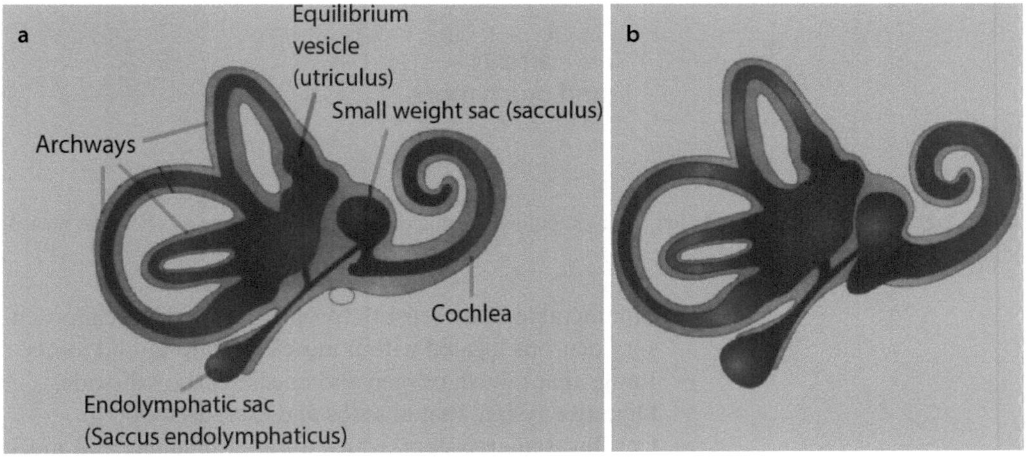

◘ **Fig. 2.1** Schematic representation of the endolymphatic situation. **a** Inconspicuous situation with normally wide endolymphatic ducts; **b** hydrops with widened endolymphatic ducts

2

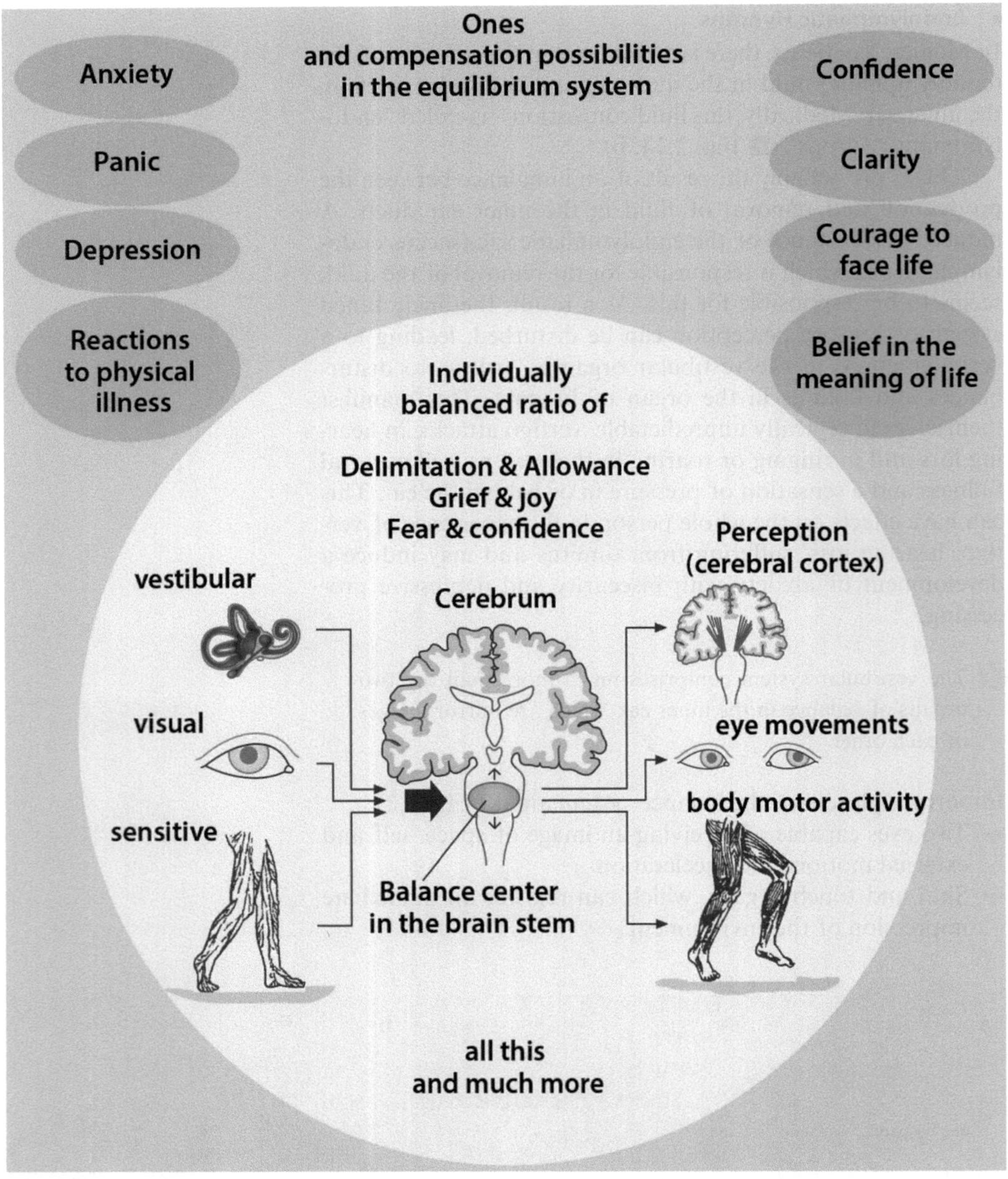

Fig. 2.2 The balance system. Incoming information, clearing in the equilibrium center (vestibular nuclei), outgoing information

- Innumerable body sensors (proprioceptors), mechanosensory neurons located within muscles, tendons, and joints
- Lungs that take in oxygen and release carbon dioxide,
- Digestive system that absorbs and excretes food,
- Cardiovascular system, which allows exchange, and much more to keep the organs alive

- Nervous system that transmits the perceived impressions to the brain (afferent) and the impulses from the brain (efferent) to the end organs.
- Brain that, on a long evolutionary basis, coordinates all sensory impressions in the brainstem and responds with reactions and movement
- Courage, hope and confidence, so that what is feasible can also be wanted and tackled.
- Fellow human beings who can make life possible, difficult and beautiful in the first place

The Balance: Constant Interaction of Many Individual Components

What we experience as "balance" is the result of the continuous interplay of demands and a meaningful reaction to them, *which* must be constantly maintained and renewed. In addition, there must be their integration at all levels of the central nervous system. An acute failure of a component can upset the balance and cause vertigo, dizziness, unsteadiness or others forms of missing balance.

If this short explanation is sufficient as a first orientation, you can "skip" the following deepening into the topic and read on directly in ► Chap. 3.

For many, however, it is important to understand as precisely as possible what is organically known so far, in order to gain as much clarity as possible. For these and those who may want to know more later, the basics of the vestibular system, the structure and functioning of the inner ear will be presented in its basic features.

This initially leads to a – despite efforts to the contrary –, to a sometimes not so easy walk up to the "labyrinth", as the inner ear structures are called.

2.1 The Vestibular Organ

2.1.1 Orientation Via Gravity

Those who want to orient themselves in space depend on getting "an impression" of gravity and a picture of their immediate and nearer surroundings. Even single-celled sea dwellers incorporated limestone particles into their organism. Although this made them less mobile, it enabled them to orientate themselves about "below" and – thus automatically – also "above" (◘ Fig. 2.3).

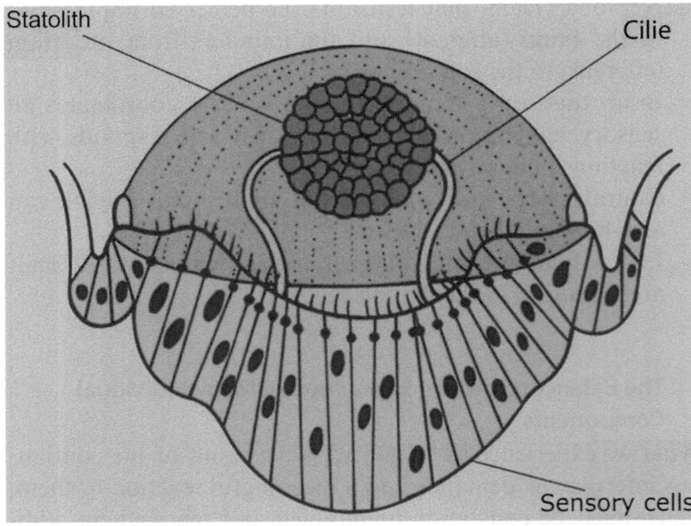

Fig. 2.3 Image of a hollow animal about 600 million years ago. A calcareous body in the middle of a gelatinous mass shows connections to simple sensory cells. (From: Scherer 1997)

Here, as so often in life, an initially obviously "severe" disadvantage compared to the others ultimately turned out to be an opportunity for development. Thus, the perception of gravity via the increase of density in the cell system was a first step in the development towards an increasingly complex equilibrium system. After perception surfaces for above and below had been established, it was only a smaller step to develop the same sensitive perception surfaces – perpendicular to them – for left and right as well.

- **Limestones Point the Way**

This principle of perception of above and below as well as left and right has proved so successful that this basic element of the limestones is also found in highly complex vestibular systems of birds and mammals.

2.1.2 Otolith Organs – Utricule and Saccule

In the human vestibular organ, two small "sacs" are found.

The evolutionary oldest part is called utricle (utriculus (lat. small tube)) because of its somewhat tubular appearance, the later added saccule (sacculus (lat. small bag)). Utricle and saccule are placed approximately in a parasagittal orientation (plane). With 12–16 mm^3 they take up just the space of a coffee bean (Lang 2003).

▪ Protected in the Hardest Bone of the Human Body

In humans, about 30,000 calcium crystals (*otoliths*) are embedded in a gelatinous membrane (macula) in both organ parts. Due to these crystals, the density of the membrane is considerably higher. In the gelatinous wall, an association of sensory hair cells (med.: maculae) receives the impulses of the otoliths, which change depending on the movement in space (◘ Fig. 2.4).

Humans have about 33,000 sensory cells in the macula utriculi and about 18,000 sensory cells in the macula sacculi. Two different types of vestibular sensory cells can be distinguished according to both their appearance and their function: Type I, which is amphora-shaped in appearance, is surrounded by thick relay fibers and tends to mediate high frequencies (phasic dynamic). The elongated cylindrical-looking type II is coupled by thin fibers and transmits slow (tonic) frequencies (see ◘ Fig. 2.4).

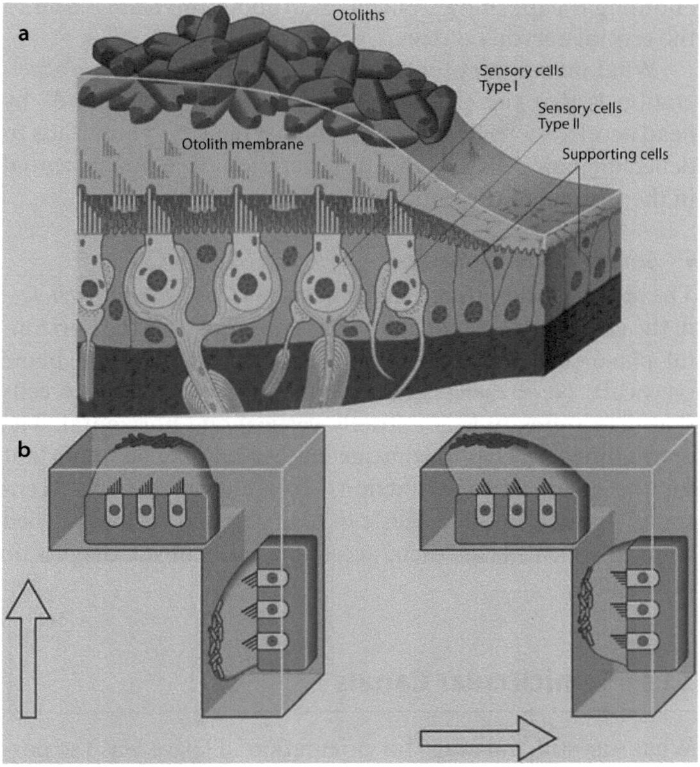

◘ **Fig. 2.4** **a** Macula in the otolithic organs saccule and utricle; **b** deflection of the sensory hairs of the macular organs in saccule and utricle by displacement during linear accelerations, vertically in saccule, horizontally in utricle. (From: Boenninghaus and Lenarz 2007)

The sensory cells also react in the vestibular part to acoustic stimuli and differently depending on the frequency. Thus, the vestibular evoked potentials can be derived from a broad spectrum in a frequency spectrum of approximately 100 Hz to 4000 kHz (Walther and Cebulla 2015). In this context, the sensory epithelium in the vestibular organ not only contains nerve pathways that report external impressions to the central nervous system (afferent), but nerve pathways from the central nervous system to the vestibular organ (efferent) are also found. The ratio of afferent to efferent fibers is 500–10,000; this corresponds to a ratio of 1:20 (Lang 2003). This means that these sensory organs are also subject to control from the central nervous system and certainly also the "limbic system", in which, the emotional parts of perception are controlled and responded to, usually without this being conscious in detail.

The Balance System Never Sleeps

The "gravity" of the earth's is conveyed via the small crystals in the utricle and the saccule sacs as basic information ("resting tone"). Even when the body is at rest, i.e. when actually "nothing is happening", information about this state is sent to the central nervous system.

What makes the otolith hair cells sensitive to linear acceleration is that the gelatinous membrane is "left behind" by head accelerations because of its higher density. Thus, leads to deflecting hair cells and this to generation of action potential in the vestibular afferents (◘ Fig. 2.4).

Sensory Cells "Deflected"

The sensory fields are arranged in such a way that the *utricle* – in the case of an upright gait – sense accelerations the horizontal plane (left *and* right) and the *saccule* the upright plane (vertical). Nevertheless, the orientation of the sensory cells that detect gravity is not strictly vertical and horizontal. The orientations overlap to some extent, which may be important for the compensatory functions. In addition, the two "centrally" located sensory cells can also respond to low-pitched sounds, which makes them accessible for acoustic diagnostic procedures.

2.1.3 Semicircular Canals

What was still "missing" for orientation in space was the possibility to detect rotational movements. For this purpose, a construction consisting of three fluid-filled tubes has been established in the course of evolution. In humans, these are designed as "semicircular canals" (◘ Fig. 2.5).

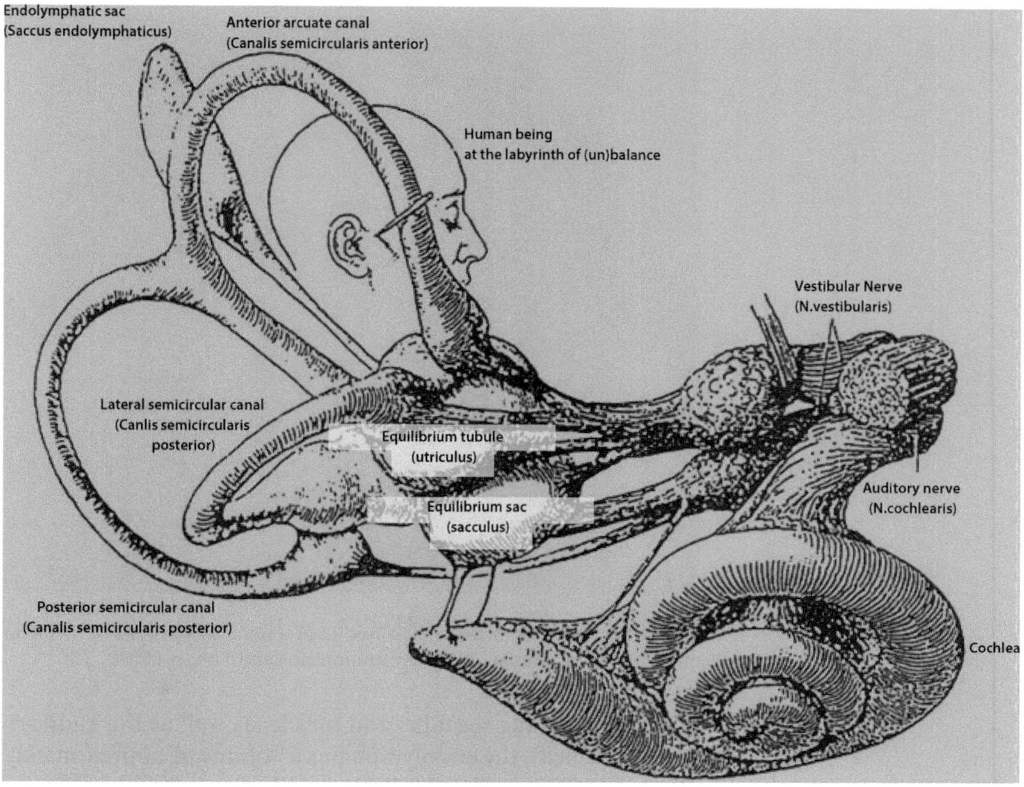

Fig. 2.5 Right membranous labyrinth and the associated human being

There are three semicircular canals on each side, one horizontal and two verticals. They are positioned approximately orthogonally and so they can sense angular movements in any plane and direction. These semicircular canals are complementary on each side of the head, so that head movements are complementary signaled by a pair of functional canals (Bronstein and Lempert 2017).

Endolymph and Perilymph

The semicircular canals take about 0.2 × 0.3 mm in diameter. Each canal has an open end, which communicates freely with the vestibule, and an enlarged ampullary end, where the sensory epithelium, the cupula, is housed (Fig. 2.6).

The cupula is a gelatinous conglomerate of sensory hair cells. It is the bending of the cupula, and therefore of the hair or cilia, that generates impulses to the vestibular nerve.

The fluid in this tube is called endolymph, and the surrounding fluid is called perilymph.

The semicircular canals are filled with a total of 3–5 µl of endolymph (lymph = fluid; inside = endo) (Michel 1998).

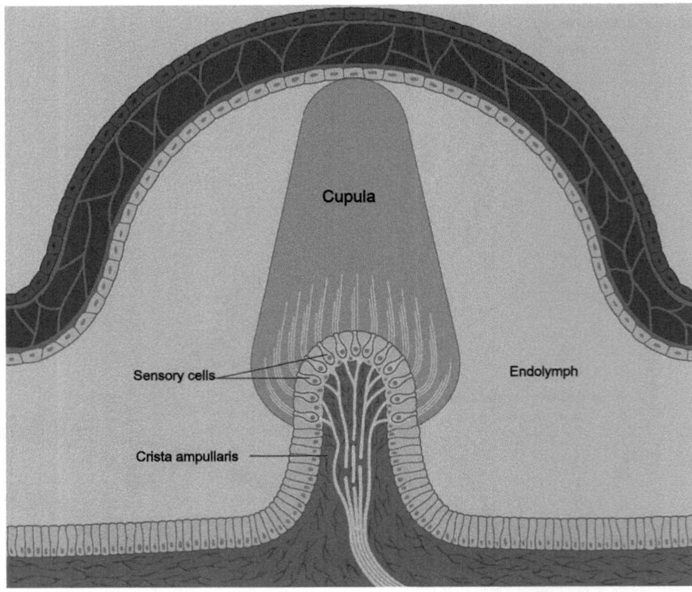

■ **Fig. 2.6** Section through the ampulla of a semicircular canal with crista ampullaris and cupula. (From: Boenninghaus and Lenarz 2007)

Together with the sacculus and utricle, as well as the auditory canal (cochlea), the endolymph has a volume of approximately 20 µl. This can triple in full-blown Meniere's disease (Morita et al. 2009). The endolymph fluid is rich in potassium (about 145 mmol/l) and resembles the fluid in cells. The endolymph is produced in a small area (in the planum semilunatum) by the so-called vascular strip (the stria vascularis) at the base of the ampulla. The perilymph surrounding the membranous canal has a volume of 12–16 µl. Its composition is similar to that of the fluid in the blood vessels and it contains a lot of sodium (about 140 mmol/l).

What make the cupula bend is the pressure exerted by endolymph during head rotation?

If, for example, the head is rotated from its resting position, the semicircular canals, which are firmly anchored in the skull, are also rotated. The fluid in the arcades, however, initially remains at rest because of its inertia. This causes the sensory cells, which are firmly attached to the canal wall, to be oriented in the opposite direction like a taut membrane.

One can imagine the semicircular canals simplified as three spirit levels aligned in all directions of space. Instead of an air bubble in the spirit level, there is a gelatinous body in the ampoule – as a movable "reading unit".

The movement of the sensory cells produces a change in the nerve impulses compared to the rest signal, which is sent towards the brain. This happens simultaneously in the three arcades, which are placed in the main directions of the room.

▪ Acceleration Leads to Increased Pulse Rate

At the beginning of a movement, the forces acting on the sensory cells are greatest. But when an acceleration becomes a sustained speed, as in the case of a vehicle that starts quickly at first and then continues "at the same speed", the semicircular canal with its fluid is turned just as quickly as the gelatinous dome. Then the uniform movement is perceived just like a rest position.

> The five parts of the vestibular organ can react to the smallest and fastest accelerations, but they adjust to uniform movements.

A movement triggers a change in the rest pattern (potential) in the semicircular canals of the two – opposite – vestibular organs. These behave mirror-inverted to each other:

- An angular momentum to the same side triggers an increased momentum rate in the responsible arcade ("*on*").
- An angular momentum to the opposite side, on the other hand (and compared to the resting tone), causes a reduced signal rate ("*off*").

Thus, a horizontal acceleration of the head to the left triggers

- an increased pulse rate of the left and mirror-inverted
- a reduced pulse rate of the right horizontal arcade

This gives the brainstem two pieces of information: something is moving towards one side *and* something is moving away from the other. This is also important for compensation in the case of balance damage. Each of the six arcades (three on each side) has a fixed direction of rotation.

The ability of each semicircular canal to react differently to changes in its side and the opposite side provides a basis for the phenomenon of equilibrium compensation.

2.1.4 The Saccus Endolymphaticus and the Sinus Endolymphaticus

The saccus endolymphaticus is normally responsible for endolymph clearance and reabsorption. Moreover, according to Plontke and Gürkov (2015), animal data indicate a capacity of the saccus endolymphaticus for secretory activity at low endolymph volume. That is, the portion of the vestibular organ responsible for removing endolymph could also help compensate for lack of volume. Different cell types are activated in the saccus endolymphaticus. In addition, it now seems sure that immunological processes of the inner ear take place here (Rudack 1995).

In the event of a locally excessive or reduced endolymph pressure, the directional valve systems in the endolymph ducts restore the balance by longitudinal flow of the endolymph. In addition, the hormone vasopressin and natriuretic peptide appear to influence pressure regulation (Salt and Plontke 2010).

Anatomically, the endolymphatic sinus corresponds to a membrane structure at the initial part of the endolymphatic duct, where the duct from the utricle and the duct from the sacculus meet.

▪ Pressure Equalization Between Endo- and Perilymph

Depending on the current endolymph volume and the associated pre-expansion of the sinus, a greater or lesser amount of endolymph can be transported via the endolymphatic duct into the endolymphatic saccus via this structure – as with a valve with flow limitation – in the event of low-frequency pressure fluctuations (e.g. caused by swallowing or contractions of middle ear muscles). Thus, when endolymph volume is low, endolymph transport into the endolymphatic duct may be limited. Conversely, more endolymph could be transported into the endolymphatic duct when endolymph volume is high. Thus, according to Plontke and Gürkov (2015), the endolymphatic sinus could be involved in the regulation and control of aberrant endolymph volume.

Westhofen (2009) points out that in healthy individuals at rest there is almost no pressure difference between endolymph and perilymph.

2.2 Auditory Part

2.2.1 From Sound to Nerve Impulse

Hearing means receiving, processing and recognizing sound signals. Sound waves first pass through the outer ear to the eardrum. The impulses to the eardrum are transmitted via small ossicles to the inner ear. In the process, the sound impressions are amplified 18–22 times (▪ Fig. 2.7).

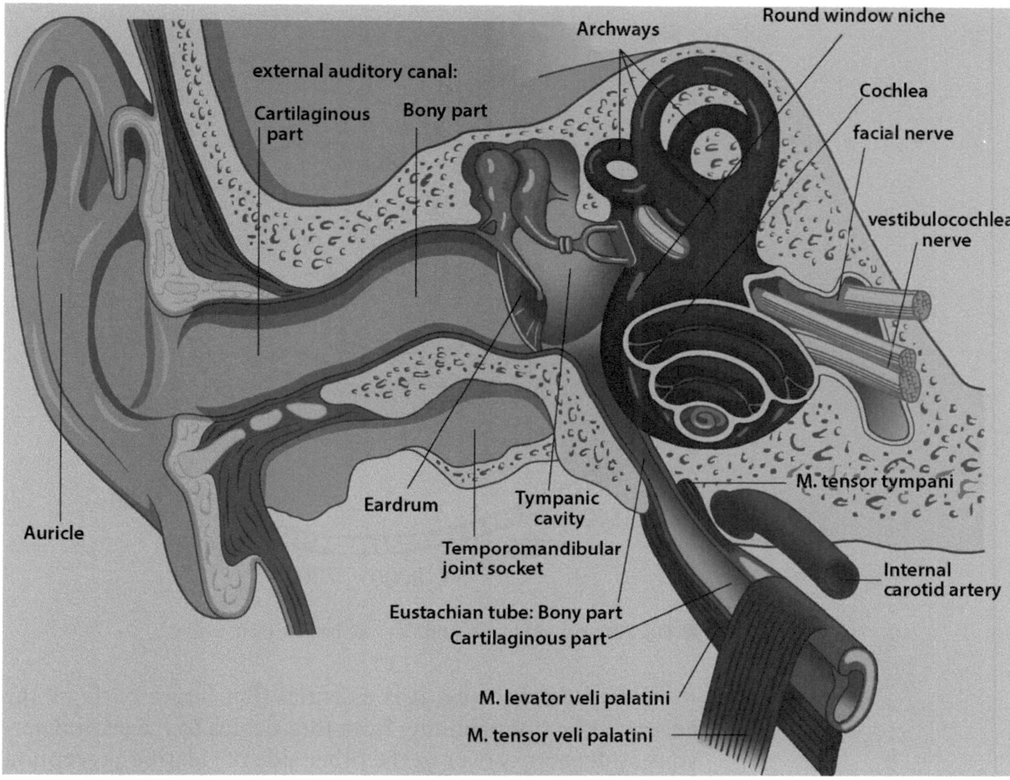

Fig. 2.7 The ear. Overview (From: Boenninghaus and Lenarz 2007)

▪ Cochlea

Depending on the pitch (frequency), the sound waves reach different places in the cochlea, which is named after its outer shape.

Vibrations with a high frequency, i.e. bright tones, are reflected in the first turn of the cochlea near the middle ear. Low-frequency tones, i.e. low and dull tones, are imaged at the end of the cochlea turn near the "cochlea hole" (helicotrema). Thus, each frequency has a specific location in the cochlea depending on its quality (Fig. 2.8).

▪ Organ of Corti

The conversion of the mechanical energy coming from outside into nerve impulses takes place in the organ of Corti, the sensory organ. Only (!) 3000 inner hair cells are the receiving stations; the 12,000 outer hair cells usually have a moderating amplifying or weakening influence. The inner hair cells convert the auditory impression from the outside into a nerve impulse. This is then transmitted to the auditory center in the brainstem.

2

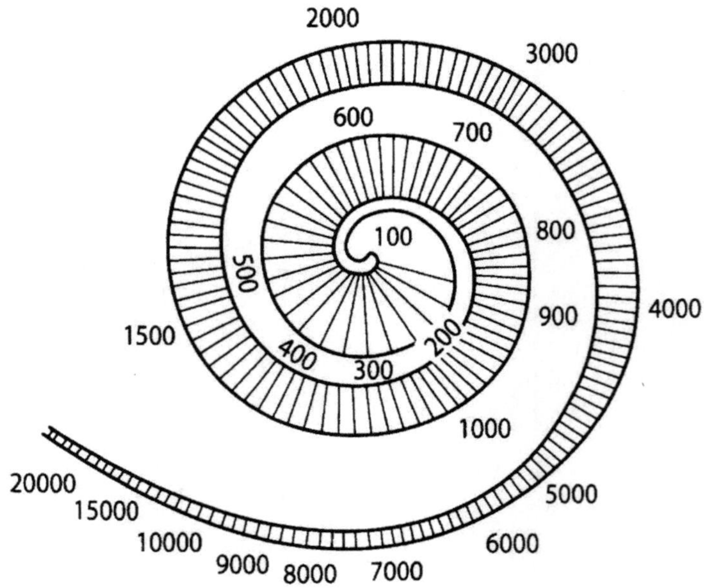

Fig. 2.8 Sound localization on the basilar membrane

For spatial hearing, it is essential that larger parts of the nerve conductions running from the cochlea to the central nervous system cross over to the other side of hearing perception and the brainstem at a very early stage, from the second nerve node onwards. In this way, time differences can be perceived and evaluated as spatial impressions in the auditory center.

Complex Networking and Communication in the Hearing System

Already during the recording of the auditory impression, many regulating influences take place. These are active and very individual processes. On the way from the inner ear to the perception of the auditory impression, the information from the outside is processed by many regulatory processes in fractions of a second, amplified or weakened and – in the vast majority – not allowed to enter further perception. Only what is important for the individual reaches it, be it frightening or pleasant, but in any case, of interest and preferably "new". Here, too, the limbic system plays a major role. Thus, any sound, no matter how objectively measurable, will be perceived differently depending on attention and mood. In this way the outside world that penetrates "into us" via objectively measurable sound impulses, becomes a highly individual reality.

2.2.2 From the Otolithic Organs to the Cochlea

In terms of evolution, the cochlea represents a late-forming offshoot of the saccule (Ritter 2003). In addition to its vestibular function, the saccule reacts to very low tones, whereby the transition from perceptible vibrations to low tones is smooth.

▪ Early Warning System Hearing

While on the basis of the utricle three semicircular canals for the detection of rotational movements have developed, an offshoot has developed from the sacculus, which in the course of development from fishes via reptiles to mammals became increasingly sensitive also to higher vibrations, i.e. sounds. This is why in principle the structures of the sensory cells and the endolymph fluid are also found in the cochlea as in the semicircular canals. This has become of vital importance on land, where sounds are transmitted through air. Those that can hear early on whether danger is imminent or prey is approaching were able to react better.

▪ Different Resonance Behavior

One problem in processing is that sound impulses enter both the auditory and the vestibular part. However, only the auditory part should "respond" to the sound and react with meaningful nerve impulses, while the vestibular part should not show any reactions to acoustic impulses. The necessary and decisive development of nature was described in 1934 by de Burlet and again in 2006 by Carey and Nivee on the basis of comparative anatomical and physiological investigations. Thus, the vestibular part is bony, i.e. "walled in" in solid material, while the auditory tube is softly embedded. This results in different resonance behavior, which is essential for the separate perception of sound waves in the auditory part and the lack of reaction in the vestibular part.

If gaps occur in the bony envelope due to a congenital or accidental condition ("so-called third window", often in the upper semicircular canal), the vestibular organ reacts to sound impulses, which triggers vertigo ("Tullio phenomenon").

▪ Where are the Functions Found in the Anatomical Structures?

Ménière's disease is a disorder of the inner ear (◘ Fig. 2.7). The outer ear includes the auricle (pinna), the external auditory canal and the eardrum – the borders to the middle ear. The eardrum is a highly sensitive and painful membrane. In a healthy state, the middle ear is filled with air. It contains three ossicles in a "tympanic cavity", which are named after their appearance hammer (malleus), anvil (incus) and stirrup (stapes).

▪ Transition From Air to Water

The stapes rests on the oval window, the boundary to the inner ear. Here the sound waves, which were previously transmitted via air, are converted into fluid movements in the perilymph of the inner ear duct. The second boundary is the round window, which releases the pressure waves initiated via the oval window back to the middle ear.

In upright standing humans, the vestibular organ is found in the upper part of the inner ear and the organ of hearing in the lower part. It is no coincidence that the inner ear is also called the labyrinth, which we – with Ritter (2003) and Lang (2003) – want to walk through in millimeter steps for orientation.

The evolutionary basis of the tubular system, surrounded by fluid (perilymph), is the approximately 5 mm long utricle. It is firmly anchored in the bone and accommodates a perception surface (maculae) of approximately 2–3 mm loads with calcium crystals (otoliths) in its gelatinous membrane.

Via a small canal, the "Canalis utriculus-saccularis", the utricle is connected with its teammate for vertical alignment, the saccule, and the canal towards the saccus endolymphaticus in a duplication of the meninges (dura, ◘ Fig. 2.5). The canal is called Ductus endolymphaticus in Latin.

The connecting path between the two otolith organs, utricle and saccule, and the endolymphatic sac acts like a valve in the tubular system due to its angular arrangement and kinking: the so-called "Bast valve".

▪ Tube and Flap Systems

The three semicircular canals with a diameter of 1.2 mm arise from the utricle. They are positioned in the three main directions of the space – each perpendicular and arranged in mirror image to the opposite side.

Each canal has an open end, which communicates freely with the vestibule, and an enlarged ampullary end, where the sensory epithelium, the cupula, is housed (◘ Fig. 2.6).

There are only five openings in the utricle, because the upper and the posterior semicircular canals merge before they enter the utricle.

▪ Bone-Fixed: The Otolith Organs

The roundish saccule with a transverse diameter of approximately 2 mm and a longitudinal diameter of approximately 3 mm is also firmly attached to the bone. Like the utricle, it accommodates perceptual area (macula) covered with otoliths, measuring approximately 1–2 mm.

The sacculus is connected to the cochlea, the organ of hearing, by a "unifying" duct about 0.7 mm long and 0.2–0.5 mm in diameter, the ductus reuniens. The cochlear duct (auditory canal) winds 2.5 times in a spiral around an axis (modiolus) that contains nerves and blood vessels.

In the cross section, three definable units are found: the auditory canal and two surrounding floors filled with perilymph. These are in turn named after their spatial location: the tympanic staircase (scala tympani) is close to the middle ear, the tympani, and the vestibular staircase (scala vestibuli) is close to the vestibular organ (vestibulum).

The upper wall of the auditory canal, the Reissner's membrane, separates the endolymph, which comprises only about 2 µl, from the 8 µl of perilymph fluid in the vestibular staircase. The lower wall, the basilar membrane, separates the auditory canal from the perilymph of the tympanic staircase.

2.2.3 Organ of Corti

▪ Hearing Organ with 15,000 Sensory Cells

On the basilar membrane sits the hearing organ, the "organ of Corti" named after its first describer, with about 15,000 sensory cells (12,000 outer and 3000 inner hair cells; ◘ Fig. 2.9).

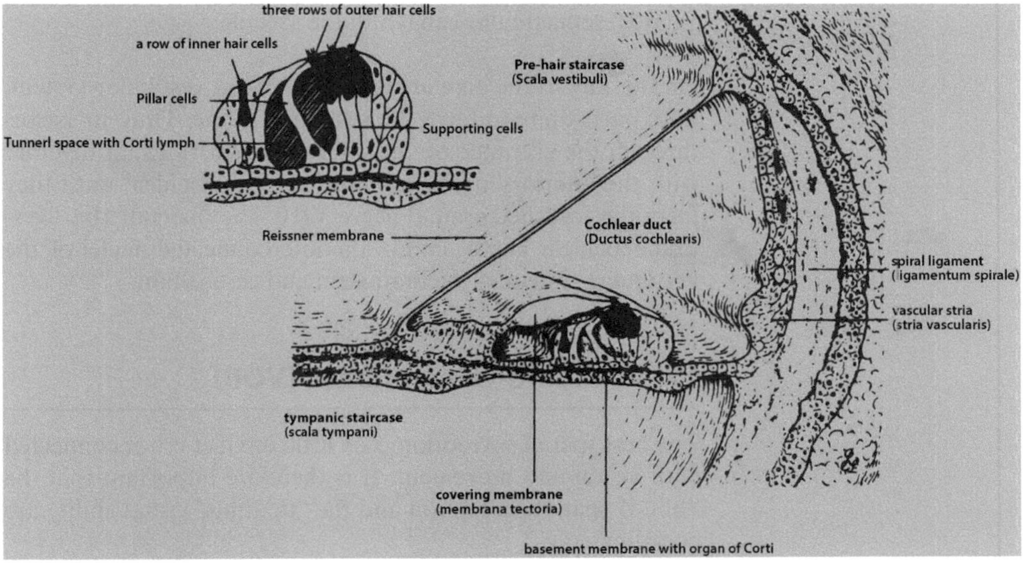

◘ **Fig. 2.9** The organ of Corti in cross section. (From: Boenninghaus 1990)

The organ of Corti is covered by a membrane, the covering membrane (membrana tectoria), which is connected to the sensory cilia. The outer wall of the auditory canal, the spiral ligament (ligamentum spirale), carries the lateral vascular strip (stria vascularis), which plays an important part in the production of the endolymphatic fluid.

The perilymph is surrounding the membranous labyrinth is. The perilymphatic space is connected to the surrounding fluid of the cerebral cavity via the perilymphatic duct (Ductus perilymphaticus, but also named Aquaeductus cochleae) with an average diameter of 0.09 mm (1–2 mm) and a length of 6.3 mm.

The perilymph duct starts from the scala tympani just in front of the round window, runs in the shape of an "S" and ends in a triangular mouth at the posterior edge of the petrous bone. In adult humans, it is usually traversed by a network of fine connective tissue fibers (Michel 1998).

2.3 Vestibular Nerve

■ Initially Divided Into Two Parts: The Vestibular Nerve

Each of the three semicircular canals and the two otolith organs transmit their information (afferent) to the vestibular nerve (■ Fig. 2.6). This is initially still divided into two parts:

- The upper part contains the fibers of the superior (anterior) and lateral (horizontal) semicircular canals and those of the utricle – and a minimal portion of the saccule
- The lower part contains the fibers of the inferior (posterior) semicircular canal and the saccule.

On the way to the core areas of the central vestibular system, both parts unite to form the vestibular nerve. Thus, its passes through the entrance of the internal auditory canal together with the auditory nerve coming from the cochlea, until they form the so-called cranial nerve VIII. The fibers of this "vestibulocochlear nerve" end in the interconnected nuclei of the vestibular system in the brainstem and cerebellum.

2.4 Vestibulo-Ocular Reflex (VOR)

The best spatial perception is of little use if it is not connected with vision and movement. It is therefore important that the "blind" spatial perception and the "floating" visual ability are coordinated.

When walking, it makes sense that the eyes always look forward in order to detect possible stumbling blocks early enough at an angle of 150° downwards.

In addition, it is important that we can fixed an object even during a movement. To do this, when we move our head, the movement of our eyes must simultaneously shift by the same angle against the direction of movement – without us having to think about it first.

▪ Three-Neuron Reflex

Thus, in only three steps (three-neuron reflex), the information is transmitted – *reflexively* – via the node in the vestibular nucleus (nucleus vestibularis).

- *Step 1*: The vestibular organs pick up movement impulses via the changes in the three movement detectors (cupula) in semicircular canals and the displacement of the small calcium crystals in the otolith organs and send them to the core area of the eye muscles.
- *Step 2*: In the core area of the eye muscles, the responsible third, fifth and sixth cranial nerves (III, IV, VI) inhibit the muscles attaching to the eye on the side of the rotational movement and activate them on the opposite side.
- *Step 3*: If the head turns to the left, the eyes move to the right with the same angular velocity.

The reduced neuronal arrangement between the vestibular organs (vestibulo) and eye movement (ocular) is the vestibulo-ocular reflex (VOR), which guarantees fast and efficient ear-to-eye transmission.

One of the characteristics of the VOR is that its optimum working range is at high frequencies and fast velocities of head movement. VOR is specialized in stabilizing the eyes during fast/high-frequency movements, in sharp contrast to visuomotor mechanisms such as pursuit or optokinetic eye movements, which only work at relatively slow movements of visual stimulus.

If you experimentally oscillate your head up and down (e.g. in the "no-no" or "yes-yes" orientation) while looking at the book in front of you, you will still be able to fixate the writing. Your semicircular canals transmit speed information to the eye nerves and muscles via short pathways with few switches. In response, the eye muscles respond with appropriate speed. The speed of eye movement is measured in angular degrees per second (°/s). Thus, movements up to an angular velocity of 40 °/s can be compensated.

2.4.1 Suppression of the VOR – a Central Achievement

The VOR can be suppressed voluntarily and unconsciously. This can be useful and necessary if,

When you want your eyes focus on an object that rotates with you. For example, when "going around the corner", one does not want to see the surroundings in focus, but an object that is also moving, e.g. the wristwatch. The VOR must be suppressed, so that the gaze can remain on the moving object and does not move in the opposite direction to the head movement. This suppression is an achievement of the central nervous system in the "oculomotor nucleus" of the cerebellum (flocculus).

2.5 Oculomotor System

The eyes must be able to follow not only their own movements, but also those of other people and moving objects. For this, the interaction of eye movements on what is seen had to develop (oculomotor system). Information received by the eyes is transmitted as nerve impulses from the retina to various nodes in the brain – the "visual cortex". Via core areas of the visual cortex and the cerebellum, the information can both be transmitted to the nodes of the vestibular organ (vestibular nuclei) and compared with the information from the vestibular organ.

The result of this comparison is transmitted back to the oculomotor nuclei to guide the movement of the eyes to the target object.

▪ Optokinetic Nystagmus, Smooth Pursuit and Saccades

The path from vision via the brain back to the eye movements is more complex and thus also slower than the fast "three-neuron reflex" described above. If the movement of large visual targets results in slow but still compensable eye movements, relatively slow voluntary reset movements (saccades) may become necessary.

With continuous rapid movements, regular resetting movements of the eyes occur. The pattern of an **optokinetic nystagmus** – triggered by vision – develops.

▪ Optokinetic Nystagmus Is Not Exhausted

The optokinetic nystagmus cannot be influenced voluntarily, does not become exhausted and cannot be suppressed by the vestibular system. Unlike the vestibular organ, constant uniform movements do not lead to habituation, so we always remain "optically" on it, except in the case of – mostly unpleasant – pharmacological influences.

If you want to see the result of such a multi-step process in comparison to the small experiment when testing out the VOR, then please hold the book in front of your eyes.

Please first move it slowly in front of your eyes to the left and to the right or up and down.

With slow changes, "slow following movements" allow you to keep a moving object in your visual field. You will still be able to recognize what is written without actually wanting to read it.

If you move the book faster (over 45 °/s), perhaps as fast as you moved your head before, the image becomes blurred. Now the eyes can no longer follow accurately: Fast "resetting movements" (saccades) become necessary to catch it in the field of vision again, the letters become blurred.

Smooth pursuit allows following an object that moves in visual field. If the moving object covers a large area in the visual field, it can be called optokinetic stimulus. This is mediated largely by the cerebral cortex and the cerebellum. These systems work optimally at low frequencies (<0.5 Hz) and low velocities (<50 °/s). As the target velocity increase, the eye velocity cannot keep up, a small saccade is produced to catch up the target.

Saccades are fast refixation eye movements with velocities up to 500 °/s. Their velocity is directly proportional to the size of the saccade, but velocity is not under voluntary control. They can be automatic or reflexive, for example in response to an unexpected visual target or voluntary in responds to commands: right – left during examination.

2.6 Nystagmus

▪ Reflective Jerk Movement

If things move too quickly, for example when looking out of a moving train or on a merry-go-round, the possibilities of a compensatory countermovement of the eyes are exhausted. Then the eyes have to be moved back again and again in a quick reflexive jerking movement that is not perceptible to the person affected. This rhythmic sequence of slow and fast movements of the eyes of the opposite person is medically called "nystagmus".

The term nystagmus comes – like so much in medicine – from the Greek: Nystagmos (literally: νυσταγμός "sleepiness" and nystazō "nodding", "slumbering") refers to uncontrollable, rhythmic movements of an *organ*. If this concerns eye movements, nystagmus is usually understood to mean "eye trembling".

In nystagmus, two components of movement are found:

- a *slow* component, i.e. a movement triggered by the head movement and corresponding to its speed, but directed in the opposite direction, with speeds of up to approximately 100 °/s, and
- a *fast* component, i.e. a reflexive restoring movement in the same direction as the head movement, with speeds of up to approximately 700 °/s.

The classification of nystagmus is based on shape, direction, speed, amplitude, duration and intensity. Because of the better recognizability for the observer, the direction of the nystagmus in clinical diagnostics is called after the fast phase.

2.7 Who Is Able to Do What!

The constant and always active effort to achieve sufficient spatial orientation, posture regulation and gaze stabilization takes place in a dynamic range of low-, medium- and high-frequency signals. The strain changes permanently "in motion". From low to high strain there is a spectrum of about 1–10 Hz. Under stronger physical strain, the dynamic demands increase. Higher-frequency signals are then generated, e.g. during locomotion (walking, running), while at the same time low-frequency signals are required to store the distance ("navigation"). The frequency increases even further with shocks and vibrations (Walther et al. 2012).

Each of the three systems for the perception of external and intrinsic movements has an optimal working range in which the impulses can best be processed.

In equilibrium system of healthy people, stimulus processing complements and overlaps each other.

- With the eye (following) movements, we can best capture very slow and slow movements up to 0.2 Hz and "keep our eyes on them".
- The perception stations in the semicircular canals (cupula) already react to slow movements. From frequencies of 0.2 Hz onwards, they depict reality better than the eye tracking movements. They reach their optimal range between 0.5 and 16 Hz. This also represents the optimal working range for the reflex arcuate to the eye muscles (VOR) (Walther et al. 2012).

- After that, the semicircular canals can still react up to 20 Hz, but they no longer reproduce the effective forces quite exactly.

The utricle and saccule are in an intermediate position. They work from the slightest movement from an acceleration of 0.05 m/s^2 (Stoll et al. 2004) – optimally up to a frequency of 1.5 Hz.

In normal circumstances these sensory inputs are activated simultaneously, rather than individually, and this covering information interacts at virtually all levels in the neural axis.

If, however, the function of the semicircular canals is permanently impaired, this deficiency can be compensated for to a large extent by the ocular movements and the function of the utricle and saccule. However, the "quality" for the special subarea of their functions is no longer completely achieved. As a result, very fast movements can then only be followed up with resetting movements of the eyes (saccades). At the same time, it becomes more difficult to distinguish one's own movements from those of the environment. However, with practice, confidence and the activation of conscious association (thinking), the vast majority of everyday tasks can be adequately mastered.

2.8 Other Conditions for Equilibrium

2.8.1 Information from the Skin, Hands and Feet

Spindle-Shaped Nerves (So-Called Body Sensors): Proprioceptors

An important source of information about the position of the joints in relation to each other, as well as about the tangible environment, is obtained by touching and feeling with our hands and feet, as well as with our so-called *body sensors (proprioceptors)*, mechanosensory neurons. These are tiny nerve spindles in the muscles that inform us about the state of tension, the position and the length of muscles, tendons and joints. The *neck receptors*, which provide information about the position of the head in relation to the trunk, play a special role in the upright gait.

The enormous importance of the proprioception can be illustrated as follows: even people *without* vestibular organ function can, if they have practiced this long enough, still stand with their eyes closed and even, with appropriate restrictions, walk.

2.8.2 The "Belly Feeling"

Closely connected to the vestibular nuclei is the vomiting center. If an ingested substance tastes foul (perishable), it makes sense to vomit it. This happens regularly in the case of "nausea". This reflex is very old and can still be seen today in simple jellyfish. Probably the connecting path to be found in humans between the balance centers and the cranial nerve X, the vagus nerve. As a "roving" nerve of the autonomic nervous system, the vagus nerve reaches as far as the stomach. It often gives us a "belly feeling" among many other non-conscious tasks. This can be consulted when "something is bothering you".

2.8.3 Heart, Lungs, Food and Drink

Active Maintenance of Balance

Normal equilibrium is the product of a constantly active interplay between diverse information from the environment and its reception and processing at all levels of the central nervous system. To make this possible, it needs: Inhalation and exhalation

- Heart and circulation
- Supply and removal of calories and fluids
- Stable metabolic state
- Appropriate hormone balance
- Transmission through functional nerves from the feet to the brain and vice versa
- People and fellow human beings
- Friends and enemies, counterpart and opponent

2.8.4 Implementation in Motion

Movement Experiences and Reactions

Mostly unconsciously and within milliseconds, the new information from the environment is compared and evaluated with previous movement experiences. If the comparison of the different information results in a difference to the balance, reactions usually follow immediately and "involuntarily" in the form of muscle activities and eye movements, which are supposed to restore a stable state. This requires (almost) all muscles of the musculoskeletal system.

Most of the fixed nerve connections to and from the muscles originate from the spinal cord pathways and also meet again there. Among other things, they regulate the fine balance and interplay of the complementary flexor and extensor muscles.

2.9 Interface Points in the Brain

Balance is usually only consciously perceived when it is on the wane. Contrary to what we think, we function overall without having to consciously "think" about it all the time. The body and the brain have the most work to do with themselves in order to organize its maintenance. Information and irritations about the environment take up only a small part, and very little of it is perceived "consciously". Nevertheless, the development of brain abilities has led us to get as far as we are now, for better or for worse.

▪ Alignment of Inherited and Learned Patterns

The core of the vestibular system is located in the brainstem in the so-called vestibular nuclei and in the cerebellum. There, the incoming information from the various sensory organs (visual, vestibular, proprioceptive) are integrated into a coherent impression. To a very large extent, they are – for the sake of survival – also already stored in the brainstem as basics and rough concepts. One cannot even think about the multitude of patterns and action sequences necessary for survival, perception and movement without becoming incapable of action. Like (almost) everything that works well or has to work, this happens mainly unconsciously.

▪ Brain Stem Interprets Without Thinking

Due to the mirror-image arrangement of the total of six semicircular canals *and* the otolith organs, which are also opposite to each other, every conceivable position *in space* results in a different information pattern for the brain. This is evaluated in the brain as a spatial impression. Decisive for the perception in the brain is not the individual value left or right, but what arrives in the brainstem as a balance between activation in one direction and inhibition in the other. The brain stem interprets – without "consciously thinking" – a difference between right and left as movement.

2.9.1 Advantages and Disadvantages

▪ Double Backup

Advantage: In the case of healthy people with balance, the information is doubly secured. Therefore, vestibular compensation is possible as an adaptive process, whereby symptoms and signs of a lesion (for example from an acute peripheral vestibular lesion) may be diminished and disappear. It depends on visual, proprioceptive and remaining vestibular inputs as well as a plasticity from the central nervous system. Sensory reweighting allows adequate balance control when on sensory input is unavailable or unreliable.

■ Awareness Requested Only When Unexpected

Disadvantage: The more complex a system is assembled, the more vulnerable it can become. Thus, the possibilities for malfunctions, increase with the number of elements. Single parts can fail, but it can also happen that all parts can no longer be adequately integrated to another. For example, the right semicircular canals transmit differently than the left one. Perhaps the eyes see something that the vestibular organ sense quite differently. This leads to a confusion of information, although they all do their job well.

When new questions arise or when the old answers do not allow satisfactory solutions, the process can be conscious and – partly – changed. If I want to know whether something of the "equilibrium" is working, I have to challenge it, for example through new balancing exercises.

2.10 Balance of the Soul

Like as there is a physical balance, there is certainly a psychological or "soul" balance. This is not easy to describe, however, because there are hundreds of conflicting ideas and theories throughout human history about what "soul" and "psychic" are. One agreement, however, is that emotions interact with orientation and balance in various ways.

■ Limbic System

An important interface lies in the so-called limbic system. There, emotional impulses are perceived, interpreted and "automatically" converted into actions – mostly before the consciousness "learns" what has happened.

If one looks at the development of the "soul", it is noticeable that the most important feelings or emotions in the infant and toddler are still expressed very physically. When a toddler is content, he beams; when he is hungry or thirsty, lies uncomfortably or needs to be changed, he cries. In the course of the normal, healthy growth process, an ever-widening range of emotional qualities develops. Pleasure is differentiated into contentment, joy, trust, faith, love, hope, tenderness; unpleasure into anxiety, fear, shame, guilt, disgust, sadness, helplessness and hopelessness.

Since people – except for hermits – are always in contact with other people, their emotional development always takes place in close interaction with their social environment. In this process – as it becomes clear in mental illnesses – the soul also needs its own balance. In the meantime, neurophysiologists can name some important conditions for the successful maintenance of mental balance in the face of ever new stresses and challenges.

■ Secure Bonds Help

According to this, even in the earliest years, those children who have established a secure attachment to at least one adult caregiver explore their environment significantly more, courageously and curiously than those children who have an insecure attachment. This means that a secure attachment is the crucial basis for engaging with the stresses and risks of new situations and actively dealing with them. This enables us to stand on our own 2 feet, have our own experiences and find the way in the world.

■ Inner Beliefs

Those who were able to have basic experiences of emotional security and their own competence are later able to develop their own ideas about themselves. These ideas are inner images that offer a person support and security, and to which he or she orients himself or herself in the course of his or her further development.

They are inner convictions that have grown in the course of one's own development and have been reaffirmed again and again, from which a person in difficult situations always finds new courage for a new beginning.

■ Dealing With Fear

Always endangering, but also bringing forward in the sense of a challenge, fear in the case of real or fantasized danger is the life theme of man par excellence. Anxiety becomes an existential issue very early on when trust in the bond with at least one parent cannot be established or when conditions are placed on "being allowed to be there". This can be quite dramatically when the newcomer to the world does not fit in with its environment, be it,

- because it was not wanted;
- because it is of its own character "unruly" or
- because parents may not be able to provide loving, caring behavior because they may not have learned it themselves.

Why might this be important for understanding Ménière's disease? One important reason is that every Meniere's patient deals with the disease differently. Thereby, the acquired and/or learned processing structure, which has been passed on until the onset of Meniere's disease, also has an influence on the symptom expression and the possibilities of coping (even if the origin of the vertigo disease is to be found in the inner ear).

Depending on the developmental stage of the injury, ascertain way of dealing with fear is solidified, which also could become effective in dealing with the dizziness. For example, well- to highly structured people may be more likely to "obsessively" push for a mechanistic solution – or try to suppress the disease. They sometimes have to take long detours with many disappointments before an acceptance of realistic coping options can occur.

People with a depressive mood mode may be more likely to withdraw, or cling, and possibly – also – process the illness guiltily.

Those who are more "emotionally active" could involve their environment in the changeable ups and downs of suffering and hope – and often let it despair along with them.

In any case, Ménière's attacks can thoroughly upset what is taken for granted and probably for this reason not infrequently evoke fears of death and destruction.

Literature

Boenninghaus HG (1990) Hals-Nasen-Ohrenheilkunde. Springer, Berlin, Heidelberg/New York

Boenninghaus HG, Lenarz T (2007) Hals-Nasen-Ohren-Heilkunde, 13th edn. Springer, Berlin, Heidelberg/New York/Tokio

Bronstein A, Lempert T (2017) Dizziness. A practical approach to diagnosis an management, Cambridge clinical guides, 2nd edn. Cambridge University Press, p 200

Lang J (2003) Anatomie des vestibulären systems. In: Haid CT (ed) aus interdisziplinärer Sicht. Thieme, Stuttgart, pp 4–16

Michel O (1998) Morbus Menière und verwandte Gleichgewichtsstörungen. Thieme, Stuttgart – nicht mehr lieferbar

Morita N, Kariya S, Farajzadeh Deroee A, Cureoglu S, Nomiya S, Nomiya R, Harada T, Paparella MM (2009) Membranous labyrinth volumes in normal ears and Meniere disease: a three-dimensional reconstruction study. Laryngoscope 119(11):2216–2220

Plontke SK, Gürkov R (2015) Morbus Menière. Facharztwissen HNO. LRO 94:530–554

Ritter K (2003) Die Entwicklungsgeschichte des Innenohrs. In: Haid CT (ed) Schwindel aus interdisziplinärer Sicht. Thieme, Stuttgart, pp 1–3

Rudack C (1995) Immunologie des Innenohres. Ein Überblick. HNO 43:275–281

Salt AN, Plontke SK (2010) Endolymphatic hydrops: pathophysiology and experimental models. Otolaryngol Clin North Am 43(5):971–983

Scherer H (1997) Das Gleichgewicht, 2nd edn. Springer, Berlin, Heidelberg/New York

Stoll W, Most E, Tegenthoff M (eds) (2004) Schwindel und Gleichgewichtsstörungen, 4th edn. Thieme, Stuttgart

Walther LE, Cebulla M (2015) Frequenzdynamische Analyse der Otolithenfunktion mittels vestibulär evozierter myogener Potenziale (VEMP). Laryngo-Rhino-Otol 94:153–155

Walther LE, Hörmann K, Blochin M, Blödow A (2012) Rezeptorfunktion der Bogengänge Teil 1: Anatomie, Physiologie, Diagnostik und Normalbefunde. HNO 60:75–88

Westhofen M (2009) M. Menière. Evidenzen und Kontroversen. HNO 57:446–454

Pathophysiology of Ménière's Disease

What Is the Damage?

Contents

3.1 Vertigo from the Inner Ear – 49
3.1.1 Stadium Classification According to Jahnke (1994) – 54

3.2 Eye Tremor (Nystagmus) During an Acute Attack – 54

3.3 Impaired Balance After Vertigo Attacks – 55

3.4 Hearing Loss – 57

3.5 Dysacusis (Distorted Hearing) – 57

3.6 Lack of Loudness Compensation and Noise Sensitivity (Hyperacusis) – 58

3.7 Hearing Impressions Without External Sound Source – Tinnitus – 59
3.7.1 Forms of Tinnitus – 59
3.7.2 Psychological Conflicts – 61
3.7.3 Tinnitus in Endolymphatic Diseases Such as Ménière's Disease – 61

3.8 Feeling of Pressure in and Behind the Ear – 62

3.9 Sensory Sensations (Paresthesia) – 63

3.10 Lack of Compensation and Double Inhibition – 63

3.11 Reactive, Psychogenic Vertigo – 67
3.11.1 How Can Organic Vertigo Become Psychogenic Dizziness in Ménière's Disease? – 68

H. Schaaf, *Ménière's Disease*, https://doi.org/10.1007/978-3-662-63610-7_3

3.11.2 Maintenance of Vertigo in Cases of Previous Mental Illness – 74
3.11.3 Can Fear and Panic Cause Ménière's Attacks? – 79

Literature – 81

■ Endolymphatic Hydrops

Medically, this congestion in the inner ear is called endolymphatic hydrops. It affects the membranous ducts of both the vestibular and auditory organs. ◘ Figure 3.1 schematically shows the narrow, canals in healthy individuals and the dilated endolymphatic ducts in Ménière's disease. This is the organic core of the disease's effects.

During the early stages of the disease, hardly any noticeable organic changes are observed (Plontke and Gürkov 2015). Over time, changes in the membranous labyrinth are caused by the dilated endolymphatic space with impairments and increasing damage to the sensory cells.

Morgenstern (1985) describes strong expansions and bulges, first the sacculus and later also the utriculus membrane. The expansions of the sacculus and the utricle can finally fill the whole narrow space, with the walls of the endolymphatic space leaning against the bony wall of the cochlea. Sometimes the wall of the sacculus is arched up to the ossicular chain (stapes footplate) or fibrotic traits are formed between the membrane of the sacculus and the stapedius plate.

3.1 Vertigo from the Inner Ear

■ Congestion in the Saccus Endolymphaticus

The expansion of the endolymphatic space occurs, when the ratio of production and removal is no longer balanced and

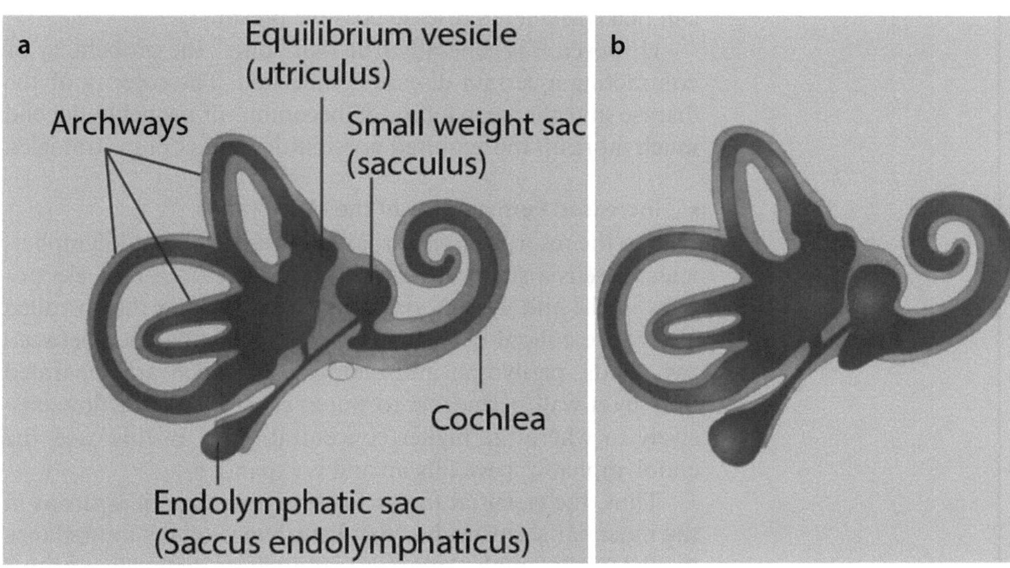

◘ **Fig. 3.1** Schematic representation of the endolymphatic situation. **a** Inconspicuous situation with normally configured endolymphatic ducts; **b** hydrops with dilated endolymphatic ducts

more is produced than can be removed. This seems to be mainly due to a reduced function of the resorption cells of the saccus endolymphaticus.

This could be due to the fact that the endolymphatic sac is overburdened with immune defense tasks for which it is probably also responsible (Rudack 1995; Paparella and Djalilian 2002), so that it cannot sufficiently take over this double task.

The observation that the endolymphatic sac in Ménière's disease often looks smaller (shriveled) and shows signs of fibrosis fits this assumption (Jahnke 1994). In this case, an earlier mumps infection, an inflammation of the middle ear, an inflammation of the labyrinth by bacteria as well as a viral infection are possible triggers. However, this is hardly verifiable – just as little as the assumption of Gacek (2015) regarding a herpes infection. Trune (2006) points out that an inflammatory reaction in the petrous bones of Ménière's patients has not been observed. This is an argument – against the often expressed assumption, that Ménière's disease is due to an autoimmune disease of the inner ear (Plontke and Gürkov 2015).

▪ Inherited or Acquired?

Meanwhile, some studies suggest that there is some predisposition for inner ear weakness with Ménière's symptoms. Ménière's disease may be more common in families (Frykholm et al. 2006) and may also be inherited in part (Arweiler et al. 1995; Morrison et al. 2009). An autosomal-dominant inheritance is assumed, that is when two genes meet, the gene that can make Ménière's disease possible prevails.

However, it is generally true that "only" the probability of contracting a certain disease is inherited. The severity of the disease and the probability of becoming ill probably depend much more on the acquired possibilities and coping strategies.

▪ Increased Permeability of the Membranes

Due to the resorption disturbance in the saccus endolymphaticus, there is a slight increase in the concentration of electrolytes in the endolymph and thus an increase in the so-called electrolyte colloid osmotic pressure. This imbalance between two fluids, perilymph and endolymph, which are separated only by a wall permeable to water, causes water to flow passively to where the higher concentration is. In this case, the endolymphatic space fills up and is expanded.

Thus, the essential factor for the formation of hydrops in the inner ear seems to be "the disturbance of the ion balance in the endolymph between production and absorption" (Morgenstern 1985, p. 22).

> While it has long been assumed that the attacks occur mechanically through ruptures of membrane portions, electron microscopic investigations suggest that the Ménière's attacks can also be explained by an overall increased permeability of the barrier between endo- and perilymph fluid (Jahnke 1994; Morgenstern 1985); also ruptures of the Reissner membrane can be detected in this context.

Because the endolymph contains much more potassium than the perilymph, an increased permeability of the membranes leads to a flooding of the perilymphatic spaces with potassium. This is poison for the sensory cells and nerve endings of the auditory and vestibular organs and leads to functional restrictions or even loss of function. But also, the flooding of the endolymph with sodium also has consequences: The environment of the sensory cells gets mixed up and it seems, that the sensory hairs will be separate from the sensory cells.

In medical terms, this sounds like this, here explained by Jahnke (1994, p. 428):

» *The increased entry of potassium-rich endolymph into the perilymph ... reduces the formation of the action potential of afferent neurons, but also reversibly damages the hair cells. Also, the formation of the receptor potential of the hair cells, the mechanoelectrical transduction mechanism, which depends on the ion environment of the endolymph, is impaired by a sodium ion influx into the endolymphatic space. Furthermore, according to animal experiments, the increase of sodium and especially calcium ion concentration in the endolymph leads to a decoupling of the of the sensory cells from the tectorial membrane.*

▪ Pressure-Sensitive Calcium-Dependent Potassium Channel

Specifically with regard to the role of potassium, a research group led by (Düwel et al. 2005) demonstrated a pressure-sensitive calcium-dependent potassium channel in experiments with isolated hair cells from the utricle of guinea pigs. A change in the hydrostatic pressure of the endolymph, as in endolymphatic hydrops, is believed to lead to an increase in potassium outflow. If this experimental result in the test tube is transferred to a living person, this could be one way of explaining an increase in the frequency of transmission of the vestibular nerve on the affected side, which would then lead to the nystagmus in an acute attack.

▪ Functions Get Out of Balance

In summary, this means that the finely tuned and sensitive system of balance is massively disturbed during the attack. The functions of the vestibular and hearing organs are thrown off balance. Irreal but highly threatening information of a circling environment are then reported to the brainstem: A disturbance of in the inner ear is whirling through the head. This causes rapid reflex eye movements (nystagmus) and leads often to nausea and vomiting, if the vomiting center near the vestibular nuclei is also affected.

However, the presence of endolymphatic hydrops alone is not sufficient to explain the dizzy spells. Out of 541 deceased with a proven hydrops in the temporal bone, only 276 could be reliably assigned to Ménière's disease according to the criteria of the Committee on Hearing and Equilibrium (1995) (Foster and Breeze 2013). Thus, there are people with proven hydrops without Ménière's disease. Furthermore, hydrops also exists during the periods without any Meniere attack.

It is also important to note with regard to the pathophysiology of Ménière's disease that the simplified hypothesis that hydrops is caused – alone – by a blockage of the endolymphatic duct or a reduced absorption in the endolymphatic sac is not sufficient. A significant continuous longitudinal flow of endolymph from the cochlea into the saccus endolymphaticus could not be measured so far. Regulation of the endocochlear fluid volume is controlled locally, via radial flow of endolymph trough the perilymph and then recycled back into the scala media via spiral ligament and stria vascularis (Salt et al. 2012).

Westhofen (2009) states that

> » *In the meantime, it is now uncontested that endolymphatic hydrops is a consequence of morphological and functional changes in the inner ear and the base of the skull, but not the sole cause of the progressive functional impairment of the cochlea and the labyrinth that occurs in attacks.*

This conclusion is also drawn by Ruckenstein (2010):

> » *Thus, the concept of endolymphatic pressure buildup leading to a periodic rupture of Reißner's membrane cannot be supported by the experimental literature.* (Ruckenstein 2010)

▪ Additional Trigger Necessary

Because of this: Excess pressure in the fluid spaces of the inner ear can result from changes in the organic basis or the functioning of the inner ear organs and the surrounding bone base. However, this is "only" the observed condition for the increasing loss of function of the organs of hearing and balance. Something must be added to make it pathologically.

This is an invitation to a lot of speculation. So it happens that almost everything (too little or too much liquid, bacteria and viruses, allergies and many other things that occur frequently) has been associated with the development of Ménière's disease (► Chap. 5).

▪ Trigger

Jahnke (1994) assumed – without reliable evidence – as triggers that could induce an attack:

- Inflamed foci, especially of the maxillary sinus and teeth
- Stress-related functional disorders of the autonomic nervous system
- Psychological factors
- Metabolic disorders (rarely hypofunction of hormone-producing organs such as the adrenal cortex)
- Immunopathological changes

The duration of the Ménière's attack seems to depend on the regeneration of the barrier between endo- and perilymph. Active transport mechanisms seem to filter the excess sodium ions from the endolymph and excess potassium ions from the perilymph.

▪ Course Unsecured

How the damage of the labyrinth in Ménière's disease is progressing is not yet known.

From an evolutionary point of view, I would assume, that the evolutionary "youngest" parts of labyrinth are the most untested and thus also the most vulnerable. This would mean that first the cochlea with the auditory functions would be affected. Then a restriction of the sacculus functions would be suspected earlier than the utriculus function (Düwel et al. 2005).

Whether the semicircular canals – as protuberances of the evolutionary very old utricle – are the last to be measurably restricted in their function, will have to be shown by means of diagnostics that have now been significantly improved. Caloric irrigation alone will not be decisive.

It can be assumed that with each attack, a part of the function of the vestibular and hearing organs is reduced.

To see it positive, this means that the next attack may not be as severe – at least in the long run: On average after 9 years, in 75% of the untreated and non-surgically treated patients (!), Ménière's disease seems to "burn out", that is the dizzy spells become weaker or disappear completely (Stahle et al. and Kitahara in: Huang 1991).

The price for the decrease of attacks is an increasing impairment of hearing and function of one vestibular organ. This means that each time a new – more or less significant – loss of balance occurs, which can usually be compensated again and again, unless – as described below – additional processing problems occur.

3.1.1 Stadium Classification According to Jahnke (1994)

The ENT physicians, when they were still in charge of the guideline of Ménière's disease themselves, made a stage classification. The scheme is mainly based on the severity of the hearing loss.

- **Stadiums of Ménière's Disease**
  - *Stage 1*: Fluctuating (unsteady) hearing. In this stage, hearing can completely normalize after a dizzy spell
  - *Stage 2a*: Dizziness and fluctuating hearing, which spontaneously improves but does not return to normal
  - *Stage 2b*: Dizziness and fluctuating hearing, which only improves after osmotic therapy (through "draining, diuretic substances")
  - *Stage 3*: Significant hearing loss without fluctuation, further attacks of dizziness
  - *Stage 4*: "Burn-out" of Ménière's disease

It is noticeable that the changes in balance function have been included inaccurately in the stadium classification. This is probably also due to the fact that at that time, the diagnostic possibilities were not yet available as they are today. But surprisingly, a panel of experts within the American Academy of Otolaryngo-Head and Neck Surgery opposed "routine vestibular testing" in a broad-based consensus finding (Basura et al. 2020).

Ménière's disease can go through all stages but can also stop at stage 1. In stage 4, Ménière's disease is organically on a par with people, who have lost a vestibular organ for other reasons. However, this may have been preceded by dramatic experiences of long-lasting uncertainty, which may have left scars.

3.2 Eye Tremor (Nystagmus) During an Acute Attack

Ménière's attacks are typically associated with a nystagmus, a "tremor of the eye". This is based on involuntary, rapidly following, rhythmic eye movements, which are caused by the direct connection of the inner ear with the eye muscles. "Normally", this is very useful, because the information about the body position is directly coordinated with the line of sight (► Chap. 2).

In the case of a Ménière's attack, the disturbed nerve impulses imitate real, rapid changes in space, so reflexively an attempt is made to align the eyes accordingly. This leads to the rapid eye movements that are no longer up to the task, which ultimately only cause dizziness.

▪ Stimulus Nystagmus, Failure Nystagmus

In classic Ménière's attacks, a change in the direction of rotation typically occurs. This is related to the degree of potassium poisoning of the perilymph. First, the inflowing potassium from the endolymph causes the nerve cells in the perilymph to be stimulated (stimulus nystagmus). This triggers eye movements in the direction of the affected ear. Afterwards, the potassium concentration leads to paralysis of the nerve cells; this results in a failure nystagmus.

These experimentally well-documented observations explain the very different eye flickering movements during an attack, but if there is a strong mixing of peri- and endolymph, the stimulus stage can be passed through so quickly, that only the failure stage can be observed (Morgenstern 1994).

3.3 Impaired Balance After Vertigo Attacks

▪ Deviation from Permanent Information

What happens in the case of repeated, more or less severe failures of an organ of balance? As described in ► Chap. 2, both organs of equilibrium are constantly active, even in a state of rest. They also show the permanent earth's gravity as permanent information (basic pattern). The brainstem "understands" a deviation from this permanent information as movement to the side where the information rate has increased. If the brain stem moves to the left, it means: Now the eyes and the body must make compensatory movements to the right!

If one side fails temporarily or permanently, such as the right side, the activity of the left side predominates – without the latter having actively contributed anything. Under normal circumstances, this corresponds to a left turn of the head. This means for the brain stem: Now the eyes and the body must make compensatory movements to the right! If the person was still standing up to this point, he will tip over to the right side.

The VOR Cannot Distinguish

Via the vestibulo-ocular reflex (VOR), which is unable to distinguish between real movement and dysfunction in the vestibular organ, the eyes try to compensate the apparently continuous movement of the head. Consequently, they turn to the right as best they can. However, since there is no end "in sight", they must always quickly turn back to the left in order to try again to balance to the right. The result is a nystagmus, which is clearly visible from the outside. The fast movement part – when the irritation has subsided during the actual Ménière's attack (see above) – strikes in the direction of the healthy organ.

Viewed from the inside out, the image of a rapidly rotating environment is created. If "real head movements" are added to the healthy side, the symptoms intensify. Therefore, the patient is usually lying on the affected side, which causes the least additional complaints. Finally, the continuous rotary movement also irritates the vomiting center, which is located very near in the brainstem.

With each loss of function on one side, the opposite organ, in combination with the other components of the balance system, attempts to take over the functions of the failed part as far as possible. If this happens gradually, the adaptation process takes place step by step – and remains often unnoticed.

Constant Pressure Seems at First to Restrict the Low Frequencies in the Vestibular Organ

Orientation in space, posture regulation and stabilization of the field of vision require different signal strengths and frequencies. According to Reiß and Reiß (2015), the low-frequency signals are responsible for storage and navigation. The higher frequency signals are generated during movements such as walking and running.

As described in ► Chap. 2, two types of vestibular cells can be distinguished. Type I is tending to transmit high frequencies (phasic and dynamic). The elongated cylindrical type II is coupled at thin fibers and conveys slowly (tonic) slow frequencies. It is conceivable that they, as the cells with the thinner nerve fibres, are the first to suffer damage when exposed to increased pressure in Ménière's disease.

This could explain why in Ménière's disease the response to low-frequency stimuli, as exerted in the caloric (cold-warm flush) test, is more likely to be reduced than the response to rapid stimuli, as in the head impulse test. This would also explain why the limited processing of low-frequency movement stimuli in everyday life can cause a feeling of insecurity and dizziness.

But maybe this thought is too simple.

3.4 Hearing Loss

Hearing loss during an attack is explained by poisoning of the hair cells by potassium (Zenner 1989). In the early stages of the disease, a full recovery of function is still possible.

> Irreparable damage occurs if the potassium poisoning lasts too long or is repeated too often. Then the cell architecture of the surrounding membrane is damaged permanently, so that the lymph can no longer be segregated.

In addition, and also during the attack -free period, the increased fluid load, caused by endolymph congestion, has an effect on hearing. In particular, the contact of the sensory hairs with the tectorial membrane shifts (◘ Fig. 2.9); in extreme cases, covering membrane and sensory hairs can be completely disconnected (Zenner and Ernst 1993). The consequence is that the sensory cell can no longer be excited by sound stimuli.

The preference for the low-frequency range in this hearing disorder can be explained by a material composition of the basilar membrane, which in turn can be expressed in a different physical "stiffness gradient". Thus, the acute additional volume load has the most serious effect at the tip of the cochlea.

▪ Unilateral Increasing Hearing Loss

However, the frequent ability to regress and the fluctuations indicate that the function of the affected hair cells has not ceased for a long time but has only been temporarily impaired. Only when a long-lasting, chronic volume overload occurs, all areas in the ear tube and thus all frequencies are affected. The result can be increasing hearing loss. However, this only rarely seems to lead to complete deafness, usually it finds its limit at 60–80 dB hearing loss.

3.5 Dysacusis (Distorted Hearing)

The hearing disorder is perceived unpleasantly, especially in the speech area. Sounds can be distorted, and music can be heard dissonantly. This is due to the fact that the acquired hearing impression, we are familiar with, is based on the interaction of both ears. If this state changes, for example by passing less information from one ear, distortion or reverberation effects are the result. In this process, the two different auditory impressions from the right and left are perceived as understandably unpleasant and distorted until the next higher region can compensate for this "centrally".

Normally, compensation in perception occurs even if the hearing loss is severe. The brain learns to adapt to this new hearing situation and then no longer interprets the new situation as a distortion. This process normally occurs "by itself", but it can be improved and supplemented by hearing therapy exercises (Schaaf and Hesse 2012). However, compensation can be inhibited by "clinging" to hearing that often cannot be restored.

3.6 Lack of Loudness Compensation and Noise Sensitivity (Hyperacusis)

Volume and loudness modulating processes take place at almost every level of auditory processing. Of all the sensory organs, the auditory system has the highest (absolute) sensitivity: the difference between the smallest sound that can still be heard and the loudest sound that can still be tolerated has a factor of 10 million units of sound pressure.

▪ Stapedius Reflex Provides Noise Reduction

In the middle ear, the so-called stapedius reflex – with a direct feedback between the brainstem and the stapes muscles (Mm. stapedii) – ensures that subjectively and even more objectively loud sounds, the eardrum stiffens so much that the sound impulses are damped.

The so-called outer hair cells in the inner ear (in the organ of Corti) have a pronounced modelling function. In the case of very weak sound stimuli, they can increase the deflection of the basilar membrane or, in the case of very strong stimuli, reduce the deflection. In this way, acoustic signals are attenuated or amplified in the inner ear depending on the (objective) volume and (subjective) central feedback.

▪ Special form of Noise Hypersensitivity (Recruitment)

As a result of the weakening and damage the sensory cells for hearing, a special form of noise sensitivity can also occur in Ménière's disease. This is the lack of loudness compensation for hearing loss: "recruitment".

The cause is a restricted function, especially of the outer hair cells. If these hair cells are affected, it is no longer possible to understand quiet sounds, but loud sounds cannot be attenuated either. The result is hypersensitivity in the affected frequencies, depending on the severity of the hearing loss. This special form of noise sensitivity diminishes more and more, the more a compensation can be achieved in further hearing processing by increasing habituation. This normally happens “by itself” over time – in concrete terms, the higher levels of the hearing processing system ensure, that the subjective consequences of the peripheral damage are centrally compensated.

The opposite occurs when the noise sensitivity is experienced as so great that this induce a permanent escape from noise. Then a special hearing therapy can be useful, which – under guidance – introduces the patient carefully and cautiously to his or her noise sources.

3.7 Hearing Impressions Without External Sound Source – Tinnitus

Tinnitus is the term for hearing impressions without an external sound source. “Tinnitus” derives from the Latin “tinnire” and means “to ring, hum, buzz”. Although objective form of tinnitus exits, tinnitus is mostly subjective noises.

▪ Objective Ear Sounds

Objective ear noises are audible and measurable not only for those affected, but also for examiners. Thus – in the case of good hearing – tension and tenseness of the middle ear muscles or jerky opening movements of the auditory trumpet can be heard. In the case of a pathologically altered auditory trumpet, breathing sounds can be heard.

In very rare cases, vascular malformations can be the cause of tinnitus. These knock to the rhythm of the heartbeat. A simple test can help to detect and usually rule out this suspicion:

Pinch your arm so hard that it hurts.

If the frequency of your tinnitus does not change now, this very rare cause of objective tinnitus can be excluded with almost complete certainty.

▪ Subjective Tinnitus

Subjective tinnitus can occur at all levels of auditory processing from the middle ear to the perception of the sound in the cerebrum.

3.7.1 Forms of Tinnitus

The subtypes mentioned below are especially important for Ménière’s patients.

Outer Ear: Ear Plug

Not rare but harmless accompanied by a slight deterioration in hearing, a block in the outer ear may cause tinnitus. Earwax can expand into a plug after a shower, for example. This also happens through frequent use of ear sticks, which usually achieve the opposite of what they are supposed to: They plug the earwax further and further towards the eardrum.

Loss of External Auditory Perception

Due to the loss of external auditory perception, the background noise in hearing that is always present, becomes audible as tinnitus. Once the cause has been identified by a specialist, the obstacle can be quickly removed, and you have gotten away with a fright.

Inner Ear

▪ Loss of Inner Perception

In most cases, the causes of tinnitus are found in the inner ear. The frequency of tinnitus gives an important indication of the exact location of the event. Thus, in the case of noise damage, which mainly affects the high-frequency range, we usually also find high-frequency tinnitus noises; in the case of the mostly congenital middle tone weaknesses, we usually find ear noises around 1000–2000 Hz; and in the case of problems with the inner ear fluid, we mainly find low-frequency noises.

Damage to the sensory cells results in leads to a loss of information in the affected frequencies. If signals from the cochlea are missing, the superior control center does not passively "wait" for information, but "requests" it, which then increasingly drives the outer hair cells. This increases their activity, but without the usual amplification of auditory stimuli. A pathological regulatory cycle is created. The excessive activity of the outer hair cells could in turn permanently excite the still intact parts of the inner hair cells, so that these release nerve impulses, which are again interpreted as tinnitus in further hearing processing.

Central: In the Hearing Processing System

▪ Electrical Discharges

A harmless and frequent phenomenon are the impressions, that are often perceived for seconds, such as crackling, crackling, twitching, etc. Since the nerve impulses are to be regarded as electrical phenomena, this seems to be a form of discharge or natural "skip phenomenon", which occur quite naturally in an (electrical) network. Nevertheless, these can also be perceived as tinnitus. Most of the time, however, these phenomena are so short that one cannot decide in a hurry whether it was the heating or the CD system after all.

■ The Tinnitus Bites the Top of the Head

Even a peripherally generated tinnitus can become centralized. It is assumed that this happens as a result of "circulating electrical excitation". It then literally gets stuck in the hearing-processing system, but, as with all subjective types of tinnitus, never louder than 10–15 dB!

The ringing in the ears can also be felt (!) on the unaffected side without the need for a new hearing impairment on this side. This is due to the transmission of hearing information to the other side, which is the basis for bilateral hearing. This makes it "possible" to perceive tinnitus on the other side of the ear as well.

If the tinnitus has already become independent, it remains perceptible even in cases of deafness, caused by illness or surgery – at 10–15 dB above the hearing threshold. This may occur after of gentamycin (► Chap. 7). Therefore, tinnitus usually remains, or its character changes with an even wider range.

3.7.2 Psychological Conflicts

■ Tinnitus as a Warning Sign

Not seldom, tinnitus occurs in a crisis and is therefore assumed – often erroneously and certainly without "conscious intention" – to be the cause of the problem. Here, all attempts to solve the problem must also fail if they miss the problem. Frequently, there are various forms of exhaustion, anxiety disorders or depressive processes. We assume that this tinnitus perception is caused by a weakening of the central hearing filter functions.

3.7.3 Tinnitus in Endolymphatic Diseases Such as Ménière's Disease

■ Hair Cells Whirl

The typically low-frequency tinnitus in Ménière's disease can be explained by the endolymphatic hydrops. In contrast to noise damage and sudden deafness, in which the sensory hairs are directly damaged, the increased fluid load leads to more distance between the sensory cells – that is the hair cells – and the tectorial covering membrane, covering them.

This changes the working point of the outer hair cells, at the same time mechanical turbulence occurs. Both mechanisms lead to an increased irritation of the outer and inner hair cells. This can result in an auditory impression: the low humming sound (Preyer and Bootz 1995). Thus, in accordance with the clinical picture, the hair cells also whirl.

A "material property", the different physical stiffness gradient along the basilar membrane, is responsible for the fact that an acute additional volume load has the greatest effect at the end of the cochlear duct (helicotrema).

Sometimes other, usually high-pitched tones are added in the course of the treatment, if the high-frequency range is also affected by the hearing impairment.

3.8 Feeling of Pressure in and Behind the Ear

■ Pressure Sensation Through Sensitive Auditory Nerve

The feeling of pressure often described in Ménière's is usually felt behind the ear or like water in the ear. However, this is not actually the case. This perception of pressure corresponds essentially to a sensation of pressure on the sensitive auditory nerve, which is stimulated by the endolymphatic changes. This phenomenon can be explained in a similar way as a phantom pain in the ear, which is also possible but very rare.

The ear – like many other organs – knows only a few answers to very different stimuli. These are essentially:

- Hearing or not hearing
- Tinnitus – in case of hearing disorder
- Sensation of pressure and pain as an experience or reminder of the middle ear infections, that are common in most people during childhood

As we can remember painfully, the latter are often accompanied by a full middle ear. Fortunately, since the availability of antibiotics, no more suppurations in the bones or brain space are rare. The endolymphatic pressure increase could trigger these sensory impressions and thus give the feeling of a full ear.

Ruckenstein (2010) explains the feeling of ear pressure or "full ear" thus:

Middle ear infections, common in adolescence, are usually associated with low-frequency hearing loss and aural fullness, for example because of otitis media (inflammation in the middle ear).

Exacerbations of Menière's disease typically are associated with acute deteriorations of hearing in the low frequencies, which are the same frequencies affected by a conductive hearing loss. Therefore, it would seem reasonable to conclude that Menière's disease evoke a sensation of aural fullness based on prior learned associations.

Accordingly, a low-frequency hearing loss is also reminiscent of ear pressure. In terms of learning theory, this corresponds to "classical conditioning" (see ► Sect. 3.11).

3.9 Sensory Sensations (Paresthesia)

▪ Hyperexcitability and Tension

Sensitive sensations of one half of the face must be explained differently. These cannot be mediated via the auditory or vestibular nerve, but via the large fifth cranial nerve (N. trigeminale). This cranial nerve transmits sensations from the facial skin around the eyes, upper jaw and ears as well as from the lower jaw and the dental area to the brain. The sensations described as tingling, hypersensitivity, numbness or even pain could be interpreted as hyperexcitability and can usually be significantly alleviated by relaxation techniques such as progressive muscle relaxation according to Jacobsen. Here there may be a connection between the core areas of the vestibular and auditory nerve and the trigeminal nerve. However, the symptoms may be the expression of a general tension with the main expression in the area of the ear, and this can spread to the entire affected side in the course of the disease.

3.10 Lack of Compensation and Double Inhibition

▪ The Concept of "Persistent Perceptual and Postural Dizziness" ("3P-D")

Persistent postural-perceptual dizziness (PPPD) was defined for the International Classification of Vestibular Disorders in 2017. It is a chronic vestibular disorder that manifests with waxing and waning symptoms of dizziness, unsteadiness, or nonspinning vertigo that last for 3 months or more and are exacerbated by upright posture, active or passive motion of self, and exposure to environments with complex or moving visual stimuli (Staab 2020).

Triggers of PPPD include a wide variety of conditions that may cause vestibular symptoms or disrupt balance functioning, including neuro-otologic and other medical conditions and psychological distress.

While diagnostic tests and conventional imaging usually remain negative, patients with PPPD present in a characteristic way that maps on to positive diagnostic criteria. Patients often develop secondary functional gait disorder, anxiety, avoidance behavior and severe disability.

Once recognized, PPPD can be managed with effective communication and tailored treatment strategies, including specialized physical therapy (vestibular rehabilitation), serotonergic medications and cognitive-behavioral therapy (Staab 2020).

- **Missing of Re-adaptation**
- Prolonged uncertainty and dizziness
- Double inhibition
- Absence of compensation

If one source of the balance system provides confusing information, such as in a Ménière's attack, this requires a quick reaction (adaptation). Therefore, an attempt is made to inhibit the transmission of the confusing impulses from the damaged vestibular component to the central nervous system. This leads to a reduction in reception from the troubled organ.

At the same time, Ménière's vertigo is – mostly – accompanied by understandable feelings of fear.

To reduce this component, the connections between the anxiety cycle in the limbic system and the central processing pathways also make it possible to raise the threshold for impulses from the afferent perceptions (Balaban et al. 2011).

> This means: Both for organic reasons (inhibition of the confusing organic impulses) and due to the fear reaction ("psychic"), the flow of information from the affected vestibular organ can be inhibited (double inhibition).

If one part is reduced in the vestibular system, the remaining parts of the vestibular system automatically predominate. When the information from the vestibular system is pushed back, a (relative) predominance of impulses from the visual perception and the proprioceptors (the visual and proprioceptive system). This leads to a partly conscious, but predominantly unconscious concentration on these two systems and to a subordination of the information from the vestibular organ.

Purely organically, in the case of damage in semicircular canals of the vestibular organ, faster movement frequencies than 0.2 Hz must be reproduced via the eye movements. But these are not able to do this exactly. This – suboptimal – solution can lead to the fact, that it is no longer possible, reliably to differentiate between one's own movements and movements from the environment. This can result in a restricted movement and posture behavior (careful movements, possibly with supports) and a high level of attention for the moving environment.

> Adjustments make sense in the acute stage – and have to be abandoned when the acute event is over.

These adjustment efforts are useful in the acute stage. However, they must be abandoned when the disorder is over! In the acute attack of Ménière's disease, this happens "relatively" fast – unlike a loss of balance that lasts for weeks.

In Ménière's disease, after recovery from the organic event, a complete recovery in movement behavior is usually possible. The respective loss of balance, which usually remains after the individual attacks, is usually so (low) that it can be compensated during the seizure-free period. It is then important that the adaptation efforts are not inhibited or even suppressed by fear or an anxious avoidance behavior.

> If the adaptive behavior after the attack cannot be abandoned, there remains a maladaptation due to the failure to re-adapt (Staab 2012).

A persistent inhibition and thus a persistent feeling of dizziness can remain, for example, if one fears, that the "Ménière" as an attack – or in its effects – has not yet come to an end after all, or if one permanently fears, that the next attack will come soon. A concatenation of organic and emotional reactions can lead to an unfavorable loop of sustained securing behavior and increased reaction to movement stimuli.

Then a limited tolerance for postural changes often develops, whether they are caused by movements or by the visual environment. This results in high-frequency, small-amplitude postural corrections and often leads to postural control strategies, that would be appropriate to compensate for a high (fall) risk (e.g. when walking on black ice).

Staab (2012) describes the factors, that promote persistent dizziness and dizziness behavior:
- high anxiety levels,
- high attention to the symptoms of balance,
- catastrophic thoughts about the possible development.

This is "reinforced" by real repeated organic events, which often occurs in a Ménière's disease.

"Mortal Sins" in Compensation

In addition, the development towards a re-functioning balance may be delayed in the case of

- too much avoidance or too little practice,
- little own and professionally conveyed confidence in success of the possible efforts,
- anti-vestibular drugs "against dizziness" instead of balance exercises,
- overlooking a possible pre-existing or developing mental impairment.

What Can Remain Purely Organic Over Time – At the End of the Disease

As the Ménière's disease progresses, the Ménière's attacks over the years usually lead to a one-sided hearing loss with tinnitus and a one-sided failure of the affected vestibular organ. In most cases, the hearing performance can be supported with a hearing aid or a cochlea implant. The loss of balance can also be compensated to a large extent. This means that most of the vestibular skills necessary for daily life can be provided by one vestibular organ.

Thus, as *a* reaction to the loss of balance in the brainstem as a new basic impulse rate for the information REST has been established. This has approached both sides in a compensatory way and thus decreased in the result.

Gaze Leaps (Saccades)

When moving to the sick side, the information rate on the healthy side is reduced. Even then the impulses to the moving side "outweigh" the "new" resting state. However, the difference is not as great as if the impulse rate of the healthy organ had been added. This means that changes to the sick side cannot be recorded as precisely as those to the healthy side. This can lead to a saccade (gaze leap).

Therefore, in very fast movements to the sick side, the compensatory eye movement is no longer able to keep up. In this case, a sudden gaze leap ("saccade") must be added in order to fix the target.

Possible Function Reduction for Too Fast Movements

This means that even after a long period of loss of balance, certain extreme situations can only be mastered with "eye jumps" or "double vision" (i.e. apparent movements of the surroundings). For the affected person, this means, that in these situations, feelings of dizziness and unpleasant memories may occur. Here, knowledge and an appropriate foresight can help, without avoiding further action.

3.11 Reactive, Psychogenic Vertigo

In more frequent attacks, vertigo affects not only the vomiting center, the eye-movements and muscle activity, but also the entire condition of the affected person. Then the vertigo can also seize the soul and manifest itself as constant dizziness. This is called psychogenic dizziness. If Ménière's disease appears first and then the psychogenic dizziness, it is called reactive psychogenic dizziness.

It should be pointed out that this is not an inevitable process. There are life circumstances that protect against this additional development (protective factors) and also factors that promote it.

▪ Constant Dizziness

The reactive psychogenic dizziness is described rather unpacifically by those affected. One is dizzy, not stable, shaky, teasing, confused in the head, has a booming feeling and fear, often very much fear. Whole days are now "Ménière days". In certain situations, this feeling, combined with fear and panic, can be experienced like a Ménière's attack, although there is no trembling of the eyes (nystagmus) and the sufferer can stand.

How can an organic illness develop into psychogenic dizziness?

▪ Fear Can Become a Disease Component

Those who lose their balance unpredictably and often massively, usually lose their footing and security. To make matters worse, the typical attacks of rotational vertigo are often accompanied by fear of death and destruction. If this existentially threatening event occurs more often, the fear of its repetition understandably grows. In the process, fear can become so great, that it itself is perceived as insecurity and dizziness up to a feeling of vertigo. So it can become a disease component of its own.

The mechanism of action of the reactive psychogenic dizziness acquired as a result of the disease is easily explained in many cases.

Often salivation starts at the sight of food; this is an extremely sensible, biologically important reaction. If the bell is rung at the same time as the meal, after a certain time the ringing alone is enough to make salivation.

What happened? – A stimulus that until then had been completely insignificant in connection with food is coupled with a biological reaction that has always been present. The consequence is that this previously insignificant stimulus triggers the same reaction as the biologically meaningful one. This corresponds to a "classical conditioning" (Pawlow 1927). If the new connection between stimulus (ringing) and reaction (salivation) proves successful, the ringing can also become increasingly unspecific. Consequently, more and more similar stimuli can trigger the above reaction if this is in turn "rewarded". In this case, this is the case when the "stimulus" is followed by the expected food. This leads to a "stimulus generalization".

▪ Learnable and Forgettable

Since we cannot "consciously" occupy ourselves with such and other learning processes and results that take place again and again all day long, much of it disappears into the unconscious. For example, after a certain period, it can seem completely "hazy" and incomprehensible to us why our mouths always salivate at a certain ringing. However, this process can be explained – and also "forgettable" (!) and thus erasable.

3.11.1 How Can Organic Vertigo Become Psychogenic Dizziness in Ménière's Disease?

Vertigo attacks are usually accompanied by violent feelings like:

- Uncertainty
- Fear and panic
- "Vegetative" symptoms (e.g. sweat, changes in blood pressure, palpitations, etc.)

Of course, these do not take place in an isolated, airless room, but under certain "concomitant circumstances", that preceded the attack or in which the attack occurred (◘ Fig. 3.2).

▪ Accompanying Circumstances Become Triggers

With corresponding, individually different sensitivity, these concomitant circumstances or parts thereof can subsequently trigger the same symptoms as an organically caused Ménière's attack completely unconsciously.

These accompanying circumstances are often:

- A spatial situation in which the attack occurred or was repeated
- A situation that is frightening, depressing or "pulling the rug from under your feet"
- Tinnitus increasing in loudness, which had preceded the organically induced attack

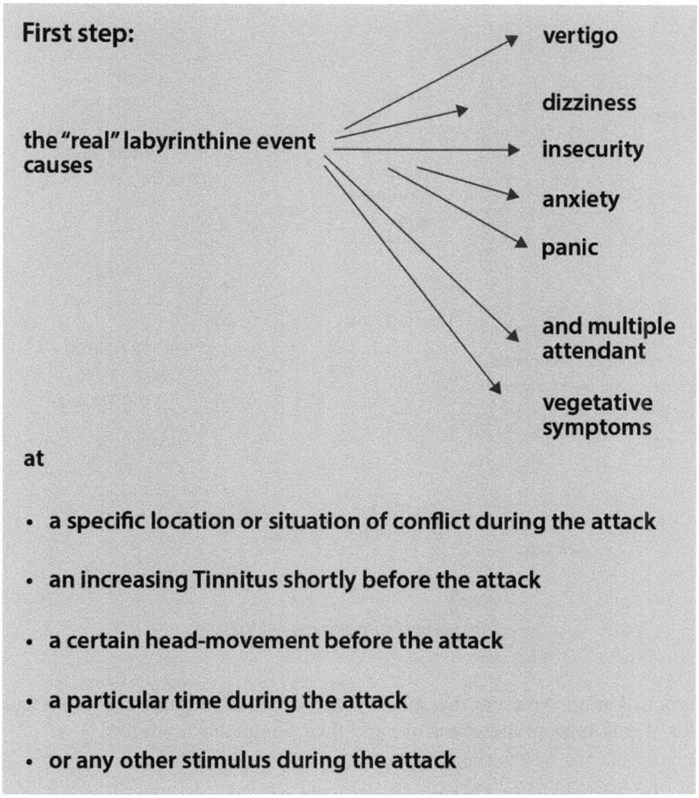

Fig. 3.2 First step of classical conditioning. An event that initially only occurs simultaneously to vertigo can itself become a triggering stimulus, if it is appropriately sensitive and then adequately reinforced

- A head movement
- The time

To put it clearly: These concomitant circumstances do not trigger an organic evoked Ménière's attack, as can be seen in a vertigo with falling down and especially with eye tremors (nystagmus).

But the feelings of

- insecurity,
- fear and panic,

as well as "vegetative" symptoms like:

- sweat,
- blood pressure changes,
- heart palpitations, etc.

can be experienced in the same way *as* a Ménière's attack (**Fig. 3.3**).

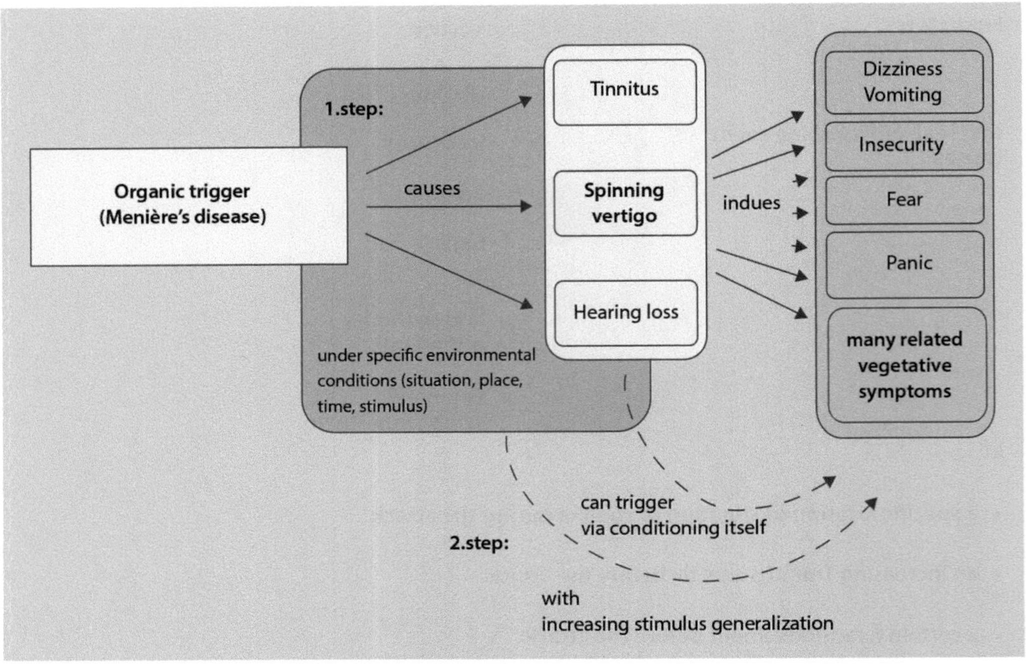

Fig. 3.3 Second step of classical conditioning. An event that initially only occurs simultaneously to vertigo can itself become a triggering stimulus, if it is appropriately sensitive and then adequately reinforced

In addition, in this vicious circle of:
- fear
- misjudging fear as a dizziness
- increasing feelings of dizziness in certain – again with fear – accompanying circumstances
- increasing fear of the increasingly frequent and prolonged dizziness
- experienced fainting during the attacks and "indefinitely" afterwards

even the stimuli that trigger them become increasingly unspecific. Consequently, similar situations or phenomena can trigger the sensation of dizziness, a process known as stimulus generalization.

Maintaining Factors

Unfavorable Cognitive-Emotional Processing

Yet we humans do not (only) react like Pavlov's dog or Skinner's pigeons. Therefore, further processes at the level of cognitive-emotional processing must be added, which help us to understand why reactive dizziness may be established in some affected persons, but not in others.

Unfavorable Assessments

These include:
- A low assessment of once own coping skills
- Unfavorable attention processes and evaluations that focus more on the disease than on health
- Catastrophic assessments
- Avoidance behavior that can arise from the fear of attacks that have already occurred and the fear and uncertainty of new attacks
- The fear (fed by the fear of new vertigo) of having new and corrective learning experiences
- An impairment of social communication
- Lack of social networks

In addition, unfavorable basic assumptions and cognitive distortions can be added. At the level of basic assumptions, persistent attitudes that are challenged by the dizziness can be "pushed up", for example "I am not good enough". Cognitive distortions such as absolute thinking ("I must always be able to work under unrestricted stress".) can cause pressure and tension and thus make coping just as difficult as irrational assessments (e.g. absolute demands) and "systematic errors of thought".

Basic Categories of the Evaluation

Four basic categories of irrational evaluation can be distinguished according to Ellis (1977):
- *Absolute requirements:*
  - "I must be unassailable and get recognition from all".
  - "Everything has to go smoothly".
  - "I must be in perfect health".
- *Global negative external and self-assessments:*
  - "I'm not good enough".
  - "All others do better, etc."
- *Catastrophic thinking:*
  - "The swindle will destroy my life".
- *Low frustration tolerance:*
  - "If the dizziness doesn't go away, it would be unbearable".

Tables of Thinking Errors

Systematic errors in thinking according to J. Beck (1997) are:
- Arbitrary conclusions: "You can't be efficient with Ménière's disease".
- Selective generalization: "I'm not taken seriously".
- Overgeneralize: "Yesterday something unpleasant happened to me again. It'll keep getting worse".

- Personalize: "The Ménière is there to make me down", "What am I being punished for?"
- Thinking in "black and white": "Either you're good or you're bad" or: "Either I'm fit and able and 100% healthy or I'm on the ground and unable to do anything".
- Minimize and maximize: "The Ménière is the worst thing that can happen to me".

In this sense, Wirth (2000) has been able to identify many thoughts in his dizziness patients that increase "dizziness" and fear.

Ménière-Related Thoughts

So, patients report unfavorable thoughts like:

- "What will people think of me if I waver like this?"
- "Maybe I have to die now!"
- "I feel like something's broken in my head!"
- "I'm sure I'll fall down and get hurt!"
- "I can't take any more of this dizziness!"
- "The dizziness never ends!"
- "I can't get over this dizzy spell!"
- "I'm being thrown off track!"
- "The ground is being pulled out from under my feet!"
- "I'm losing my grip on the world!"

Sustained Feelings

The most often feeling accompanying a dizzy reaction is fear. Specifically, it can be fear that

- the dizziness doesn't end or will soon return,
- once suddenly feel nauseous and vomit, which is very real with Ménière's disease,
- something bad happens,
- the dizziness is a sign of a yet undiscovered threatening disease.

Feelings unfavorable to the habituation are

- Helplessness
- Anger
- Grief over the sometimes lost balance

Experienced Helplessness

The feeling of control and feasibility can get lost during the course of the illness, even to the point of experienced helplessness.

The conviction to get the disease under control and to be able to influence the course of the disease also depends on the experienced or not experienced therapeutic support. The conviction can refer to the person "who cannot be helped" or to the illness "that cannot be cured". In the unfavorable case, an attitude develops in which patients believe that they are completely dependent on the doctor or "medicine" or are at the mercy of an unknown fate.

The lower the conviction becomes that they can control their own lives, the more likely they are to fall into fear and depression, as Wirth (2000) observed.

■ Anxiety and Vertigo

There is also another phenomenon. Even anxiety, which occurs almost naturally during dizzy spells, can itself be experienced as dizziness and vertigo. This can initiate a permanent process of anxiety and vertigo.

This "vicious circle" can continue even if the vestibular organ has long since lost its function. It is important to know that these mechanisms take place mainly unconsciously and are often "monstrous" in their effect for those affected – and usually also for their relatives, friends and neighbors.

■ Unpredictability Is a Major Factor in Persistent Anxiety

The main factor for persistent anxiety in Ménière's patients is the unpredictability of the attack, as Kirby and Yardley (2009), based on psychological questionnaires, have empirically demonstrated. The perceived embarrassment and shame of being observed by others in their own misery and the feeling of being handicapped also play an important role (Arroll et al. 2012), which patients are reluctant to talk about without being asked. This fear fed by insecurity and shame can, in our experience, be addressed by

- The best possible understanding of the disease and its triggers
- The distinction between psychogenic and inner ear vertigo
- A good preparation for the possible event in order to be able to deal with it

In addition to this "learning-theoretical approach", there is also a "psychodynamic interpretation" of the reactive psychogenic dizziness in Ménière's disease.

Lamparter (2002) sums up:

■ Illness Becomes Stress

> *In the course of the disease, the further triggering of the attacks seems to become increasingly detached from the extent of the subjectively experienced "stress". The disease itself becomes more and more "stressful", because the affected patient can*

never be sure not to experience an existentially shattering attack in the next moment. .... These can in turn lead to an increase in inner tension and intensify the general emotional defense, which is generally predisposing for psychosomatic reactions. This, in turn, can lead to an increase in intrapsychic tension, the removal of which no longer takes place as a reaction to tangible external events, so that an organic event – albeit only apparently – independent of psychic influences results. The patient often feels bitterly alone with this relatively rare but dramatic disease, especially as its severity is often not sufficiently recognized by the environment.

▪ **Risk of Mental Illness Increases**

More than one third of patients with (chronic) dizziness are described as having clinically significant psychological problems (Staab 2012). Patients with repeated dizziness are even more likely to suffer from anxiety or depression than patients with temporary vertigo. Thus, mental illness is seen significantly more often in Ménière's disease patients than in the general population: Coker et al. (1989) found 70% significant depression in patients with active Ménière compared to 32% in a calmed (burnt out) Ménière's disease. Both values are significantly higher than the approximately 6–9% depression in the general population. Also phobic syndromes (anxious avoidance behavior) are significantly more frequent in patients with Ménière's disease (Celestino et al. 2003; Takahashi et al. 2001; Levo et al. 2010).

In the large British study – with comparison group! – the Morbus Ménière group showed a significantly increased incidence and longer duration of depression, fatigue, tension and dejection (Tyrrell et al. 2015). Ménière's patients visited a doctor more often for depression or anxiety disorders and took antidepressants more often.

3.11.2 Maintenance of Vertigo in Cases of Previous Mental Illness

The Mainz research group led by Eckhardt-Henn et al. (2009) was able to show in a prospective longitudinal study over 1 year in 68 vertigo patients, that a pre-existing mental illness contributes significantly to the development of reactive psychogenic dizziness.

> Mental illness increases the risk of reactively psychogenic dizziness. This is especially true for diseases with – unpredictable – recurrent character such as migraine and Ménière's disease.

On the other hand, the extent of the organic disturbance in the organ of balance had no influence on the development of mental illness. Consequently, Eckhardt-Henn et al. (2009) also call for a psychological diagnosis and corresponding psychological test diagnostics in cases of persistent dizziness. In 1996, Savastano found higher values in "neuroticism level" and for "psychological stress", higher subjective values for physical symptoms, a higher cognitive focus on the feeling of illness and a higher disease behavior.

Anderson and Harris (2001) concluded – certainly very questionable – from results of *a* "Quality of well-being" scale that Ménière's patients – at the time of the study – ranked between Alzheimer's patients and AIDS and cancer patients 6 days before death.

Celestino et al. (2003) observed (without wanting to explain this) the development of an additionally psychogenic proportion more often in middle-aged women, poor education, longer lasting Ménière's disease and a large number of Ménière's attacks. Rarely did this increase occur among men of young age and with higher vocational training.

Yardley et al. (2003) described an influence of organic factors such as several severe dizziness attacks (which could not be separated from the psychological component, however), hearing loss and tinnitus on the self-assessed state of health in 370 respondents of the English Ménière support group. It showed up however of its independent components such as:

- Youth age
- Female sex
- Living alone
- Poor employment status
- The assumption, that the behavior of the doctor is not helpful

In Savastano et al. (2007), described increased anxiety values in the psychological test in 77 Ménière's patients as well as in 133 patients who showed "only" one of the symptoms dizziness, tinnitus and hearing loss. Ménière's patients differed from the other patients only with regard to elevated values in the "extroversion" scale.

Arroll et al. (2012) examined 74 patients using the "Dizziness Handicap Inventory" with regard to dizziness intensity. With the "Illness Intrusiveness Ratings Scale", they estimated the influence on the lifestyle, on the development of depression and on the uncertainty caused by the disease. It was found that dizziness has the greatest negative influence on lifestyle. Only 2 patients were symptom-free, 6 showed moderate symptoms, while 66 patients showed significant depression.

Between 1994 and 1997, we examined a total of 96 Ménière's patients who were admitted as in-patients for 6–8 weeks. We found:

- 41% (n = 39) well-compensated patients with a sufficient handling of the dizziness for them. They suffered more from hearing loss and/or tinnitus.
- 59% (n = 57) with reactively psychogenic dizziness, which dominated the clinical picture.

Lahmann et al. (2015) examined a collective of 547 patients with a wide spectrum of organic and non-organic vertigo syndromes in an interdisciplinary vertigo consultation. The investigation included a detailed neurostatus, a structured clinical interview for mental disorders (SCID-I) and a questionnaire for self-assessment of vertigo symptoms, depression, anxiety, somatization and quality of life. The neurological examination revealed organic vertigo in 80.8% of cases and non-organic vertigo in 19.2% of cases.

In 48.8% of all patients, psychological abnormalities, mostly anxiety and phobias, as well as somatoform and affective disorders were observed. In patients with confirmed organic dizziness, 42.5% of all patients showed psychological abnormalities. Thus, almost half of the patients with vertigo showed psychological abnormalities, even if – as in most cases – an organic reason for the occurrence of the vertigo could be found!

▪ Too Less Information Maintains Dizziness

In addition, we found in our patients that the psychogenic dizziness forms are to be expected the more frequently, the less the affected persons are comprehensibly informed about the organic events and their effects.

▪ "Spiral Phase Model"

Reineke (2002) examined examines the possibility of "coping" with this "critical life event" according to Schuchardt's "spiral phase model". Schuchardt presents the coping with crisis events as a processing process in eight phases, which ideally passe through one after the other, so that a successful coping can take place.

Reineke found that all ten remained in the first phase, defined as "uncertainty", for a very long time after the first attacks. This uncertainty prevented them from being able to deal with the illness in a "real" way, leaving plenty of room for anxiety and uncertainty, which increased the feeling of dizziness.

Already in Yardley et al. (2001), and her colleagues were able to show that unfavorable assumptions and unquestioned thoughts (cognitions) about the consequences of vertigo have a negative influence on the course of the disease. This includes fears, wrong assumptions about the course of the disease and possibly also wrong or misunderstood (therapeutic) instructions. This can – independent of the organic causes – lead to the fact, that necessary activities are avoided or the environment, that could subjectively intensify the symptoms, is no longer visited.

■ **What Can Maintain (Almost Any) Dizziness Is Avoidance and to Less Activity**

To less activity and avoidance behavior inhibit central compensatory mechanisms from being set in motion. As a result, those affected can lose the ability to deal with the situation, with the result that neuropsychological adaptation fails to occur.

A vicious circle of unfavorable cognitions, fears and sparing behavior develops, which can lead to a hardening of the symptoms.

If vertigo patients are then left with the feeling of deception, the remaining security and reliability in relationships often dwindles dramatically. A state of loss of control and helplessness can develop with fear of expectation and subsequent avoidance, which usually increases the problem and leads to social isolation and/or dependence. Consequently, although the development of a psychological process such as "reactive dizziness" is not primary dependent on the extent of the organic damage, it does depend on the way in which the organic process is experienced and on the way in which the environment and the practitioner are understood. For the affected persons themselves, the usually gradual expansion of vertigo to the mental area is hardly noticeable on its own.

■ **Clues Searching for a Fixed Point, Pedal Attempts**

However, certain clues can be helpful:

In order to be able to distinguish even psychogenic dizziness from a vertigo caused by the inner ear, it is useful to choose one or more surely immovable points or objects **before** the next vertigo event and to fix one of these in the attack. Then you can check for yourself whether the world is moving around you or whether the object can be held in place. A further criterion for differentiation is to stand up, stamp firmly and check, whether walking and pedaling attempts can achieve stability and whether the dizziness in the head subsides.

In the case of an organically caused Ménière's attack, fixing an object and getting up are not or hardly possible – and also not useful. On the other hand, psychogenic dizziness can

Table 3.1 Possible distinction between psychogenic vertigo and inner ear vertigo

Clues		Inner ear-related vertigo	Psychogenic dizziness
Own recognition	Fixation of a solid object	Not possible	Possible
	Heavy stomping	Not possible, increases dizziness	Reduces the sensation of dizziness and leads to more stability
	Familiar people	Without direct influence on vertigo	Can significantly improve recovery from dizziness
Medical examination	Eye tremor (nystagmus)	Identifiable (Frenzel glasses)	Not present
	Description of the vertigo	Vertigo, the space moves around the person	Diverse, permanent, for days, always …
	Audiogram (hearing test)	Repeated low frequency losses and fluctuations	Without change

subside with increasing activity – and often with the help of a familiar person (Table 3.1).

Despite the increased risk that the soul, along with the organ of balance, also weakens, a Ménière's disease does not automatically lead to a mental illness.

Thus, mental comorbidity is not equally pronounced in all patients with Ménière's disease. Cluster analyses of disease perceptions showed that some react like a healthy group and others show very striking values (Savastano et al. 1996). Much depends on the processing possibilities, the knowledge about the disease, the handling of the disease and last but not least the environment.

As described in ► Chap. 1, Tyrrell et al. (2015) and coauthors found in a large number of Meniere's disease patients that mental health and well-being showed a significant correlation with the duration of the disease. Patients with longer-lasting symptoms of Meniere's disease turned out significantly better than those with a recent onset. This indicates that there may be adaptive strategies. The authors suggest increased social support and social interaction, which could contribute to a satisfying way of dealing with life in spite of the symptoms (Tyrrell et al. 2015).

Accordingly, support from the social environment is seen as very important, and it is logically advised that relatives be also be involved in the counseling process.

3.11.3 Can Fear and Panic Cause Ménière's Attacks?

▪ Semi-conscious and Especially Sensitive?

An exciting question, even if it can only be answered speculatively, is to what extent mental distress can be involved in the development or manifestation of Ménière's disease. One of the first to assume that the psyche could express itself in balance and muscle tension was a psychoanalyst of the first hour, Paul Schilder (1942). He even suspected that changes in the psyche could lead to organic changes in the vestibular organ. The basis for this was his observation, that this organ is a sensory organ, that receives only semi-conscious impressions, to which it reacts with mostly unconscious, "instinctive, primitive movements".

A neurophysiological substantiation of this seemingly daring assumption could be provided by the fact that the vestibular sensory epithelium is also influenced at least by the central nervous system and thus also by the limbic system.

▪ Trigger "Stress"

If one looks at the connection between "stress" and Ménière's fits, opinions differ.

While Soderman et al. (2004) identified emotional – not physical – stress as a possible trigger in 46 patients with a total of 153 seizures (reported by the patients themselves), Andersson et al. (1997) could not confirm this in 20 patients over a period of 193 days. The individual characteristics of the individual factors were too great to be able to make a reliable statement.

▪ Explosive Voltage Dissipation

Especially for the triggering of the first attack in Ménière's patients, psychoanalytic authors have made assumptions. Thus, Fowler and Zeckel (1952), Hinchcliffe (1967), Basecqz (1969), Groen (1983), Landino (1985) and Lamparter (2002) believe to have found a significant psychologically mediated component. They suspect that an explosive dissipation of tension occurs during a seizure, as the persons affected have often been unable to express an existential shock in any other way.

Above Average Diligence?

Groen (1983) reported on 21 Ménière sufferers in whom he believed to find common personality traits. He described for them an above-average intelligence, which he attributed to job descriptions(!), a pronounced tendency towards seclusion, perfectionism in work and hobby and a pronounced "super-ego". He suspected a "key-lock mechanism" with three essential influencing factors in these patients:

- A more or less specific personality structure
- An interpersonal conflict that is particularly frustrating for a personality with just this structure
- An inhibition or impossibility of emotional expression

Landino (1985) examined eight patients from rural areas. These also showed self-contained characteristics, which, however, differed significantly from the characteristics reported by Groen.

After all, the psychologist Rüster was able to examine 30 Ménière patients from the psychosomatic clinic in Hamburg-Eppendorf in 1989. He described them – in the language of psychologists – as yielding, considerate and aggressively inhibited people. They presented themselves as moderate, balanced and extremely conscientious. No wonder that these people were also easily irritable and had "aggressive-sadistic" traits, which were, however, repressed.

As an essential result of his extensive literature work, Rüster (1989) points out that several psychological characteristics are noticeable in patients with Ménière's disease. In the foreground were anxieties due to and during the dizzy spells, but also a constant anxiety-depressive mood. In addition, aggressive inhibitions and a vegetative instability were frequently described. Typical personality structures and the essential criterion of the existence of emotional triggers were repeatedly found.

After a mailing survey of Japanese patients with fluctuating hearing with and without vertigo, a Japanese working group around Onuki et al. (2005) suspects that these patients

- are "tied" to their work – perhaps they also mean over-enthusiastic in their work,
- would inhibit themselves and feel pressed by time,
- were intransigent towards themselves.

At the same time, they saw a clear difference in their daily life-style (compared to the other Japanese). Nevertheless, they interpret the committed behavior and self-restraint as a desire to be rewarded by others. If this reward does not come, the patients would get a great internal stress, which they interpret as a possible Ménière trigger.

De Valck et al. (2007) also suspected a higher "sense of duty" (compulsiveness) in Ménière's patients, but found no deviating values in a questionnaire designed for this purpose compared to other ear and balance patients.

- **Few Studies, Different Results**

The problem of all available studies is that although they show great unity in themselves, they differ from each other in important points. There is always a lack of meaningful comparison groups with other psychosomatically ill patients, for whom similar typical structures are often described, and there is always a lack of statistically convincing case numbers.

So, there will probably not be a specific type of Ménière; everyone reacts differently to the very differently developed disease. Wexler and Crary (1986) describe that where comparison groups have been included, the differences become smaller and approach zero when the comparison groups approach Ménière's disease in their symptomatology. They assume that each disease produces its own psychopathology.

My own experience and Schilder's assessment have led me personally to call the first German edition of this book in the subtitle "War in the Inner Ear". The image of two seems to me to be themselves – unconsciously! – fighting forces in many Ménière's patients often seems to be coherent. Nevertheless, the majority of mental distress, as mentioned above, is probably a reaction to the organic illness. There are probably many mixed forms in between.

For scientific purposes, it is therefore necessary to distinguish between psychogenic and organic vertigo in order to evaluate the success of therapy.

Literature

Anderson JP, Harris JP (2001) Impact of Meniere's disease on quality of life. Otol Neurotol 22:888–894

Andersson G, Hagnebo C, Yardley L (1997) Stress and symptoms of Menière's disease: a time-series analysis. J Psychosom Res 43(6):595–603

Arroll M, Dancey CP, Attree EA, Smith S, James T (2012) People with symptoms of Meniere's disease: the relationship between illness intrusiveness, illness uncertainty, dizziness handicap, and depression. Otol Neurotol 33(5):816–812

Arweiler DJ, Jahnke K, Grosse-Wilde H (1995) Meniere's disease as an autosomal dominant inherited disorder. Laryngol Rhinol Otol 74:412415

Balaban CD, Jacob RG, Furman JM (2011) Neurologic bases for comorbidity of balance disorders, anxiety disorders and migraine: neurotherapeutic implications. Expert Rev Neurother 11(3):379–394. https://doi.org/10.1586/ern.11.19

Basecqz G (1969) Psychodynamic aspects of Menière's disease. Laval Med 40:838–843

Basura GJ, Adams ME, Monfared A, Schwartz SR, Antonelli PJ, Burkard R, Bush ML, Bykowski J, Colandrea M, Derebery J, Kelly EA, Kerber KA, Koopman CF, Kuch AA, Marcolini E, McKinnon BJ, Ruckenstein MJ, Valenzuela CV, Vosooney A, Walsh SA, Nnacheta LC, Dhepyasuwan N, Buchanan EM (2020) Clinical practice guideline: Ménière's disease. Executive summary. Otolaryngol Head Neck Surg 162(4):415–434

Beck JS (1997) Practice of cognitive therapy. Beltz PVU, Weinheim

Celestino D, Rosini E, Carucci ML, Marconi PL, Vercillo E (2003) Ménière's disease and anxiety disorders. Acta Otorhinolaryngol Ital 23(6):421–427

Coker NJ, Coker RR, Jenkins HA, Vincent KR (1989) Psychological profile of patients with Menière's disease. Arch Otolaryngol Head Neck Surg 115(11):1355–1357

Committee on Hearing and Equilibrium (1995) Guidelines for the diagnosis and evaluation of therapy in Menière's disease. Otolaryngol Head Neck Surg 113:181–185

De Valck CF, Wuyts FL, Vanspauwen R, Walravens S, Van de Heyning PH (2007) Conscientiousness in patients with Meniere's disease. Otol Neurotol 28(3):365–368

Düwel P, Walther LE, Haasler T, Westhofen M, Lückhoff A (2005) New concepts towards a pathophysiology of Meniere's disease at the cellular level. Laryngorhinootology 84:412–417

Eckhardt-Henn A, Tschan R, Best C, Dieterich M (2009) Somatoform vertigo syndromes. Nervenarzt 80:909–917

Ellis A (1977) Principles and method of rational-emotive behavior therapy. Pfeiffer, Munich, p S.256

Foster CA, Breeze RE (2013) Endolymphatic hydrops in Meniere's disease: cause, consequence, or epiphenomenon? Otol Neurotol 34:1210–1214

Fowler EP Jr, Zeckel A (1952) Psychosomatic aspects of Menière's disease. JAMA 148:1265–1271

Frykholm C, Larsen HC, Dahl N (2006) Familial Meniere's disease in five generations. Otol Neurotol 27:681–686

Gacek RR (2015) Recovery of hearing in Meniere's disease after antiviral treatment. Am J Otolaryngol 36(3):315–323

Groen JJ (1983) Psychosomatic aspects of Menière's disease. Acta Otolaryngol 95:407–416

Hinchcliffe R (1967) Emotions as a precipitating factor in Menière's disease. J Laryngol Otol 81:471–475

Huang TS (1991) Menière's disease: recent advances in basic and clinical aspects. Acta Otolaryngol Suppl 485:7–154

Jahnke K (1994) Stage-appropriate therapy of Menière's disease. Dtsch Arztebl 91:428–434

Kirby SE, Yardley L (2009) Cognitions associated with anxiety in Menière's disease. J Psychosom Res 66(2):111

Lahmann C, Henningsen P, Brandt T, Strupp M, Jahn K, Dieterich M, Eckhardt-Henn A, Feuerecker R, Dinkel A, Schmid G (2015) Psychiatric comorbidity and psychosocial impairment among patients with vertigo and dizziness. J Neurol Neurosurg Psychiatry 86(3):302–308. https://doi.org/10.1136/jnnp-2014-307601

Lamparter U (2002) Vertigo. In: Ahrens S, Schneider W (eds) Textbook of psychotherapy and psychosomatic medicine, 2nd edn. Schattauer, Stuttgart, pp 354–361

Landino A (1985) On the psychosomatics of Meniere's disease. Mater Psychoanal 11:104–147

Levo H, Stephens D, Poe D (2010) Use of ICF in assessing the effects of Meniere's disorder on life. Ann Otol Rhinol Laryngol 119:583–589
Morgenstern C (1985) Pathophysiology, clinic, and conservative therapy of Meniere's disease. Arch Otorhinolaryngol 1:1–66
Morgenstern C (1994) Meniere's disease. In: Naumann HH, Helms J, Herberhold C, Kastenabuer C (eds) Oto-rhino-laryngology in clinic and practice, vol 1: ear. Thieme, Stuttgart, pp 768–775
Morrison AW, Bailey ME, Morrison GA (2009) Familial Menière's disease: clinical and genetic aspects. J Laryngol Otol 123(1):29–37
Onuki J, Takahashi M, Odagiri K (2005) Comparative study of the daily lifestyle of patients with Menière's disease and controls. Ann Otol Rhinol Laryngol 114(12):927–933
Paparella MM, Djalilian HR (2002) Etiology, pathophysiology of symptoms, and pathogenesis of Menière's disease. Otolaryngol Clin N Am 35:529–545
Pawlow IP (1927) Conditioned reflexes. Clarendon, London
Plontke SK, Gürkov R (2015) Meniere's disease. Specialist knowledge ENT. LRO 94:530–554
Preyer S, Bootz F (1995) Tinnitus models for use in tinnitus counselling therapy of chronic tinnitus. HNO 43:338–351
Reineke M (2002) Morbus Menière – Behandlungsmöglichkeiten aus rehabilitationspädagogischer Sicht. Diploma thesis at the Institute for Rehabilitation Sciences at the Humboldt University of Berlin, 104 p
Reiß M, Reiß G (2015) Balance diagnostics. Videonystagmography and new examination methods. Springer, Berlin
Ruckenstein MJ (2010) Ménière's disease. Evidence and outcomes. Plural Publishing, San Diego, Oxford, Brisbane, p S162
Rudack C (1995) Immunology of the inner ear. An overview. HNO 43:275–281
Rüster P (1989) Psychosomatics and psychopathology of Meniere's disease. Dissertation, University of Hamburg
Salt AN, Hartsock JJ, Gill RM, Piu F, Plontke SK (2012) Perilymph pharmacokinetics of markers and dexamethasone applied and sampled at the lateral semi-circular canal. J Assoc Res Otolaryngol 13(6):771–783. https://doi.org/10.1007/s10162-012-0347-y. Epub 2012 Sep 12. PMID: 22968908; PMCID: PMC3505589
Savastano M, Maron MB, Mangialaio M, Longhi P, Rizzardo R (1996) Illness behaviour, personality traits, anxiety, and depression in patients with Menière's disease. J Otolaryngol 25(5):329–333
Savastano M, Marioni G, Aita M (2007) Psychological characteristics of patients with Ménière's disease compared with patients with vertigo, tinnitus, or hearing loss. Ear Nose Throat J 86(3):148–156. PMID: 17427776
Schaaf H, Hesse G (2012) Tinnitus-Leiden und Chnace. Profil. München 171 S
Schilder P (1942) The vestibular apparatus. In: Schilder P (ed) Mind, perception & thought in their constructive aspects. Columbia University Press, New York, pp 83–134
Soderman AC, Moller J, Bagger-Sjoback D (2004) Stress as a trigger of attacks in Menière's disease. A case-crossover study. Laryngoscope 114(10):1843–1848
Staab J (2012) Chronic subjective dizziness. Continuum 18(5):1118–1141
Staab JP (2020) Persistent postural-perceptual dizziness. Semin Neurol 40(1):130–137. https://doi.org/10.1055/s-0039-3402736
Takahashi M, Ishida K, Iida M, Yamashita H, Sugawara K (2001) Analysis of lifestyle and behavioral characteristics in Meniere's disease patients and a control population. Acta Otolaryngol 121(2):254–256

Trune DR (2006) Ion homeostasis and inner ear disease. In: Hamid M, Sismanis A (eds) Medical otology and neurotology: a clinical guide to auditory and vestibular disorders. Thieme, New York/Stuttgart

Tyrrell J, White MP, Barrett G, Ronan N, Phoenix C, Whinney DJ, Osborne NJ (2015) Mental health and subjective well-being of individuals with Ménière's: cross-sectional analysis in the UK Biobank. Otol Neurotol 36(5):854–861. https://doi.org/10.1097/MAO.0000000000000732

Westhofen M (2009) Meniere's disease. Evidence and controversies. ENT 57:446–454

Wexler M, Crary W (1986) Menière's disease: the psychosomatic hypothesis. Am J Otol 7:93–96

Wirth W (2000) Psychological possibilities in vertigo Tinnitus Forum 4/2000

Yardley L, Beech S, Weinman (2001) J Influence of beliefs about the consequences of dizziness on handicap in people with dizziness, and the effect of therapy on beliefs. J Psychosom Res 50(1):1–6

Yardley L, Dibb B, Osborne G (2003) Factors associated with quality of life in Menière's disease. Clin Otolaryngol Allied Sci 28(5):436–441. https://doi.org/10.1046/j.1365-2273.2003.00740.x. PMID: 12969347

Zenner HP (1989) Pathological motility and depolarisation of outer hair cells. Basic steps in K+ induced attacks of Menière's disease. In: Nadol JB (ed) Menière's disease. Pathogenesis, pathophysiology, diagnosis and treatment. Kugler & Ghendi, Amsterdam, pp 247–252

Zenner HP, Ernst A (1993) Cochlear-motor, transduction and signal-transfer tinnitus: models for three types of cochlear tinnitus. Eur Arch Otorhinolaryngol 249(8):447–454. https://doi.org/10.1007/BF00168852. PMID: 7680210

Special Forms of Meniere's Disease

Contents

4.1 Lermoyez Syndrome – 86

4.2 Tumarkin Drop – 86

4.3 Cochlear Form – 87

Literature – 87

H. Schaaf, *Ménière's Disease*, https://doi.org/10.1007/978-3-662-63610-7_4

4.1 Lermoyez Syndrome

■ Migraine Symptoms Often

In Lermoyez syndrome, which is not so common, hearing initially improves after an attack of vertigo. Until now, there is as no explanation for this. Also, the nystagmus in Lermoyez syndrome should only go in the direction of the sick side, without showing the alternation of stimulus and failure nystagmus (Kempf and Jahnke 1989).

In a case report, Manzari et al. (2012) examined how the functions of the parts of the vestibular organ change in an acute attack on the basis of the cervical and ocular VEMPs and the vestibulo-ocular reflex (VOR). In this case, the significantly reduced dynamics of the utricle function was striking.

Patients with Lermoyez syndrome often report migraine symptoms (Paparella in: Huang 1991, pp. 108–114). Otherwise, this form does not differ clinically from the classic picture of Meniere's disease and is also treated therapeutically in the same way.

4.2 Tumarkin Drop

Some patients with M. Meniere's disease may experience brief but violent balance attacks, usually at the end of the "natural" M. Meniere's course. The sudden fall ("drop attack") from complete well-being and with complete consciousness without any warning sign was described by Tumarkin in 1936 as an "otolithic catastrophe". This can be accompanied by a feeling as if one's head is being torn apart. This phenomenon, named after the first describer, is explained by a rupture of a balance sac, the sacculus and/or the utricle (Calzada et al. 2012; Huang and Young 2012).

There is a belief that at the end of a long history of Meniere's. the pressure of the hydrops can no longer be withstood even by the evolutionary oldest structures, the vestibular sacs saccule and utricle.

The rupture of saccule or utricle leads to a spontaneous movement of the otoliths with "abrupt loss of tone in the muscles supplied by the 'vestibulospinal' pathway" (Helling 2008), i.e. in the head it circles in a flash and the legs sag away. Pyykkö et al. (2019) speculate that sympathetic nervous system tone and the baroreflex are diminished in the process.

Typically, and fortunately, the attack is short, 10–20 s. Consciousness is preserved – an important distinguishing criterion from other diseases. However, we have also seen patients who have fainted because of the violent vegetative reaction or after hitting their head on a hard surface.

It is likely that this form of the disease, if any, only presents in late stages of Meniere's disease (Kentala et al. 2001). The few surveys with a follow-up period of more than 10 years suggest a proportion of 3–7% (Baloh et al. 1990; Pyykkö et al. 2019).

In this clinical picture, it is important to differentiate and exclude short-term circulatory disturbances ("small strokes", which are nevertheless strokes) of the brainstem. Migraine attacks must also be excluded.

Tumarkin crises cannot be influenced by medication – it is not possible to reach for a suppository or tablet so quickly. As far as can be seen, however, intratympanic gentamycin treatment (▶ Chap. 7) helps here too, if the entire labyrinth is not to be removed – as is still sometimes done (Viana et al. 2014).

4.3 Cochlear Form

Of the Meniere's diagnoses, Morgenstern (1994) has classified 2–3% as a special cochlear form, when a mostly tub-shaped, fluctuating loss of low frequencies without accompanying vertigo is observed. This is probably the clinical picture of endolymphatic events discussed in detail in ▶ Chap. 5. If – as envisaged by Gürkov et al. (2016) – the "hydropic inner ear disease" – can be established as Meniere's classification, this will then probably be named "hydrops disease of the cochlear type".

Literature

Baloh RW, Jacobson K, Winder T (1990) Drop attacks with Meniere's syndrome. Ann Neurol 28:384–387

Calzada AP, Lopez IA, Ishiyama G, Ishiyama A (2012) Otolithic membrane damage in patients with endolymphatic hydrops and drop attacks. Otol Neurotol 33:1593–1598

Gürkov R, Pyyko I, Zou J, Kentala E (2016) What is Menière's disease? A contemporary re-evaluation of endolymphatic hydrops. J Neurol 263(Suppl 1):71–81

Helling K (2008) Otolith dysfunction and treatment options. ENT 56:996–1002

Huang TS (1991) Menière's disease: recent advances in basic and clinical aspects. Acta Otolaryngol Suppl 485:7–154

Huang CH, Young YH (2012) Ocular and cervical vestibular-evoked myogenic potentials in Tumarkin falls. Otol Neurotol 33:1251–1256

Kempf HG, Jahnke K (1989) Lermoyez syndrome. Clinical aspects and follow-up. HNO 37:276–280

Kentala E, Havia M, Pyykko I (2001) Short-lasting drop attacks in Menière's disease. Otolaryngol Head Neck Surg 124:526–530

Manzari L, Burgess AM, Curthoys IS (2012) Vestibular function in Lermoyez syndrome at attack. Eur Arch Otorhinolaryngol 269:685–691

Morgenstern C (1994) Meniere's disease. In: Naumann HH, Helms J, Herberhold C, Kastenabuer C (eds) Oto-rhino-laryngology in clinic and practice, vol 1: ear. Thieme, Stuttgart, pp 768–775

Pyykkö I, Manchaiah V, Zou J, Levo H, Kentala E (2019) Association between syncope and Tumarkin attacks in Ménière's disease. J Int Adv Otol 15(1):135–140

Tumarkin L (1936) Otolithic catastrophe. A new syndrome. Br Med J 1: 175–177

Viana LM, Bahmad F, Rauch SD (2014) Intratympanic gentamicin as a treatment for drop attacks in patients with Meniere's disease. Laryngoscope 124:2151–2154

Differentiation from Other Clinical Pictures

What it Is NOT

Contents

5.1 A Misdiagnosis and its Treatment – 93
5.1.1 From Body to Soul and Back Again – 93

5.2 Fluctuating Hearing with Low Tone Tinnitus Without Vertigo – 96
5.2.1 Diagnosis – 100
5.2.2 Therapy – 100

5.3 Migrainous Vertigo (Basilar Migraine) – 101
5.3.1 Symptomatology – 102
5.3.2 Pathophysiology – 103
5.3.3 Diagnostics – 103
5.3.4 Treatment – 103

5.4 Benign Paroxysmal Positional Vertigo (BPPV) – 105
5.4.1 Diagnostics and Therapy – 105

5.5 Vestibular Neuritis – Acute Unilateral (Idiopathic) Vestibulopathy – 107
5.5.1 Possible Causes – 107
5.5.2 Diagnostics: Complete or Partial Failure? – 108
5.5.3 Therapy – 109
5.5.4 Balance Training – 110
5.5.5 Lack of Compensation – 111
5.5.6 Possible Functional Reduction for Too Fast Movements – 111
5.5.7 Hearing Impairment and Ringing in the Ears – 112
5.5.8 A Subsequent Paroxysmal Positional Vertigo – 112
5.5.9 Confusion in Experience – 112

H. Schaaf, *Ménière's Disease*, https://doi.org/10.1007/978-3-662-63610-7_5

5.6 Perilymph Fistula – 113
5.6.1 Diagnostics – 115
5.6.2 Therapy – 115
5.6.3 Excursus: Influences of Air Pressure on the Ear (Tullio Phenomenon) – 116
5.6.4 Tube Ventilation Disorder – 116

5.7 Vestibular Paroxysmia – 116

5.8 Isolated Otolith Dysfunction – 117

5.9 Psychogenic Dizziness – 118
5.9.1 Dizziness Instead of Unpleasant Feelings – 118
5.9.2 The Problem of Understanding – 120
5.9.3 Where Does the Psychogenic Dizziness Take Place? – 121
5.9.4 From the "Phobic Postural Vertigo" (PPV) to "Persistent Perceptual and Postural Dizziness" (3P-D) – 121
5.9.5 Dizziness in Sociophobia (Social Phobia) – 128

5.10 Multiple Sclerosis – 129

5.11 Central Vestibular Vertigo Syndrome – 130
5.11.1 Diagnostics – 130
5.11.2 Prevention – 131

5.12 Blood Pressure Fluctuations – 131

5.13 Acoustic Neuroma – 132
5.13.1 Diagnostics – 132

5.14 Bilateral Loss of Vestibular Function – 132

5.15 Head-Extension Vertigo: Cervicogenic? – 133
5.15.1 Diagnostics – 134
5.15.2 Therapy – 134

5.16 Drug-Induced Dizziness – 135
5.16.1 Gentamycin for the Elimination of Ménière's Disease – 136

Literature – 137

There Is a Great Risk of Confusion

Vertigo and Dizziness are very common symptoms with over 300 possible causes. Hearing loss and often associated tinnitus are equally common.

In a study from Finland, based on a survey and partly also on the examination of a sample from the general population, it was found that the number of respondents who reported dizziness and additionally a hearing disorder as well as tinnitus (i.e. the classic symptoms also exhibited by Ménière's disease) was 14 times higher than the number of actual Ménière's patients (Havia et al. 2005). Two Common Second Causes of Dizziness in Patients with Menière's Disease are "benign paroxysmal positional vertigo" and psychogenic dizziness (van Esch et al. 2016).

> Dizziness, hearing impairment and tinnitus often occur together, but are rarely Ménière's disease.

This makes it clear how important it is to make a precise diagnosis and to distinguish it from other clinical pictures, which may have to be treated in a completely different way.

> The diagnosis "Menière disease" may only be made if an endolymphatic event is accompanied by inner ear-related vertigo.

In addition, once the diagnosis has been made it is still important to check whether each new episode of dizziness is a Ménière's attack. Thus, the rare Ménière's disease can be joined by common vertigo disorders such as:

- Benign positional vertigo (BPPV)
- Migraine
- Psychogenic vertigo and dizziness
- Circulatory problems

Then these additional components are often misdiagnosed as Ménière's vertigo. The consequence is that adequate therapies are omitted.

For this reason, some types of vertigo, which are either difficult to distinguish from Ménière's disease and/or may occur in the course of Ménière's disease, are discussed in more detail below.

5.1 A Misdiagnosis and its Treatment

5.1.1 From Body to Soul and Back Again

How organic and treatable findings mix with psychogenic images and then the "necessary" therapies can be omitted is to be shown by the cases described in the following.

■ Case 1: Benign Paroxysmal Positional Vertigo (BPPV)

A retired 74-year-old priest was diagnosed with Ménière's disease 8 years ago. Just after his retirement, a severe attack of vertigo had occurred. This resulted in long-lasting helplessness, fainting and nausea. The ENT physician also diagnosed bilateral hearing loss. The simultaneous presence of vertigo and hearing loss had led to the suspicion of Ménière's disease. In the last 7 years, the attacks of vertigo had recurred more frequently; the severity had not diminished in any way. However, despair and fainting have increased. Also, an unsteadiness of gait had often remained for days.

In the anamneses with us the patient described that the vertigo always occurred in certain movement situations. His idea was therefore that the cervical spine caused the vertigo. Therefore, he constantly tried to avoid head movements to the left. In doing so, he had visibly adopted a protective posture. He himself had further noticed that the vertigo attacks had always occurred in situations with great psychological pressure.

After a thorough examination of the cervical spine, there was indeed a clear hardening of the left neck muscles. However, the X-ray examinations did not reveal any conspicuous findings. The auditory findings showed a significant decrease in the high frequency range, but not in the low-frequency range, as would have been expected in Ménière's disease. Tinnitus was not present.

After a specific questioning, it became apparent that the dizziness could be divided into two parts in terms of time and character: The first part was made up of vertigo attacks lasting for about 30 s to (subjectively appearing much longer) 2 min with a tendency to fall to the left. This "whirled" him to the floor. Thereby the room spun for him, he got a feeling of annihilation – with preserved consciousness. This was followed in the second part for a long time by a solidifying feeling of powerlessness, despair, "being depressed" and insecurity. Then he could only walk staggeringly and also only visit his doctor "supported". This feeling of dizziness lasts for more than 6 h, in some cases even for 2–3 days.

Positioning examination During a positioning examination, vertigo and eye tremor (nystagmus) could be induced when the patient was positioned on the left side. Subjectively, he expressed a – familiar – violent onset of dizziness, which subsided after 30 s. In contrast, neither vertigo nor nystagmus occurred when the patient was positioned on the right side.

It turned out that the patient did not suffer from Ménière's disease but from a – misdiagnosed – benign positional vertigo of the left side. In this disease of the vestibular organ, small calcium crystals (otoliths) have "strayed". Spontaneously or after a head injury, they have been deposited from one part of the vestibular organ (utricle) into another (lower semicircular canal), where they do not belong. When the patient changes position, they move in direction of gravity, causing a brief, but intense vertigo. These attacks are accompanied by specific eye tremors (nystagmus), which can be well examined.

In this patient, Ménière's disease could be excluded. However, the second part of the prolonged vertigo and the bilateral high-frequency hearing loss remained to be clarified. This could be clarified by the patient's history.

▪ Predominant High-Frequency Hearing Loss

Born in Gdansk (Poland) in 1928, as a teenager he was exposed to bombing raids first by the German and later the Soviet army. The multiple noise could explain the high-frequency hearing loss, that the patient consciously did not notices. While his father was deployed as a soldier far outside of Gdansk, the son had to witness the attacks on his mother at home, powerlessness in an adjoining chamber.

As far as it was possible in this conversation, the positional vertigo seemed to have triggered an earlier psychological experience of powerlessness, despair and depression. This triggered the long-lasting – psychogenic (!) – vertigo that lasted for hours or days. This had nothing to do with the organic disease itself.

Thus, without knowing the background of the patient's life, the practitioner is quickly inclined (or seduced) to believe that the patient is "acting up." This can result in the patient not being understood and, above all, not being treated in the way that would be possible.

Therefore, it is to understand on which personal history "objective" disease is based.

Then one can understand,

- what triggers it,
- how to deal with it and
- what could bring about recovery.

The therapy consisted of:

- Positioning maneuvers, which could eliminate the organic symptomatology
- Physiotherapy to correct the almost shortened neck muscles

- Prescription of two hearing aids that improved the patient's ability to communicate, and
- Short-term psychotherapy, which focused on the processing of the experiences in the war

▪ Case 2: Ménière's Disease and Positional Vertigo

A 67-year-old female patient suffered – indeed – since many years from Ménière's attacks of several hours with low-frequency tinnitus at 250 Hz on the right and a low-frequency hearing loss on the right up to 70 dB. However, her vertigo symptoms had changed significantly over the past 4 years. Thus, none of the vertigo symptoms lasting for hours with vomiting had occurred, but short, violent attacks had (on demand dependent from movement-!). Now she is afraid to move much at all. She does not dare to go outside anymore; this is experienced as very oppressive by the husband and the daughter's family.

▪ First Menière Disease, Then Positional Vertigo

An inpatient stay in a psychosomatic clinic as well as a psychologist, who was consulted because of the increasingly depressive symptoms, could not help her. Here, the positional test showed a positional vertigo to the left, so that in this patient two different (!) organic diseases were present, both of which subsequently resulted in an increasing psychogenic dizziness component.

The experience of vertigo corresponds to the accompanying vegetative symptoms of the Ménière's attacks that have taken place. These then run as an "as-if" event. The therapy consisted of course also in positioning maneuvers, which let the symptomatology recede completely.

These examples should be also sensitized to the fact that A noise-impaired person with tinnitus and blood pressure fluctuations with vertigo has two easily treatable diseases, but not Ménière's disease.

- Elderly people with hearing loss, tinnitus and otherwise unclassifiable dizziness do not have to suffer from Ménière's disease.
- People in whom fluctuating hearing is accompanied by fluctuating low tone tinnitus without signs of balance impairment do not necessarily have Ménière's disease. However, psychogenic vertigo may accompany their ear symptoms if they wait – possibly with their doctor – for the onset of Ménière's disease.

Although the exact diagnosis of Ménière's disease is not always easy, the differentiation from other clinical pictures (◘ Table 5.1), which often have deceptively similar symptoms, is important, as this usually results in different therapeutic consequences.

Important clinical pictures that can be confused with Ménière's disease are explained below.

5.2 Fluctuating Hearing with Low Tone Tinnitus Without Vertigo

A usually buzzing, roaring, deep-frequent tinnitus, often associated with repeated hearing fluctuations in the low-frequency range, is a relatively common disorder of the inner ear (◘ Fig. 5.1). In many cases, it occurs with a feeling of pressure or aural fullness. Sometimes it is accompanied by sensory disturbances on the same side of the face.

▪ Special Form of Hearing Impairment

This special form of tinnitus and hearing is often misjudged as a precursor to Ménière's disease. However, it is very likely that it is an independent clinical picture that can be distinguished from other tinnitus diseases. In this case, so-called endolymphatic fluctuations in the "auditory duct" of the cochlea form the organic final pathway of this disease (Schaaf and Hesse 2012; Teranishi et al. 2009).

With the help of MRI, it is now possible to prove that this special form, limited to the hearing part, exists. If one follows the classification proposal of Gürkov et al. (2016), this will then be named as "***Hydrops disease of the cochlear type***".

Endolymphatic hydrops is presumably not exclusively typical of a particular cause of disease (Zenner 1994), but the ear reacts similarly to many different stresses and diseases, for example with increase pressure endolymphatic fluid. This means that in principle mechanisms are present, which can lead to an unbalanced supply and removal of the endolymph. This is – within the normal range – certainly the case with everyone; after all, humans do not function like machines. Probably the evolutionary younger hearing organ reacts much more sensitively even to minor changes, while the much older vestibular organ can probably compensate for far more fluctuations.

It is true that Ménière's disease can start with endolymphatic fluctuations before the full-blown symptoms of Ménière's disease develop, often within a year. However, it is also true that only very few people with endolymphatic fluctuations develop Ménière's disease.

Table 5.1 Points of reference for distinguishing the most important clinical pictures in suspected Ménière's disease

Disease	Symptoms	Possibility of confusion	Difference to Menière's disease	Other therapy
Ménière's disease	Attacks of vertigo for at least 20 min to several hours Fluctuating, usually progressive hearing loss (usually low frequency) Tinnitus, aural fullness	–	–	–
Cochlear endolymphatic fluctuations	Low-frequency hearing loss	Progressive hearing loss may be misdiagnosed	No vertigo, no pathological balance findings	Enlightenment, PMR
Vestibular migraine (Greatest risk of confusion with Menière disease)	Symptoms similar to those of Ménière's disease during an attack: vertigo, (central) hearing loss, tinnitus, usually with additional neurological symptoms such as facial numbness, headache and neck pain.	Attacks of vertigo and episodes of dizziness	In the long run: no (progressive) hearing loss despite many attacks, no other neurological symptoms, no pathological findings of the vestibular functions	Prophylaxis possible, e.g. with beta-receptor blockers
Benign paroxysmal positional vertigo (BPPV)	Vertigo after movement for about 1 min; possible: long-lasting insecurity, fear and avoidance behavior	Vertigo people with hearing impairment and tinnitus due to other causes	Can only be triggered after movement	Correct positional maneuvers usually provide relief
Vestibular neuritis (single loss of balance) with habitual deficit or additional BPLS	Vertigo over days, mostly without hearing involvement	Dizziness and residual unsteadiness and "eye jumps" – in case of extreme movements and/or symptoms as above in BPV	No recurrent vertigo from the inner ear, no progressive hearing loss	Balance exercises In additional BPPV: Positional maneuver
Psychogenic dizziness especially in panic attacks	Vertigo of any kind	No (progressive) hearing impairment	No "eye tremor" (nystagmus): Fixation possible! Walking and standing possible	Enlightenment psychotherapy, if necessary systematic desensitization

(continued)

Table 5.1 (continued)

Disease	Symptoms	Possibility of confusion	Difference to Menière's disease	Other therapy
Perilymph fistula, e.g. due to dehiscence of semicircular canal	Vertigo Fluctuating hearing	Vertigo Illusionary movements of the environment with increased pulse beat, pulse-synchronous tinnitus	Triggered by pressure changes, very loud noise	Surgery, if necessary
Middle ear vacuum	Dizziness	Dizziness Hearing impairment	Improvement after pressure relief	Tympanostomy tube, if necessary

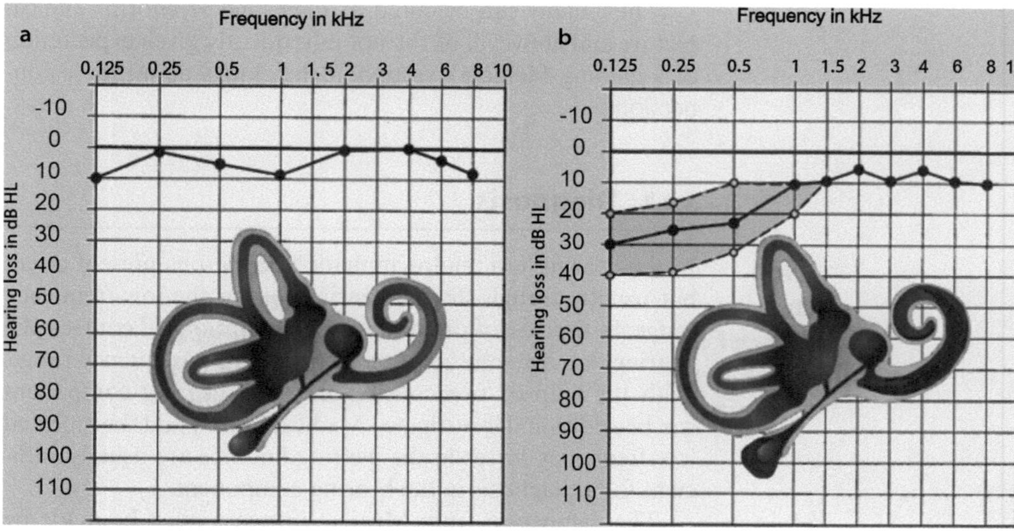

Fig. 5.1 Endolymphatic auditory fluctuations. **a** Inconspicuous; **b** with low-frequency fluctuation in endolymph hydrops in the cochlear portion

In our own longitudinal study started in 1995, we were able to follow up a total of 81 patients with repeated low-frequency hearing losses without symptoms of vertigo in 1999. In 2005, after a further 6 years, 46 of these original 81 patients (57%) accepted a renewed invitation for a follow-up examination, now mostly after more than 10 years (Schaaf and Hesse 2007).

A total of 12 patients (26%) reported symptoms of vertigo, but only four patients (9%) developed the typical signs of Ménière's disease with the typical vertigo over the course of 10 years. We conclude that only a few patients with recurrent low-frequency hearing loss develop Ménière's disease. However, it was clearly shown in our study that many patients with recurrent hearing loss become increasingly anxious and, out of anxiety, develop psychogenic dizziness in fearful anticipation of Meniere's disease.

After more than 10 years, 26% of the patients continued to have good hearing (bilateral normal acuity) in the low-frequency range. 34% showed unilateral hearing loss and 39% bilateral hearing loss. No patient became deaf.

In a similarly structured study from Japan, Yamasoba et al. (1994) were able to show that approximately 10% of patients admitted with this clinical picture develop Ménière's disease. Junicho et al. (2008) observed development to Ménière's disease in 14% of 127 low-frequency patients in a retrospective study.

This clearly refutes the fear often expressed by patients that fluctuating hearing in the low-frequency range is the precursor to Ménière's disease.

Thus, many can be cured of their "menièreiform" clinical picture and above all of the not infrequently given expectation of a coming Ménière's vertigo, if they know about these connections.

5.2.1 Diagnosis

In the hearing test, endolymphatic fluctuations present a flat, but usually trough-shaped hearing loss in the low-frequency range. In the case of often repeated and prolonged courses, the hearing damage may also spread to the high-frequency range. With the help of otoacoustic emissions hearing component can be additional investigated Medical history and the repeated low-frequency losses in the hearing findings are usually sufficient for a diagnosis in the hearing component.

The distinction from Ménière's disease must be made by vestibular examinations. In the meantime, with the help of imaging in MRI after administration of a contrast agent into the middle ear, it can be shown that a congestion of the endolymph can be seen limited to the auditory part (Gürkov et al. 2016). However, this examination can only be performed in a few centers.

5.2.2 Therapy

The therapy of endolymphatic events should start with a good clarification. When taking the patient's history, it is not uncommon to find that an endolymphatic event often depends on the situations, which frequently are caused by psychological stress. Thus, 3 days are to be regarded as a reasonable observation period for a spontaneous healing that often sets in. In this case, removal from a possibly stressful environment will be just as useful as a supportive medical explanation, and possibly also the implementation of a relaxation procedure such as Progressive Muscle Relaxation according to Jakobsen (PMR).

▪ Cortisone Trial for Significant Hearing Loss

If the hearing loss remains significant or one considers an immune-related process at the endolymphatic sac as a *possible* cause of the endolymphatic congestion, an infusion treatment with cortisone may make sense as a *trial.*

We give – if there are no other concerns, such as diabetes – 250 mg in the morning for 3 days.

If success is achieved, we give Decortin as a tablet 16 mg in the morning for 1–2 weeks.

Symptomatically, we additionally recommend the implementation of a relaxation procedure (guided by CD) such as Progressive Muscle Relaxation according to Jakobsen. In the meantime, there are good reasons to give the cortisone (in a small amount) directly (through the eardrum) into the middle ear, so that it can reach the inner ear directly from there. (for detailed information on the technical procedure, see ▶ Chap. 7).

If success is achieved, we give Decortin in *the morning* as a tablet as follows:

- 2 days 32 mg
- 2 days 16 mg
- 1 week 8 mg
- 2 days 4 mg

The result is regression rates of 70–80%.

However, this should not prevent us from reflecting and, if necessary, from pursuing fundamental conflicts that may cause the ear to react in a therapeutically accompanying manner. Short-term, sometimes very limited interventions with symptomatic aids can also be useful.

In the long run and in repetition, infusions – even with cortisone – do not make sense. An assessment conveyed to the patients that they are suffering from an incipient or "monosymptomatic" Ménière's disease is usually neither helpful nor conducive to therapy.

Possibilities of Differentiation from Ménière's Disease

If the endolymphatic activity is limited to the auditory part, neither vertigo from the inner ear nor dysfunctions in the vestibular apparatus are found.

Examinations such as the Klockhoff test and electrocochleography, which can only examine the hearing component, or caloric testing are not sufficient to diagnose Ménière's disease.

5.3 Migrainous Vertigo (Basilar Migraine)

▪ Most Important Risk of Confusion with Ménière's Disease

Migrainous vertigo is a common cause of episodic vertigo or disequilibrium (Bronstein and Lempert 2017). Thus, migraine with vertigo is one of the most important possibilities for confusion with Ménière's disease.

5.3.1 Symptomatology

▪ Migraine Can Cause Any Form of Vertigo and Dizziness

Migraines are usually characterized by attacks of headache on one side, sometimes on both sides. These can last up to 2 days and are often accompanied by nausea and vomiting, sensitivity to light and noise. Quite a few patients also experience a so-called migraine aura shortly before or during the migraine attack. The most common symptoms are flickering visual field defects, less common are tingling sensations, paralysis, speech disorders, confusion, "double vision" and unsteady gait. The cause is thought to be a temporary vasoconstriction in the affected areas of the brain. Many migraine sufferers report dizziness as an occasional or frequent companion to their headaches. For others, however, the dizziness occurs alone, even without a headache. Then it is a purely "vestibular migraine". Here the dizziness can occur in three variants, as:

- Rotational vertigo
- Positional vertigo or
- Diffuse dizziness without signs of movement

These different manifestations may occur alone, simultaneously or consecutively. Prolonged attacks over hours or days may begin with spinning vertigo and vomiting, which is aggravated by changes in position and head movement. The symptoms manifest themselves with varying degrees of severity.

The duration of attacks ranges from a few seconds to days. Consequently, patients may experience a series of short attacks of vertigo over several hours with a rather moderate disturbance of balance and (persistent) nausea in the background. This pattern is similar to migraine with headache symptoms accentuated by short attacks of severe headache.

▪ Symptoms May Change

The symptomatology of migraine can also change for each individual within the years. For example, migraine vertigo may last long after the migraine headache has stopped. Ear symptoms such as hearing loss, tinnitus or aural fullness are seen in 10–40% of patients with basilar migraine, but systematic studies in unselected patients are lacking to date (Bronstein and Lempert 2017).

Nystagmus examinations by video-oculography performed during attacks show different types and combinations of spontaneous and positional nystagmus. A central type of spontaneous nystagmus is often seen, as well as downbeat nystagmus, upbeat nystagmus, or torsional nystagmus. In addition, a migraine patient may have central positional nystagmus.

5.3.2 Pathophysiology

The pathophysiology of migraine vertigo is unknown. Hypothetically, vertigo that meets the criteria of migraine aura is attributed to a transient undersupply of the labyrinth.

The mechanism of a "spreading depression" of functions hypothesized for migraine, as found in aura symptoms, may then produce vertigo when the core area of the vestibular system (the vestibular cortex) is affected. Then complex nystagmus can be seen during acute migraine with vertigo.

▪ Messenger Substances Get Mixed Up

Another explanation relates to various neurotransmitters released during a migraine attack that are known to modulate balance functions. Still other hypotheses link migraine vertigo to genetic defects in ion channels found in various other diseases (see in detail Bronstein and Lempert 2017; Brandt et al. 2012).

5.3.3 Diagnostics

Neither migraine nor vertigo due to migraine can be diagnosed biochemically, neurophysiologically or with imaging techniques It must be inquired about in the medical history and – especially during the attack – examined clinically. Nystagmographies after caloric testing and audiograms can document the level of – usually transient – dysfunction.

Imaging procedures are useful to rule out damage in the posterior fossa. However, the procedures are not (no longer) necessary if a patient reports an appropriate history of migraine and repeatedly becomes completely symptom-free.

5.3.4 Treatment

Treatment of acute attack is necessary if the dizziness lasts longer than 1 h, considering the time between taking the drug to its onset of action. For symptomatic relief of dizziness and vomiting, any dizziness-suppressing drug is useful in this regard. However, the patient should be warned of the sedative side effects.

As an alternative, you can try triptans, which could eliminate not only the migraine headache but also the migraine vertigo.

Migraine Prophylaxis

Most experts – according to Bronstein and Lempert (2017) – believe that patients with frequent severe attacks can benefit from pharmacological migraine prophylaxis, such as:

- Beta-blockers such as propranolol 40–240 mg and metoprolol 50–200 mg or
- Antidepressants such as amitriptyline 75–150 mg, flunarizine 5–10 mg, topiramate 50–100 mg

The treatment decision should be discussed individually with neurological expertise. Realistically, a symptom reduction can be achieved in approximately 50–70%. Adverse side effects can be reduced by starting with the smallest dose and then slowly increasing the dose.

A positive effect of the treatment can take 2–3 months and is most likely to be secured if the patients also write down their vertigo attacks.

After 6 months, treatment can be discontinued on a trial basis, as the course of the disease is unpredictable. Long-lasting regression of symptoms is also possible and drug treatment is no longer necessary.

Non-pharmacological prophylaxis includes exercise and muscle relaxation according to Jacobsen (PMR) as well as – usually useful – improved stress management.

Possibilities of Differentiation from Ménière's Disease

About 5% of migraines with accompanying ear symptoms are misdiagnosed as Ménière's disease. However, links between migraine and Ménière's disease are also suspected, especially since migraine symptoms can be found significantly more often in Ménière's disease patients than in a comparison group. However, it is also possible that this link is found so often because it is ultimately so difficult to differentiate.

If migraine vertigo occurs without a headache, the accompanying circumstances that are otherwise typical for a migraine point the way to the diagnosis. This is, for example, a simultaneous sensitivity to light or noise.

Vestibular migraine – as opposed to Ménière's disease – is supported by:

- central eye disorder during the interval
- Absence of progressive hearing loss despite many attacks
- Especially the association with other neurological symptoms, such as facial numbness and head and neck pain.
- Response to prophylactic treatment with beta-receptor blockers
- Duration of attacks (20 min to several hours in Ménière's disease, any duration of vertigo up to 2 weeks in migraine)

Nevertheless, the distinction from Ménière's disease occasionally remains so difficult that, according to Brandt et al. (2012), only in the course of therapy, for example, gradual prophylaxis can bring a little more clarity.

5.4 Benign Paroxysmal Positional Vertigo (BPPV)

▪ Violent, but Treatable

"Benign" paroxysmal positional vertigo (BPPV) is one of the most common causes of organically induced balance disorders – and unfortunately also one of the most frequently misdiagnosed. Patients in the second half of life are predominantly affected. BPPV is usually easier to treat than any other type of vertigo, as the cause can be eliminated within a few minutes.

Short spinning attacks with specific eye tremors (nystagmus) after certain head movements are typical, but also when bending over or lying down. These hardly last longer than 30 s. Usually, a few seconds pass after the change of position before the vertigo sets in. Some people feel nauseous; some even vomit. There may be a slight unsteadiness of gait between attacks.

▪ Limestone in the Lower Semicircular Canal

In this disease, small calcium crystals (otoliths) have detached from the utricle spontaneously or after a skull injury. These crystals are then deposited preferentially in the nearby posterior (lower) semicircular canal, where they do not belong. When the position changes, they are moved by the earth's gravity, causing endolymph flow. This triggers the impression of a moving environment via the sensory hairs in the brainstem. The eyes are supposed to compensate for this with rapid back – movements. "Benign" paroxysmal positional vertigo usually disappears after a few weeks to months, even without treatment, but it can recur after several months or years. The spectrum ranges from a single short episode to decades of suffering. In about 1/3 of cases, "benign positional vertigo" is preceded by a craniocerebral trauma or a failure of the vestibular organ (Lempert 1995).

5.4.1 Diagnostics and Therapy

The diagnosis is already the beginning of the therapy. The following sequence of positions describes the Epley maneuver:

1. The patient begins in an upright sitting posture, with the legs fully extended and the head rotated 45° toward the side in the same direction.

2. Then the patient is lowered into a supine position (on the back), with the head held approximately in a 30-degree neck extension (Dix-Hallpike position), with the head remaining rotated to the side.
3. The clinician observes the patient's eyes for "primary stage" nystagmus.
4. The patient remains in this position for approximately 1–2 min.
5. Then the patient's head is rotated 90° in the opposite direction, so that the opposite ear faces the floor, while maintaining 30° of neck extension.
6. The patient remains in this position for approximately 1–2 min.
7. Keeping the head and neck in a fixed position relative to the body, the patient rolls onto the shoulder, rotating the head another 90° in the direction being faced. Now the patient is looking downward at a 45-degree angle.
8. The eyes should be observed by the clinician for "secondary stage" nystagmus
9. The patient remains in this position for approximately 1–2 min.
10. Finally, the patient is brought up to an upright sitting posture, while maintaining the 45-degree rotation of the head.
11. The patient holds a sitting position for up to 30 s.

These steps may be repeated twice, for a total of three times during a procedure. During every step of this procedure, the patient may experience some dizziness.

Possibilities of Differentiation from Ménière's Disease

The character of spinning vertigo, together with an unspecific description of the vertigo sensation, can lead to misdiagnosis as Ménière's disease. The likelihood of misdiagnosis increases if – independently – hearing loss is found and the patient reports tinnitus.

Important in the distinction is that a Ménière's attack:

- *Cannot* be *triggered* by a positional effect
- Unlike BPLS, is accompanied by a hearing change, usually in the low-frequency range
- Often has a fluctuating perceived tinnitus
- At least in the long run does not remain without detectable vestibular dysfunctions

However, the condition of BPPV, which is common with increasing age, can also occur in a patient with the less common Ménière's disease. In fact, there are indications (Lempert

1995) for a frequent occurrence of BPPV in the course of a Ménière's disease.

Taura et al. (2014) found in nearly 300 patients that one-third of vertigo attacks during the course of a Ménière's condition were most likely due to benign positional vertigo. It is thought that endolymphatic congestion favors the migration of the small calcareous stones (otoliths) in the utricle into the lower semicircular canal. In this case, BBPV is often (unnecessarily!) misdiagnosed as part of Ménière's disease and not treated appropriately until the correct diagnosis is made (► Sect. 5.1).

5.5 Vestibular Neuritis – Acute Unilateral (Idiopathic) Vestibulopathy

■ Dizziness Above Ground

(Unilateral) Acute failure of a vestibular organ is characterized by a sudden onset of rotational vertigo with nausea and vomiting. The vertigo is associated with a tendency to fall to the affected side when sitting or standing. Symptoms may be severe for 2–3 days, then usually improve over the next few weeks. Sometimes a failure in the labyrinth also affects the hearing organ, so that hearing restrictions and ringing in the ears can develop.

"Seen from the outside", with the eyes of the observer, an eye tremor ("nystagmus") can be notices. The fast movement part beats in the direction of the healthy organ. Viewed from the inside out, the affected person gets the image of a rapidly rotating environment. If "real head movements" towards the healthy side are added, the symptoms intensify. Therefore, the sufferer usually lies on the affected side, which causes the fewest additional complaints. Finally, the persistent rotating movement also irritates the vomiting center, which is located in the brainstem in the immediate vicinity of the balance center.

The loss of balance may recover completely or be compensated for gradually – over weeks to months. The hearing impairment may completely recover, remain completely or partially.

In the acute stage, Prosper Menière's description (► Chap. 1) also applies to the onset of a loss of balance.

5.5.1 Possible Causes

■ Neurotropic Viruses

The most probable causes are infections with so-called "neurotropic" viruses, injuries or temporary circulatory disorders of the inner ear. The "neurotropic" viruses include mumps, herpes zoster and measles viruses. These have usually nested in the body for long periods of time without causing disease. However, when the opportunity arises – usually when the body is overstrained – they can attack nerves with particular fondness. This also includes the auditory and vestibular nerves.

Traumatic and Inflammatory Events

Even though the vestibular organ is located in the hardest bone of the human body, some impacts are so violent that the bony labyrinth is also hit. Then a lifelong fracture line can usually be seen. The vestibular organs and hearing organ (cochlea) are closely connected. Therefore, diseases from the middle ear can affect both. Thus, dizziness may occur with:

- Acute middle ear infections
- Chronic middle ear disease
- Injuries of the middle ear
- Cholesteatoma as a special inflammation that "eats" into the inner ear if left unoperated
- Rare: Tumors, for example an acoustic neuroma.

In the vast majority of cases of loss of balance, however, it is not possible to say with certainty what exactly the cause was.

5.5.2 Diagnostics: Complete or Partial Failure?

As with most dizziness diseases, the description of the affected person already leads to the correct diagnosis. This must then be confirmed by the examinations. Many examinations are already possible without the use of equipment.

Thus, in acute loss of balance, the eye tremor (nystagmus) is usually noticeable. The head impulse test shows which and how many semicircular canals on the affected side can react with a vestibulo-ocular reflex and which have to help themselves with corrective saccade.

Otolith Organs Can be Recorded

Caloric testing with warm and cold water in the ear, which is usually performed in cases of vertigo, allows a statement to be made about the lateral semicircular canal.

Nowadays it has become possible to record the involvement of the otolith organs. Suitable for this purpose are the derivations of the "vestibular evoked potentials", separately recorded at the neck muscle (examination of the sacculus) and at the eye muscles (examination of the utricle).

It is possible to get a more accurate picture of the extent of the damage. This has consequences for the expected recovery time and for the understanding of the challenges for the compensation services.

The course of the compensation and thus also the success of the balance training can be checked with:

- Determination of the "subjective visual vertical" (examination of the utricle functions)
- Rotation examination on a swivel chair (interaction of both utricle functions)
- Posturography, which gives a documentable standing and stance picture depending on different balance requirements

5.5.3 Therapy

Education/Knowledge Helps

The course of recovery also depends significantly on the acute experience during the dizziness. It makes a difference whether it can become clear to those affected whether they have a benign illness or whether – often for too long – the suspicion of a heart attack or stroke remains.

If clarification fails to occur and patients are lost in dizziness, even the healthiest personality structures are put to extreme test. Beyond despair, fear can grow in the process.

Persistent anxiety is an additional factor in the reduction of balance (Staab 2012). In this context, the development of anxiety in the first days, in which mostly also depressant medication is given, does not yet seem to have any predictive value for the development of persistent vertigo (Godemann et al. 2009).

The turning point for an addition of psychological symptoms seems to occur from the tenth day onwards, when – after a correspondingly unfavorable course, with an endangered personality structure, already low resources and/or unfavorable handling – high anxiety levels can still be found.

After 6 weeks, catastrophizing thoughts seem to increase. Patients with high anxiety scores after 12 weeks are more likely to develop psychiatric comorbidity.

But what can help get back on your feet as quickly as possible?

Vestibular Suppressants Only at the Beginning

Until the symptoms subside, the loss of balance is best endured lying down, resting, and with eyes closed.

In an acute attack – during the first 1–3 days – vestibular suppressants such as dimenhydrinate (1–3 times 100 mg) can be useful if the dizziness is still too severe. From the second or third day onwards, vestibular suppressants medications should no longer be taken, as they then hinder the compensation by the remaining or recovering balance system.

Short-term treatment with cortisone (methylprednisolone, e.g. Urbason, initially 100 mg/day as a tablet, with the dose being reduced by 20 mg every fourth day) should lead to improved recovery in the vestibular organ.

The addition of antiviral drugs (valaciclovir) did not produce measurable improvements (Strupp et al. 2004).

Alcohol and other "inhibitory substances" delay central vestibular compensation!

5.5.4 Balance Training

▪ Compensation Needs Incentives

The earlier balance training (► Chap. 7) is started, the faster recovery is achieved and the less "dizziness" memory develops. This can already begin in bed, e.g. with slight head movements – even when lying down – while fixing the outstretched thumb. Central compensation is promoted and accelerated if movement stimuli always present a new challenge. So you should always practice a little more than can be achieved without dizziness.

Course:

Three messages can be taken away:

- When a vestibular organ fails, all patients improve spontaneously, even if residual symptoms remain in some patients.
- Balance exercises speed recovery by promoting central compensation.
- It is more likely to win the lottery than to experience another loss of balance on the same side.

▪ Balance Exercises Accelerate Recovery

As a rule, the symptoms of a partial loss of the vestibular organ diminish within days. Depending on the type and extent of the damage, different partial weaknesses remain, which usually disappear completely and permanently after 2–3 weeks.

In the case of unilateral vestibular loss, the restoration of balance is the product of various processes:

- Recovery of peripheral vestibular function (not always complete)
- Substitution of the loss of function by the vestibular system as well as by somatosensory and visual afferents
- Central compensation

Nevertheless, there are different courses:

Thus, the degree and speed of recovery depend on the degree of damage, but:

- A young healthy person can usually recover more quickly from a major damage than an older person from a minor one, if the latter already has other deficiencies acquired with age in the eyes, body senses or central nervous system
- People with mental health problems often suffer longer and experience more complications than those who want to get through the crisis as quickly as possible.

5.5.5 Lack of Compensation

The development towards a functioning equilibrium can be delayed in the case of (see also the comments in ► Sect. 3.3):
- too long rest or too little practice
- vestibular suppressants "against dizziness" instead of balance exercises
- little own and professionally conveyed confidence in success
- Overlooking a possible pre-existing or developing mental impairment, such as reactive psychogenic dizziness (► Sect. 5.9).

5.5.6 Possible Functional Reduction for Too Fast Movements

In the first period, damage to the vestibular organ may lead to a concentration on the detection of movements with the eyes and the proprioceptive (body's) sensors. In doing so, these two systems have to take over services that are normally performed by the vestibular organ (► Chap. 2). If we face up to this task and fear does not creep in between the adaptation services, most of the services necessary for life can also be performed with one vestibular organ.

This does not apply to very fast and extreme accelerations. This is because after an incomplete cure, a new equilibrium spectrum is provided, but this no longer covers the full width of the reception spectrum.

Thus, after a loss of one vestibular organ, in the case of very fast and very pronounced movements to the sick side, the compensating eye movement no longer keeps up. Then a jerky gaze jump (medically "saccade") must be added in order to be able to fixate again what has been taken into view.

In other words, even after a long-standing loss of one vestibular organ, certain extreme situations can only be mastered with "gaze jumps" or with "double vision" (i.e., illusory movements of the surroundings). For the affected person, this means that dizziness and memories may well occur in these situations. Here the knowledge and an appropriate pre-vision help, without omitting the further feasible.

5.5.7 Hearing Impairment and Ringing in the Ears

Sometimes, however, hearing loss or ringing in the ears can remain if the entire labyrinth, i.e. also the hearing part, was affected. Hearing aids can then help, especially with directional hearing, for which two ears are needed. Most people manage to cope with their ear noise and perhaps keep it in their ears as a reminder of a crisis they have overcome.

5.5.8 A Subsequent Paroxysmal Positional Vertigo

- **Benign Paroxysmal Positional Vertigo Possible**

In 20–30% of vestibular neuritis, the small calcium stones (otoconia) can slip out of the utricle and induce a positional vertigo. This makes the affected person and – not infrequently also the practitioner – mistakenly think of a recurrence of the event or of Ménière's disease. Then – too often and unnecessarily – curative therapy is not undertaken.

5.5.9 Confusion in Experience

What can remain unfavorable after vertigo episodes is the fear experienced during the loss of balance. Often there also remains an unpleasant memory of fainting with the feeling of having lost the ground under the feet. At worst, the loss of balance was experienced as so upsetting and threatening that previously taken for granted life securities are seen dwindling and vertiginously threatened.

However, it is not only the help or the distress experienced in the loss of balance that is important for the further future, but also the possibilities of the affected person. Recovery to "normal" can be difficult for people who had planned their lives precisely and organized them in very orderly ways before the loss of balance. People who were not afraid of anything until they experienced a vertigo attack could be "thrown off track".

As with all organic pre-existing conditions involving the experience of vertigo, a reactive psychogenic vertigo may develop that feels the same to the sufferer as the organic vertigo previously experienced – although it does not actually persist.

Here, good clarification can and must help, as well as intensive balance training that lets the affected person feel what they can do again. Often, support for the soul, i.e. psychological treatment, also helps.

"Misidentification" as Ménière's Disease

The severe rotation vertigo at the onset of the loss of balance, together with the feeling of "not getting back on one's feet properly", can lead to misdiagnosis as Ménière's disease. The likelihood of a misdiagnosis increases if – perhaps preexisting – hearing loss is found and the patient reports tinnitus.

If, in the course of time, positional vertigo also develops, one can think of a repeated occurrence, although neither the positional vertigo nor incomplete loss of balance has anything to do with each other.

Important in the distinction is:

- The unilateral loss of balance is a one-time event.
- Any hearing loss that may be present does not progress or fluctuate.
- Ménière's disease is not position-dependent.

5.6 Perilymph Fistula

The vestibular organ must be embedded in a solid, usually bony envelope so that this part of the labyrinth cannot be irritated by sound impulses. Tightly enclosed by the petrous bone are the semicircular canals, which are surrounded by fluid, the so-called perilymph (◘ Fig. 5.2).

The auditory part is surrounded by a softer material. This is an important condition, that sound effects, that reach the inner ear via the middle ear, will be processed in the auditory part, but do not trigger any impulses in the bony enclosed vestibular organ.

▪ Upper Semicircular Canal Leaking

This gets messed up when there is a gap in the bone Then the perilymph does not stay between the semicircular canal and the skull bone: the result is a perilymph fistula. However, the point at which this gap leads to the effects described below is essentially still unclear (Luers and Hüttenbrink 2013).

In the transition to the auditory part, the inner ear has two "windows" towards the middle ear, which are closed with

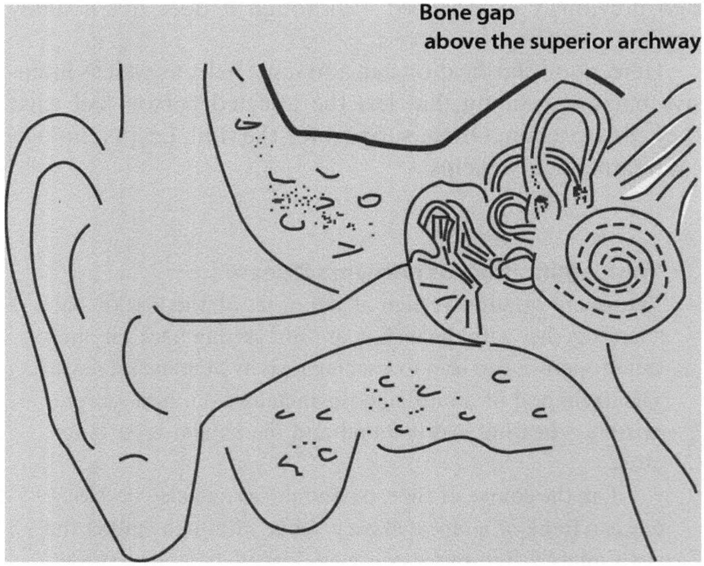

Fig. 5.2 Section through the ear. A defect (gap) in the bony capsule of the labyrinth above the superior semicircular canal is visible

membranes: the oval and round window. An additional "inner window" can arise if one of the semicircular canals is not enclosed bone-tight.

Then some may experience illusory movements of the environment due to changes in pressure. This can be caused by coughing, sneezing and pressing or heavy lifting, sometimes also by very loud noises. For the duration of the – limited – attack, nystagmus can be observed. The vertigo manifests episodically from seconds to days or chronically with fluctuations.

To test this clinically, the patient should perform a Valsalva maneuver (build breathing pressure by pressed "not exhaling") while the examiner observes the eyes for nystagmus.

Possible other symptoms include:

- Altered perception of one's own voice (autophony)
- Loud perception of body sounds (e.g. heartbeat, chewing sounds)
- Pulse synchronous ear noise

▪ Endolymph Fluctuation Due to Decreasing Ambient Pressure

Endolymph fluctuation is also possible. Unlike endolymph congestion caused by too much fluid in the interior, endolymph fistula expansion occurs in perilymph fistula because the ambient pressure of the endolymph decreases in the bony gap.

Audible "Plop"

The defects that underlie perilymph fistulas can be congenital. Sometimes they become a problem after additional stress, such as after an accident, heavy lifting or surgical procedures. Then the symptoms often start "suddenly" with an audible "pop" in the affected ear, followed by vertigo.

"Breakthroughs" with ducts remaining open can also occur after inflammatory or destructive diseases. This can be a cholesteatoma (inflammation-related "bone erosion"), but also syphilis.

5.6.1 Diagnostics

Often there is a "too good" transfer via bone conduction in the hearing test and a lowered threshold of vestibular evoked myogenic potentials (VEMPs). In particular, ocular vestibular evoked myogenic potentials (O-VEMPs) are considered an essential component for diagnostics (Luers and Hüttenbrink 2013).

Important is a high-resolution computer tomography of the petrous bone with a special imaging in the plane of the semicircular canal.,

5.6.2 Therapy

The extent of the symptoms is decisive for the therapy, not the computer tomogram. In patients with an acute fistula, for example after exertion and tension, conservative treatment can often be the most effective. This includes bed rest with the head elevated for 1 week, followed by 6 weeks during which strenuous movements should be avoided.

Sometimes a so-called tympanic tube in the eardrum is able, at least temporarily, to relieve the pressure in the middle ear.

From Conservative Therapy to Neurosurgical Intervention

Surgical correction may be attempted in patients who do not respond adequately to conservative therapy, acute pressure trauma, and direct injury to the inner ear. In the case of cholesteatoma, surgery must be performed to prevent the "bone erosion" bevor reaching the brain.

There are currently two surgical options for bone defects of the superior or inferior semicircular canal:

1. The missing bone layer is replaced in a neurosurgical procedure.
2. A plug is placed in the semicircular canal, which is glued together with a bony layer.

According to Luers and Hüttenbrink (2013), the published case series with largely positive clinical outcomes are offset by not inconsiderable risks.

> **Possibilities of Differentiation from Ménière's Disease**
> Unlike Ménière's disease, in which a vertigo attack cannot be triggered, in this clinical picture a vertigo attack can be triggered by changing the pressure on the inner ear. The resulting nystagmus can be recorded for the duration of the – limited – attack. In contrast to positional vertigo, the change in position is not the decisive impulse.

5.6.3 Excursus: Influences of Air Pressure on the Ear (Tullio Phenomenon)

- **High Sound Levels**

In 1929, Pietro Tullio described that in some people, sound stimuli can have effects on the vestibular organ. That is why today the occurrence of vertigo caused by acoustic stimuli of more than 90 dB volume is called Tullio phenomenon. Eye movements away from the side exposed to the sound can be observed. The causes of the Tullio phenomenon used to be assumed to be, in particular, deformities, which were more often caused by syphilis. The Tullio phenomenon has been described in Ménière's disease; here the reason could be the widening of the saccule (sacculus) by the endolymph congestion, whereby the inner ear structure moves closer to the middle ear.

5.6.4 Tube Ventilation Disorder

Westhofen (2009) points out that Ménière's-like symptoms can be triggered by unfavorable pressure conditions in the middle ear. Then – along Westhofen (2009) – permanent ventilation of the tympanic cavity via a tube can alleviate and sometimes eliminate symptoms. Westhofen sees the indication for this minimal intervention if a value of 50 daPa and more is found when measuring the middle ear pressure (impedance audiometry).

5.7 Vestibular Paroxysmia

Vestibular paroxysmia is a rare disorder with occasional, sudden disturbances of the vestibular nerve, primarily through the surrounding blood vessels.

The leading symptom of vestibular paroxysmia are short attacks of spinning or staggering vertigo lasting seconds to a few minutes – with or without effects on hearing. The cause of this "benign", but quite irritating, condition is thought to be compression of the auditory and vestibular nerves (cranial nerves VIII) by small arteries (Brandt et al. 2012). In this case, stray vessels in the so-called "cerebellopontine angle", some of which are also arteriosclerotically elongated and dilated – and thus pulsating more frequently – should lead to this nerve being irritated by pressure. In some patients, the symptoms are dependent on certain head positions and can occasionally be provoked by hyperventilation (heavy and increased breathing).

Triggered by False Conclusions

Symptoms are triggered by direct pulsatory compression and/or "misconnections", i.e. occasional transmission of stimuli between adjacent partially "demyelinated axons" (nerve cords that are at least partially deprived of their protective layer).

During the attack, increased balance and hearing defects may be measurable, but these are only slightly pronounced between attacks. Hearing loss and tinnitus may also occur between attacks.

It is important that an improvement or abatement of the attacks can be achieved with the antiepileptic drug carbamazepine even at low doses. Thus, a therapy trial with carbamazepine in low dosage (200–600 mg) or phenytoin is useful and part of the diagnosis.

In the positive case, this can lead to a lifelong improvement in symptoms without having to worry about a blood vessel bursting or a stroke being the result.

> But take care: Not every suspicious finding on a CT scan or MRI is associated with symptoms.

Surgical procedures can sometimes break the overly tight connection, but they should only be considered when drug therapy is insufficient (Westhofen 2008).

5.8 Isolated Otolith Dysfunction

It is unclear to what extent isolated otolith dysfunction occurs in the saccule and utricle without affecting functions of the semicircular canals. Clinical studies suggest that functional impairments of the utricle have a greater clinical impact compared to the saccule (Helling 2008).

▪ Swan and Elevator Dizziness

In the case of a functional disorder of the utricle, vertigo can be a (non-specific) leading symptom if other causes, such as an insufficient habituation or a reactive psychogenic vertigo, have been excluded.

In the past, these circumstances were rarely recognized due to inadequate diagnostic possibilities.

> **Possibilities of Differentiation from Ménière's Disease**
> The repeated attacks suggest an inner ear event, but the hearing changes are missing.

5.9 Psychogenic Dizziness

When information from different parts of the vestibular system contradicts each other, dizziness can occur. If one wants to include the soul, this also applies to emotional perceptions. This brings into consideration the unique processing and response capabilities of each person, which in turn include the interconnectedness with their social environment.

Psychogenic dizziness is a clinical syndrome characterized by vague and persistent sensations of dizziness, subjective imbalance, lightheadedness, or fullness in the head.

It can develop after and out of an organic disease or take place largely in the emotional world of the person.

Psychogenic dizziness accounts for a considerable proportion of all forms of vertigo, at least 30%. If one adds reactive dizziness after an organic disease, it can become almost half of all dizziness events or episodes.

▪ "Confusing" Affects

Psychogenic dizziness can be understood as the perception of affects that are incomprehensible and confusing for the affected person. The dizziness sensations are individually very real. Especially in the case of panic attacks the experienced vertigo is symptomatically hardly distinguishable from a Ménière's attack – except for the specific auditory phenomena and the nystagmus.

5.9.1 Dizziness Instead of Unpleasant Feelings

Mental illness is often accompanied by anxiety. Fear in itself is not bad. Thus, it is absolutely sensible to reconsider one's actions in actually dangerous situations or even to "instinctively" take flight. The same applies to fear when danger threatens the soul. But in this case one cannot simply run away.

In this framework, the dizziness can come to the fore instead of fear on the one hand, and on the other hand it can also be felt instead of pleasure, disgust or anger. This also often happens during a depressive development and as a correspondence of a depression. Especially after separations and losses, dizziness phenomena occur without the patient being aware of the depressive content.

At the same time, also psychogenic dizziness must themselves make physically noticeable, which makes it difficult to recognize for both the affected person and the examiner.

Psychogenic dizziness can be interpreted as a sign that something *in* the mental balance has not come together, is poorly integrated, is not reliable, has been overwhelmed, has become confused, or has been neglected.

Expression of an Intolerable Situation

Similarly, dizziness *can be* an expression of an intolerable situation:

- The feeling for one's own strength is lost; the firm hold is missing.
- One is not "able" to carry, on the contrary: one desires to be carried.
- Stability and control are lost, insecurity and fear become overwhelming.

Symbolic interpretations understand the mental dizziness, for example, as a *sign* of:

- Something out of joint
- Longing for support
- Transition phenomenon from one state to another in which an equilibrium is lost and a new one has to be restored

Seemingly contradictory to this, however, the mental dizziness can also lead to an – at least temporary – "hold" (in both senses of the word) for contradictions that seem insoluble. The solution, which is unsatisfactory for all sides, is that the problems continue to exist. The "relief" gained is sometimes accompanied by considerable restrictions for those involved.

Depending on the previously experienced or undergone vertigo experiences – for example after a vestibular neuritis – a psychogenic event can trigger the same symptomatology as a "purely" organic event.

Relatively often, those affected experience dizziness or diffuse dizziness (drowsiness, feeling of emptiness in the head, unsteadiness when walking, feeling of tipping over).

Psychogenic vertigo can also be experienced as attack and spinning vertigo. This would organically correspond to vertigo from the vestibular organ.

In the case of psychogenic vertigo, however, the organic findings are missing or the organic deficits found are not sufficient to adequately explain the dizziness.

> In other words: The quality of the vertigo or dizziness is oriented to the previously experienced model, which has really taken place in the sufferer or has been observed in others.

Depending on the psychogenic component, other symptoms appear such as:
- Palpitations, nausea, sweating, shortness of breath, choking, lack of appetite and weight loss.
- Disturbances in drive and concentration, loss of performance, subjectively perceived restrictions in occupational and everyday activities
- Disturbances of affect and mood as well as sleep disorders
- Anxiety symptoms

▪ Symptoms Caused by Dizziness?

Typically, the symptoms are described as if they were triggered and caused by the vertigo. Stressful situations or conflicts, which are also possible triggers of vertigo, can hardly be consciously perceived by the affected persons themselves.

5.9.2 The Problem of Understanding

▪ Soul Incomprehensible

It is in the nature of "the soul" that it does not have the possibility to express itself understandably for all, e.g. linguistically. It needs other forms to send its message. Physical illnesses reveal themselves through signs of pain, fever, paralysis or visible body changes. These are symptoms can be described with words. Many mental changes, on the other hand, are experienced as elusive intangible disorders. Thus, one must not overlook the fact that it is objectively not easy to recognize mental illnesses.

Furthermore, it is still widely frowned upon to be mentally ill. In contrast to a metabolic disorder, a broken leg or pneumonia, the question is often asked in the case of psychological problems whether the problems are self-inflicted. It is assumed too quickly that it is a case of malingering, that those affected are "acting up" or i.e. reacting over-sensitively.

5.9.3 Where Does the Psychogenic Dizziness Take Place?

Despite all the search and conjecture, the soul does not seem to have a fixed, organically tangible place in the body. Known are interfaces between soul and body. These are found in the so-called "limbic system", a small area in the central nervous system in which emotional reactions are triggered and processed.

It makes sense to approach the psychogenic dizziness through its appearance itself. Then – with all individuality – orienting clues can be found, which can be used therapeutically. The most frequent manifestations of psychogenic vertigo are anxiety disorders, phobic, depressive and dissociative disorders.

These also inversely determine the experienced character of the dizziness and vertigo (◘ Table 5.2).

One can now say in an extended way: The quality of the vertigo is oriented towards the previously experienced model, which may have taken place in the patient or may have been observed in others. The expression and the processing of the vertigo are determined by the mental component.

5.9.4 From the "Phobic Postural Vertigo" (PPV) to "Persistent Perceptual and Postural Dizziness" (3P-D)

▪ Concept of the "Phobic Postural Vertigo (PPV)"

The neurologists Brandt and Dieterich (1986) had built a bridge to organic medicine when they developed the concept of "phobic postural vertigo". They have the merit, of having made a psychological phenomenon comprehensible to physicians.

PPV is defined by symptoms of postural dizziness and fluctuating unsteadiness that are provoked by environmental or social stimuli (e.g., crossing bridges; descending staircases; exposure to busy streets, stores, or crowds). PPV may be triggered initially by vestibular disorders, medical illnesses, or psychological stress. Based on clinical observations of patients with PPV, Brandt and Dieterich included two behavioral criteria in the definition of the condition:

- presence of an obsessive-compulsive personality, labile affect, and mild depression;
- and anxiety and vegetative disturbance.

5

Table 5.2 Overview: from symptom to possible diagnosis of psychogenic dizziness

Symptom	Temporal occurrence	Perceived dizziness or vertigo
Generalized anxiety disorder	Vertigo and/or permanent dizziness	Increasing and decreasing intensity with constant inner tension and nervousness; persistent fear, also related to the fact that something could happen because of vertigo
Panic	"Attacks of vertigo" lasting from minutes to hours	"Out of the blue" attacks with throbbing, palpitations, sweating, shortness of breath to a feeling of suffocation, rise in blood pressure, nausea, diarrhea and possibly depersonalization symptoms
Phobia	Increasing before the feared situation	Fear of the situation in which a dizzy spell may occur
Depression	Continuous or diffuse dizziness	Heavy circling like "a mill wheel in the head", partial day fluctuations, social withdrawal, fear of the future and thoughts as if everything does not matter anyway and is of no use, up to giving up on life
Somatization	Diffuse vertigo/dizziness	Fixated on organic cause of vertigo, urging further diagnostic measures
Hypochondria	Diffuse vertigo/dizziness	Fear of severe, previously unrecognized disease
Dissociation	Feeling "beside oneself"	Dizziness phenomena as memory symbols for repressed/separated traumatic experiences

In triggering this vertigo, Brandt and Dietrich suspected anxious self-observation and a mismatch between what is seen and felt (afference patterns) and the previously habitual ways of acting (efference copies). Therefore, active head and body movements could be experienced as passive accelerations or illusory movements. Thereby patterns of action and perception can become blurred.

In particular, Brandt and Dieterich proposed that patients with phobic postural vertigo became consciously sensitized to transient discrepancies between predicted and actual postural movements (i.e., to differences between feedforward efferent copies of planned movements and feedback afferent measurements of actual motions). Normally, these signals are used to make instinctive (i.e., unconscious or preconscious) corrections of movements, but Brandt and Dieterich suggested that patients who became consciously aware of these signals exert more conscious effort into maintaining control of posture. These circumstances were thought to stand in the way of normal readaptation and, instead, set in motion a vicious cycle of maladaptation. In this model of illness, the expectation of dizziness and unsteadiness, which might be called an "experiential engram" from the triggering episode, is awarded disproportionate predictive strength and can then distort and even over-ride bottom-up sensory input at the preconscious level of sensory integration. This leads to subjective sensations of dizziness during everyday vestibular and visual stimulation (e.g., moving about, encountering complex visual inputs), which reinforces stiffening of stance and gait. The increased burden of abnormal self-monitoring could explain the common occurrence of dissociation and fatigue as results of mental overload; neck stiffness and functional gait disorder could develop secondary to the abnormal postural control; and a cycle of fear and avoidance could give rise to secondary phobic disorders such as agoraphobia (Popkirov et al. 2018).

In addition, they believe they have observed that affected patients often have obsessive "accentuated" personality traits, with a tendency to increased introspection and the need to "have everything under control". The central problem for patients with phobic postural vertigo is therefore also the attempt by the patient to control the balance with the development of a "self-observation spiral". This can lead to the fact that own body movements are perceived as movements from outside.

Since these symptoms were also seen after "actually expired" diseases with balance disorders, the concept was extended to include a "secondary phobic postural vertigo".

However, the concept was not without discussion and indications of open questions and limitations. Above all, Eckhardt-Henn stated (Eckhardt-Henn et al. 1997) that the group of disorders, described by Brandt and Dieterich (1986), can be traced back to anxiety disorders, depressive disorders and somatization disorders.

■ The Concept of "Chronic Subjective Dizziness" (CSD)

The group around the American psychiatrist Staab developed the concept of a CSD in an effort to combine physical and mental elements.

Staab (2006, 2012) gives *equal weight to physical and psychological events* that can be triggers of acute and persistent vertigo, for example:

- an event originating from the vestibular organ, such as a vestibular neuritis, a (repeated) benign positional vertigo or Ménière's disease,
- a (different) primary medical condition involving dizziness or fainting such as vestibular migraine or syncope (sudden loss of consciousness),
- an acute anxiety attack (panic attack). This psychogenic cause is understood as an acute interruption of mobility due to panic attacks or other intense overload ("stress").

As described in ► Sect. 3.10 for Ménière's attacks, events affecting the vestibular system require a rapid adaptation in the structure of the vestibular system. The transmission of confusing impulses from the damaged vestibular part of the central nervous system is inhibited.

At the same time, connections of the fear circuit in the limbic system with the central processing pathways enable to raise the threshold for impulses from the vestibular organs (the afferent motion perceptions) (Balaban et al. 2011). This is possible, because more than 85% of the vestibular nuclei in the brainstem and cerebellum responded by means of the neurotransmitter serotonin or its counterparts. These "neurotransmitters" are known from anxiety research.

> Thus, both for organic reasons (inhibition of the confusing organic impulses) and due to the fear reaction ("psychological"), a "double inhibition" of the information flow from the affected organ of equilibrium can occur.

This results in a relative weighting of sensory inputs about space and motion to favor visual cues over vestibular or somatosensory (proprioceptive) data.

This can result in high-demand postural control strategies such as moving cautiously or using supports to maintain safe and secure locomotion. The third is to maintain a higher level of vigilance about self-motion and movement in the environment.

These adaptations are useful in the short run but are expected to revert to normal as the precipitant resolves or compensation occurs.

> However, if the adaptation behavior cannot be abandoned, there remains a permanent maladaptation with persistent vertigo due to the failure to re-adaption (Staab 2012).

This solidifies postural control strategies that would be more appropriate to compensate for a high (fall) risk (walking on black ice).

As a result, this leads to the gap – described by Brandt and Dieterich (1986) – between the expected movement impulse (afferent copy) and the available reaction to the movement impulse (response) (efferent copy) in the brainstem.

But unlike the "phobic postural vertigo" first described in 1986, in which, in the absence of organic damage, it is primarily fear that has an irritating and inhibiting effect, an organic deficit may still be present after a loss of balance. This explains why in the concept of CSD "only" 50% of the patients show significant psychological abnormality.

Building on the considerations of a failure to readjust or a failure to re-adapt, Staab (2006, 2012) and Ruckenstein and Staab (2009) formulate three core characteristics in their model of "CSD."

- The presence of non-vestibular dizziness,which lasts longer than 3 months and usually has a recognizable beginning with a mostly fluctuating course.
- A hypersensitivity to motion impulses,maybe their own movements or movements in the environment.
- Difficulty with complex and precise visual requirements and tasks.

Staab (2012) describes as facilitating factors for persistent dizziness and vertigo:

- high anxiety levels – even before the vertigo as a "personality trait",
- high attention to the balance symptoms,
- catastrophizing thoughts regarding the possible development.

Based on a test inventory, the Revised NEO Personality Inventory (Costa and McCrae 1992), Staab (2012) has identified "anxiety and introversion" as two personality profiles that are more likely to be found in what he defines as CSD.

The (former) Mainz working group has – conversely – elaborated resilience factors that protect against a chronic course (Tschan et al. 2011). Resilience is the ability of a system to cope with change. A vivid example of resilience the ability of a skipjack: it can pick itself up again from any position.

The persistent vertigo sensation is "amplified" by real repeated organic events, which often occurs in Ménière's disease.

▪ A "Perpetuating Loop" of "Failure to Recover" and Movement-Dependent "Triggering Factors"

With corresponding, individually certainly very different "receptivity" (sensitivity), these accompanying circumstances or parts of them can then – unconsciously – trigger the same vertigo sensations as an organically caused Ménière's attack. These processes can be well explained by learning processes (classical and operant conditioning processes).

The Mainz research group (Eckhardt-Henn et al. 2009) was also able to show that a pre-existing mental illness contributes significantly to the development of reactive psychogenic dizziness. This is especially true for diseases with – unpredictable – recurrent character such as migraine and Ménière's disease.

In worst case, a "perpetuating loop" – described by Staab (2012) – of "failure to recover" and movement-dependent "triggering factors" can remain entrenched. These patients are then subjectively and chronically in a persistent state of maladaptation characterized by hypersensitivity to movement stimuli. According to Staab, the same factors simultaneously increase the risk of a concomitant psychological (comorbid) disease.

The model of the CSD – according to Staab (2012) – creates the link between neurootology and psychiatry. Behavioral elements and neurotological factors are described as key elements in the interaction. If one adds the conditioning processes, the picture of a persistent, at least to a large extent psychogenic vertigo, takes on clearer contours, on which understanding and therapy can start.

■ Concept of "Persistent Perceptual and Postural Dizziness" (3P-D)

The concept of "persistent perceptual and postural dizziness" (3P-D) (Staab 2020) may be understood as a compromise to the previous approaches of "phobic attack dizziness", "visual dizziness" and "space and motion discomfort" as well as to the theorizing around "CSD".

In addition, there may be an additional pathophysiological mechanism, namely a deficiency in cortical processes that subserve locomotion and spatial orientation at the highest levels. Although the research paradigms differed from one another and the use of imaging techniques for studying PPPD is just getting started, a pattern of results is beginning to take shape (Popkirov et al. 2018).

Activity and connectivity appear to be greater in visual versus vestibular regions of the cortex, in keeping with physiological data on visual dependence, but activity and connectivity between key cortical regions that process space–motion information (e.g., posterior insula, hippocampus) and modulate threat responses (e.g., anterior cingulate cortex) are reduced. These results suggest that underactive and insufficiently interactive cortical networks may fail to suppress the bottom-up influences of instinctive threat on postural control and spatial orientation leading to sustained use of the acute high-risk strategies (Popkirov et al. 2018).

◘ **Table 5.3** Diagnostic criteria of the Bárány Society for persistent postural-perceptual dizziness (Staab et al. 2017)

Bárány Society diagnostic criteria for persistent postural-perceptual dizziness (Staab et al. 2017)
A. One or more symptoms of dizziness, unsteadiness or non-spinning vertigo on most days for at least 3 months.
1. Symptoms last for prolonged (hours-long) periods of time, but may wax and wane in severity.
2. Symptoms need not be present continuously throughout the entire day.
B. Persistent symptoms occur without specific provocation, but are exacerbated by three factors:
1. Upright posture,
2. Active or passive motion without regard to direction or position,
3. Exposure to moving visual stimuli or complex visual patterns.
C. The disorder is triggered by events that cause vertigo, unsteadiness, dizziness, or problems with balance, including acute, episodic or chronic vestibular syndromes, other neurological or medical illnesses, and psychological distress.
1. When triggered by an acute or episodic precipitant, symptoms settle into the pattern of criterion A as the precipitant resolves, but may occur intermittently at first, and then consolidate into a persistent course.
2. When triggered by a chronic precipitant, symptoms may develop slowly at first and worsen gradually.
D. Symptoms cause significant distress or functional impairment.
E. Symptoms are not better accounted for by another disease or disorder
Source: Staab et al. (2017)

Diagnostic criteria of the Bárány Society for persistent postural-perceptual dizziness are listed in ◘ Table 5.3 (Staab et al. 2017).

▪ Diagnostic

In psychogenic dizziness, there is typically *no organic* finding that would adequately explain the symptomatology. Thus, it is likely – as a first assumption – that permanent dizziness without evidence of a gait disorder or cranial nerve impairment has at least a *mental component.*

Another clue, albeit a fuzzy one, is that the more varied the complaints experienced and described, the more likely it is that there is psychogenic dizziness. The prerequisite is that a good medical examination has *in fact* found nothing organic to explain the dizziness or the extent of the dizziness or vertigo.

The diagnosis relies on the patient history.

Dizziness, unsteadiness and vertigo are notoriously difficult to describe and patients will offer various reports of symptoms, including non-spinning vertigo ("I feel a sense of motion – it's not whirling – even though I'm still"; "I feel as if my body is swaying like I'm on a boat"), unsteadiness ("I feel I'm about to fall"), light-headedness ("I feel as if I might pass out") and mild dissociation ("I feel spaced out/as if my legs are spongy/as if I'm floating").

Unsteadiness and non-spinning vertigo tend to dominate the clinical picture.

Symptoms are exacerbated by upright posture, moving about actively or being moved passively (e.g., standing, walking or riding in a vehicle), or being immersed in environments with complex or moving visual stimuli (e.g., a hallway with complex patterned carpet, a supermarket aisle, looking at traffic).

This visual hypersensitivity, which can occur in isolation as the symptom of "visual vertigo," is a characteristic feature of PPPD, and often one of its most impairing features, especially in the modern world with its ever-growing intensity of visual stimulation.

5.9.5 Dizziness in Sociophobia (Social Phobia)

Although the fear of spiders and snakes is the most common phobia, the "social phobia" is the clinically most significant. Unlike animals, possibly great heights and elevators or other more or less avoidable things, the social environment can usually not be "avoided" without problems.

Social phobia is characterized by situational anxiety with avoidance behavior. The focus is on situations and actions that they take place under the eyes of other, more or less important people. These other people, in the perception of the affected person, not only observe, but could possibly – "perhaps even quite certainly" – also criticize their behavior.

▪ Craters Open Up

It is feared or even expected to make mistakes, to embarrass oneself, to "provoke" embarrassing situations or to be humiliated. Above all, the fear of embarrassment plays a decisive role. Confrontation with feared social situations, strangers, superiors and contact with the opposite sex can cause immediate anxiety and lead to a situational panic attack, which can occur in the experience, for example, with dizziness, as if a hole in the ground would open up.

- **Anxiety Is Not Perceived**

A social phobia can become noticeable not only in exceptional situations such as exams and public appearances, but also during everyday occasions. This is usually associated with palpitations, trembling, sweating, blushing or even dizziness. The underlying anxiety is usually not perceived. Also as the avoidance behavior is not perceived as Avoidance of fear, but as a consequence of the physical symptoms, such as dizziness or vertigo.

In most cases, the disease is only recognized when the avoidance behavior leads to withdrawal, a drop-in performance and isolation. This can begin with the restriction of the individual development and the quality of life and lead up to serious psychosocial consequential disorders, which not infrequently include alcoholism and other substance abuse.

Possibilities of Differentiation Psychogenic Dizziness and Vertigo from Ménière's Disease

Psychogenic dizziness can – in principle – appear like a purely somatic disease, i.e. also like Ménière's disease. With two diseases that are difficult to diagnose, the distinction is not easy. This is all the more true if, in the course of a Ménière's disease, a reactive psychogenic component is added to the organic impairment and, in addition, a – again organic – habitual deficit develops and perhaps also positional vertigo.

5.10 Multiple Sclerosis

- **Multiple Dysfunction Possible**

As a special form of an inflammatory damage of the nervous system, multiple sclerosis can – also unilaterally – worsen the hearing ability and cause intermittent balance disorders. Characteristic is a changing picture of functional disturbances, which can also occur only temporarily. Magnetic resonance imaging and/or a cerebrospinal fluid (CSF) sample, may confirm the diagnosis.

Possibilities of Differentiation from Ménière's Disease

Neurological examinations reveal the completely different changes in the central nervous system – in contrast to the "peripherally" located disorders in Ménière's disease.

5

5.11 Central Vestibular Vertigo Syndrome

Damage to the brainstem or cerebellum can lead to prolonged dizziness lasting days to weeks, but not to repeated attacks of dizziness. Most often, the vestibular nuclei or the vestibular-ocular pathways are affected. Here the accompanying symptoms, which in turn depend on the size of the damage and the involvement of its neighboring structures, point the way to the correct diagnosis. In older patients' infarcts, more rarely hemorrhages or tumors can be found. In younger patients, multiple sclerosis or hemorrhages into the brain may be the reason in the combination of too much nicotine, alcohol and anticonception drugs.

The causes of stroke in this region are the same as those of heart attack: smoking, high blood pressure, obesity, diabetes and lack of movement.

5.11.1 Diagnostics

■ "FAST" in Case of Suspected Stroke

A quick information about a possible stroke is given by the "FAST" test:

FAST stands for:

- *F*ace
- *A*rms
- *S*peech and
- *T*ime (fast dialing of the emergency call)

This allows even non-medical professionals to quickly check typical stroke symptoms such as hemifacial paralysis, paralysis of one side of the body and speech disorders.

■ Face

Ask the affected person to smile. In facial paralysis, the face is distorted on one side due to the weakening of the facial muscle. The smile then only shows on the unaffected side and the mouth appears crooked as a result.

■ Arms

Ask the affected person to raise both arms forward at the same time and turn the palms upwards. If a stroke is present, one arm cannot be lifted or sinks again. The person may also find it difficult to coordinate the arms so that the palms are facing upwards.

- **Speech**

Ask the dizzy person to repeat a sentence. If the person cannot repeat the words correctly, uses them incorrectly or pronounces them in a slurred manner, a stroke may be present.

- **Time**

If the person has problems with any of these tasks, the emergency should be dialed and it is essential to report that a stroke is suspected.

Individual symptoms may also be present in other diseases or alcohol intoxication. Thus, the quick test can only give clues. Nevertheless, without knowledge of the individual case, the rule remains for the time being: Better to call the doctor. Once too often than once too late.

5.11.2 Prevention

The individual risk of stroke can be reduced by a healthy diet, stable blood pressure levels and sufficient movement.

> **Possibilities of Differentiation from Ménière's Disease**
> Ménière's disease presents with dramatic vertigo attacks for the affected person, central forms of vertigo reveal themselves through failures of cranial nerve functions, but are often less noticed by the affected person.

5.12 Blood Pressure Fluctuations

"Orthostatic" vertigo is often seen with "weak" circulation and low blood pressure fluctuations.

According to Lempert (2005), circulatory disturbances in the head (transient ischemic attacks = TIA) need to be considered if they are sudden attacks of vertigo in elderly patients with vascular risks, usually lasting "only" minutes. They are usually accompanied by other brainstem or cerebellar symptoms or hearing disorders.

From a neurological point of view, if you suffer from vertigo attacks for years, you cannot have TIAs and, accordingly, you cannot benefit from the wide variety of blood flow-enhancing drugs.

> **Possibilities of Differentiation from Ménière's Disease**
> Vertigo can be mistaken for Ménière's disease, but the hearing and balance impairments are absent.

5.13 Acoustic Neuroma

▪ Benign, but Too Big

Despite its benign nature, acoustic neuroma can take up so much space in the skull bounded by bone that it displaces and damages other structures. Above a certain size (about 2 cm in diameter, as long as it does not constrict the "cerebellopontine angle"), it must be operated out or irradiated. In most cases, however, the acoustic neuroma grows so slowly that it is often possible to wait and see.

5.13.1 Diagnostics

BERA ("brainstem electric response audiometry") and balance tests usually provide sufficient information. If there is sufficient suspicion, computer and magnetic resonance tomograms are used; they can show tumors as small as 2 mm.

Possibilities of Differentiation from Ménière's Disease

Normally, the medical history already allows a clear distinction from Ménière's disease: acoustic neuromas have an insidious onset and a slowly progressing course in contrast to the violent onset and equally rapidly ending course of attacks in Ménière's disease.

5.14 Bilateral Loss of Vestibular Function

Both organs of balance can be damaged or fail completely after a severe meningitis or after too much gentamycin. This is sometimes necessary in intensive care units to save lives. It is also possible for bilateral Ménière's disease to progress to the point where both sides are completely affected. Often it is not known, then it remains "idiopathic".

▪ Eye Fluttering Movements and Gait Unsteadiness

Affected persons feel flickering eye movements or gait unsteadiness – and usually both. The flickering eye movements are caused by the absence of the vestibular reflex, consequently the patient can only see his surroundings "dim or consumed" during a head movement as if through a camera. When he shakes his head, it looks as if the opposite person jumps or moves.

The insecurity gets worse when walking in the dark, e.g. when patients have to go to the toilet at night Also is get worse, when they have to walk on rough, irregular or even slippery surfaces in the dark. Patients usually learn to avoid this or they use a stick or hold on to someone.

The most important part of treatment is rehabilitation. While many have already learned to some extent how to handle normal daily activities themselves, additional targeted rehabilitation may still be useful. It is also important to educate patients about some activities that they should refrain from and be cautious about, if possible. For example, they should not expose themselves to serious risks such as standing near a platform, snorkeling or diving.

Possibilities of Differentiation from Ménière's Disease
Balance insecurity is dependent on balance requirements and is not attack related.

5.15 Head-Extension Vertigo: Cervicogenic?

■ **Functional Limitations of the Cervical Spine**

Dizziness and balance problems are often experienced when the head is moved. This alone is not a specific diagnosis. Even healthy people get dizzy when the neck is over-moved or when the neck reclines too far. If you want to try this for yourself, try the following:

Stand on one leg with your eyes closed. You may sway a little, but you should be able to do it. Now try the same with your neck about 45° back. You will probably fall within 45 s.

This instability can be explained by the fact that the vestibular organ is bent 45° backwards outside the normal plane, which does not allow a habitual allocation, unless one trains exactly this.

Whether there is a clinically important vertigo specifically attributable to the cervical spine (CS) is highly controversial. Bronstein and Lempert (2017) point out that

- the only way to enable a new position of the head is to move it,
- the vestibular apparatus is the head movement detection system, and
- most head movements are accompanied by neck movements.

Therefore, it follows, that balance disorders can be aggravated by neck movements. Thus, most patients diagnosed with "vertebrobasilar insufficiency" or "cervical vertigo" suffer from disorders of the vestibular organs.

In case of a dysfunction of the upper cervical spine, a one-sided feeling of pressure in the temporal region may be present. Characteristic – according to Scherer 1997 – is a dizziness lasting a few seconds, but also a feeling of insecurity lasting for days, combined with a neck headache and occasionally sound perception disorders in the low-frequency range. A longer lasting spinning dizziness is not to be expected.

All in all, dizziness is too often assumed to be caused by the cervical spine or its muscles, and a much more frequent benign paroxysmal positional vertigo is probably overlooked and not specifically treated.

5.15.1 Diagnostics

■ Cervical Nystagmus

According to Hülse et al. (2005), vertigo originating from the cervical spine can be secured by placing the patient on a swivel chair and fixing the head with the hands. Then the body is rotated with the chair while maintaining the head position within 5–10 s as far as tolerated by the patient – with eyes closed. In this way, 70–80° of rotation is usually achieved. No cervical nystagmus could be registered in healthy, dizziness-free patients without cervical spine findings, but – according to Hülse et al. (2005) – in sick patients.

Regardless of the ongoing discussions, it makes sense to look for blockages, especially in the first three upper cervical joints.

5.15.2 Therapy

There are a variety of manual soft tissue and mobilization techniques to correct existing blockages. Accompanying or continuing manual physiotherapy is useful. The content of such physiotherapy is targeted active exercise treatment adapted to the condition of the overall statics of the spine. In the process, dysfunctional joints are mobilized, shortened muscles are stretched, and overloaded regions are stabilized.

> **Possibilities of Differentiation from Ménière's Disease**
> The vertigo occurs in a movement-dependent manner and no prolonged spinning vertigo is to be expected.

5.16 Drug-Induced Dizziness

■ Do Not Discontinue Any Medication Without Consulting

The following list shows some common problem areas of drug groups. However, it should always be checked on a case-by-case basis whether the experienced or feared problems with dizziness, tinnitus and hearing loss are related to the drug. This is usually determined on an individual basis. It must be weighed up whether the main effect is so important that the side effect must be endured. Certainly, no one should simply stop taking their medication, but should discuss this with the appropriate medical professional. These substances include:

- Analgesic with acetylsalicylic acid (ASS)
- Draining agents: diuretics
- Special antibiotics: aminoglycosides (streptomycin/gentamycin)
- Antimalarials: quinine and quinidine
- Antidepressants,
- Beta blocker
- Chemotherapeutic agents
- Alcohol

■ Analgesic with ASS

All active substances containing aspirin-like agents can cause – mostly reversibly – all forms of inner ear damage with dizziness, hearing loss and tinnitus. However, this depends on the amount of the active substances taken! Thus, more than 3000 mg/day must be taken in order to achieve "safe" inner ear damage. Here the risk must always be weighed against the benefit. The patient who, for example, takes ASS in amounts of 100 mg daily after a previous heart attack is certainly well advised not to skip this medication because of a tinnitus. Also, a single headache tablet does no more harm than taking analgesics every month, for example before and during the period.

▪ Dehydrating Agents – Diuretics

There are dehydrating diuretics, such as Lasix and etacric acid, which can damage the inner ear. However, this is not an inevitable and, moreover, a rare mechanism. Thus, it is still advisable to continue taking a diuretic, for example, in severe heart disease with volume overload. Therefore, a diuretic is often a permanent component of cardiac medication. Again, it must be weighed whether the usually small amounts are so harmful to the ear in the long term that other alternatives would need to be considered. The "osmotic" diuretics cause an increase in the concentration of blood constituents. They probably do not have any negative effects on the ear, but they can only be used to a limited extent.

5.16.1 Gentamycin for the Elimination of Ménière's Disease

▪ Special Antibiotics – Aminoglycosides (Streptomycin/Gentamycin)

Aminoglycosides are antibiotics that are only used in very rare, usually very severe cases. Their ear-toxic effect is known and described in detail on the package insert. They are used for tuberculosis and inflammation, especially in the abdomen or lungs, when other drugs have not been successful. They are also used "therapeutically" if, for example, the vestibular organ is to be explicitly switched off with the help of the side effects (► Chap. 7).

▪ Antimalarials – Quinine and Quinidine

Quinine can cause tinnitus, hearing impairment and dizziness, especially when given in high doses for prolonged periods. Quinidine is less likely to cause hearing loss, which is also likely to be reversible.

▪ Antidepressants

So-called tricyclic antidepressants, such as Saroten, Anafranil, Imipramin (Tofranil), can cause ears. More often, – mostly temporary – circulatory difficulties and gait unsteadiness perceived as dizziness. However, these should not prevent the depressed patient from taking advantage of the possible improvements – if it is indicated.

▪ Beta Blocker

These blood pressure and heart rate lowering agents can – rarely – cause dizziness via the desired drop in blood pressure.

■ **Chemotherapeutic Agents**
Certainly, all chemotherapeutic agents can also damage the balance system. But usually the fight against the underlying disease, usually the tumor disease, is more important.

■ **Alcohol and Other Intoxicants**
Alcohol is regularly associated with balance disorders. All intoxicants such as cocaine, marijuana, morphine and heroin can often cause people to become permanently unbalanced.

Literature

Balaban CD, Jacob RG, Furman JM (2011) Neurologic bases for comorbidity of balance disorders, anxiety disorders and migraine: neurotherapeutic implications. Expert Rev Neurother 11(3):379–394. https://doi.org/10.1586/ern.11.19

Brandt TH, Dieterich M (1986) Phobischer Attackenschwindel. MMW 128:247–250

Brandt T, Dieterich M, Strupp M (2012) Vertigo. Leitsymptom Schwindel. Steinkopff, Darmstadt

Bronstein A, Lempert T (2017) Dizziness. A practical approach to diagnosis and management. Cambridge University Press, Cambridge

Costa PT, McCrae RR (1992) Revised NEO personality inventory (NEO-PI-R) and NEO five-factor inventory (NEO-FFI) professional manual. Psychological Assessment Resources, Odessa

Eckhardt-Henn A, Hoffmann SO, Tettenborn B, Thomalske C, Hopf HC (1997) "Phobischer Schwankschwindel" – Eine weitere Differenzierung psychogener Schwindelzustände erscheint erforderlich. Nervenarzt 68:806–812

Eckhardt-Henn A, Tschan R, Best C, Dieterich M (2009) Somatoforme Schwindelsyndrome. Nervenarzt 80:909–917

Godemann F, Schuller J, Uhlemann H (2009) Psychodynamic vulnerability factors in the development of panic disorders--a prospective trial in patients after vestibular neuritis. Psychopathology 42:99–107

Gürkov, R, Pyyko I, Zou J, Kentala E (2016) What is Menière's disease? A contemporary re-evaluation of endolymphatic hydrops. J Neurol 263(Suppl 1):71–81

Havia M, Kentala E, Pyykkö I (2005) Prevalence of Menière's disease in general population of Southern Finland. Otolaryngol Head Neck Surg 133:762–768

Helling K (2008) Otolithenfunktionsstörungen und Therapieoptionen. HNO 56:996–1002

Hülse M, Neuhuber W, Wolff HD (eds) (2005) Die obere Halswirbelsäule, Pathophysiologie und Klinik. Springer, Heidelberg; Jahnke K (1977) Zur Pathogenese der akuten Symptome des Morbus Menière. Laryngorhinootologie 56:402–406

Junicho M, Aso S, Fujisaka M (2008) Prognosis of low-tone sudden deafness – does it inevitably progress to Menière's disease? Acta Otolaryngol 128(3):304–308

Lempert T (1995) Benign positional vertigo: recognition and treatment. BMJ 311:489–491

Lempert T (2005) Schwindelattacken: Differenzialdiagnose und Therapie. Fortschr Neurol Psychiatr 10:605–620

Luers JC, Hüttenbrink KB (2013) Akustische und vestibuläre Effekte bei einer Dehiszenz des oberen Bogengangs. HNO 61:743–751. https://doi.org/10.1007/s00106-013-2747-7

Popkirov S, Staab JP, Stone J (2018) Persistent postural-perceptual dizziness (PPPD): a common, characteristic and treatable cause of chronic dizziness. Pract Neurol 18:5–13

Ruckenstein M, Staab JP (2009) Chronic subjective dizziness. Otolaryngol Clin N Am 42(1):71–77

Schaaf H, Hesse G (2007) Sind rezidivierende Tiefton-Hörverluste – ohne Schwindel – die Vorstufe eines M. Menière? Eine Längsschnittuntersuchung nach 4 und nach 10 Jahren. HNO 55:630–637

Schaaf H, Hesse G (2012) Endolymphschwankungen: Stau im Höranteil – Turbulenten im Gleichgewichtsorgan. DTL, Wuppertal

Scherer H (1997) Das Gleichgewicht, 2nd edn. Springer, Berlin, Heidelberg, New York

Staab J (2006) Assessment and management of psychological problems in the dizzy patient. Continuum 12(4):189–213

Staab J (2012) Chronic subjective dizziness. Continuum 18(5):1118–1141

Staab JP (2020) Persistent postural-perceptual dizziness. Semin Neurol 40(1):130–137. https://doi.org/10.1055/s-0039-3402736

Staab JP, Eckhardt-Henn A, Horii A, Jacob R, Strupp M, Brandt T, Bronstein A (2017) Diagnostic criteria for persistent postural-perceptual dizziness (PPPD): consensus document of the committee for the Classification of Vestibular Disorders of the Bárány Society. J Vestib Res 27(4):191–208. https://doi.org/10.3233/VES-170622. PMID: 29036855

Strupp M, Zingler VC, Arbusow V, Niklas D, Maag KP, Dieterich M, Bense S, Theil D, Jahn K, Brandt T (2004) Methylprednisolone, valacyclovir, or the combination for vestibular neuritis. N Engl J Med 351: 354–361

Taura A, Funabiki K, Ohgita H, Ogino E, Torii H, Matsunaga M, Ito J (2014) One-third of vertiginous episodes during the follow-up period are caused by benign paroxysmal positional vertigo in patients with Meniere's disease. Acta Otolaryngol 134(11):1140–1145. https://doi.org/10.3109/00016489.2014.936624

Teranishi M, Naganawa S, Katayama N (2009) Image evaluation of endolymphatic space in fluctuating hearing loss without vertigo. Eur Arch Otorhinolaryngol 266:1871–1877

Tschan R, Best C, Beutel ME, Knebel A, Wiltink J, Dieterich M, Eckhardt-Henn A (2011) Patients' psychological well-being and resilient coping protect from secondary somatoform vertigo and dizziness (SVD) 1 year after vestibular disease. J Neurol 258(1):104–112

van Esch BF, van Benthem PPG, van der Zaag-Loonen HJ, Bruintjes TD (2016) Two common second causes of dizziness in patients with Menière's disease. Otol Neurotol 37(10):1620–1624

Westhofen M (2008) Die operative Therapie des vestibulären Schwindels. Verfahren und Indikationen. HNO 56:1003–1010

5

Westhofen M (2009) M. Menière. Evidenzen und Kontroversen. HNO 57:446–454

Yamasoba T, Kikuchi S, Sugaswa M, Yagi M, Harada T (1994) Acute low-tone sensorineural hearing loss without vertigo. Arch Otolaryngol Head Neck Surg 120:532–535

Zenner HP (1994) Hören. Physiologie, Biochemie, Zell- und Neurobiologie. Thieme, Stuttgart, p 16

Diagnostics and Examination Methods

Contents

6.1 Medical History – 144

6.2 Balance Examination (Vestibular Examination) – 147
6.2.1 Standing and Walking Examination – 147

6.3 Examination of Eye Movement – 149
6.3.1 Suppression of the VOR – 150
6.3.2 Head Impulse Test – Testing von the Vestibulo-Ocular-Reflex (VOR) – 151
6.3.3 Positioning Maneuvers – 152
6.3.4 Overall Evaluation of the Investigation – 152

6.4 Apparative Examination of the Semicircular Canals – 153
6.4.1 Caloric (Thermal) Test – 153
6.4.2 Rotational Testing: Examination in a Swivel Chair – 154

6.5 Examination of the Otolith Organs – 155
6.5.1 Examination of the Sacculus – 155
6.5.2 Examination of the Utricle – 158

6.6 Hearing Tests – 162
6.6.1 Pure Tone Audiogram – 162
6.6.2 Speech Audiogram – 165

6.7 Tinnitus Determination – 165

6.8 Otoacoustic Emission and Distortion Products – 166

6.9 Electrocochleography – 166

6.10 Brain-Evoked-Response Audiometry (BERA) – 167

H. Schaaf, *Ménière's Disease*, https://doi.org/10.1007/978-3-662-63610-7_6

6.11 Glycerol Load Test (Klockhoff Test) – 167

6.12 Manual Examination of the Vertebral Segments – 168

6.13 Imaging Techniques – 168

6.14 Psychological-Psychosomatic Diagnostics – 169

6.15 Psychological Questionnaires/Test Diagnostics – 172
6.15.1 Dizziness Handicap Inventory (DHI) – 172
6.15.2 Hospitality Anxiety and Depression Score (HADS) – 173
6.15.3 Patient Health Questionnaire (PHQ-D) – 173
6.15.4 University Research – 174

6.16 The Most Important Thing at the End: Evaluating and Assigning – 175

Literature – 177

It is often difficult to ensure diagnose Ménière's disease. In an effort to describe clinically meaningful criteria, important societies, including the Bárány Society and the European Academy of Otology and Neurootology, agreed on a classification in 2015 (Lopez-Escamez et al. 2015).

▪ Distinction is made between definite and probable Ménière's disease

The diagnosis of ***definite Ménière's* disease** is based on clinical criteria and requires the observation of repeated rotary vertigo syndromes (vertigo!) with - documented by audiograms - low-frequency losses (more than 30 dB between 250 and 2000 Hz) and fluctuating ear symptoms (hearing, tinnitus, ear pressure sensation) in the affected ear.

The duration of vertigo must be between 20 minutes and 12 hours.

> ***Author's comment:*** *As only very few Menière attacks occur in a doctor's office or in hospital, the symptoms can usually not be directly observed during the attack. The use of modern mobile phones presents a promising remedy. (see below).*

The assumption of a ***probable Ménière's*** includes - in the extension of the above conditions - also more unspecific, repeated balance problems with rotational vertigo, but also other "indefinite" forms of vertigo ("dizziness") with fluctuating ear symptoms lasting between 20 minutes and 24 hours.

Unfortunately, there is no *single* marker that can confirm Ménière's disease on its own. Nevertheless, in the course of the disease, a puzzle of auditory and vestibular findings is usually put together, which at least allows a more reliable assessment and therapy recommendations. This also makes it possible to distinguish Ménière's disease from the - frequent - vestibular migraine as well as from the rare perilymph fistulae and vestibular paroxysmia (▶ Chap. 5).

▪ If it were possible to make one or wishes

More certainty - at least for scientific papers - could be achieved if, in addition to the criteria in the two classifications, the following factors were also taken into account:

- The exact duration of disease (from the first vertigo attack).
- This is probably the most important factor because the "natural" course with increasing loss of function usually leads to a decreasing of vertigo - both in terms of severity and duration- over time. This is usually the case - unless Tumarkin drops develop or vertigo remains reactively psychogenically solidified - while the hearing loss usually increases.

- The number of vertigo attacks per month, differentiated between organic and psychogenic vertigo events, 6 months before and 18–24 months after a therapy under review.
- Hearing tests 6 months before and 18–24 months after therapy to be reviewed.
- An examination of a meaningful range of the various balance components. This should include both the response to low frequencies ("caloric test") and high frequencies (swivel chair and head impulse test), as well as otolith functions.
- The type of pre-treatments (medications, surgeries, hearing aids).
- A disorder-specific biographical anamnesis, in which the mental risks - perhaps already existing before vertigo - but also the effects of Ménière's disease and the patient's coping options, strategies and resources are recorded, with knowledge of the organic disease.

In a noteworthy manner, taking into account almost all of these requirements, a large study was conducted in Mainz by Eckhardt-Henn's research group (Eckhardt-Henn et al. 2009; Patel et al. 2016).

Most of the time, such a more meaningful endeavor fails because

- there are altogether only a few Ménière's patients, who moreover show an equally individual as changeable and long course, which is mostly more changeable and longer than the examination team or its institution can hold;
- usually, only one expert is involved in such an investigation;
- in "multi-center studies", standardized questionnaires and the necessary but also limiting conditions often become more important than the concrete investigation of complex events.

6.1 Medical History

The first step should be a medical history (anamnesis). This is the most important basis for vertigo and leads to a diagnosis in up to 90% of cases (Brandt et al. 2012). The type and nature of the dizziness and the temporal course play an important role.

Frequency, type and duration of dizzy spells

In Ménière's disease, the frequency, type and duration of the vertigo attacks and their accompanying symptoms, such as eye tremor (nystagmus), are indicative of this particular inner ear disease.

Typical of a Ménière's attack is a repeated, inner ear-related spinning dizziness, which is often associated with nausea and vomiting. In addition, there is hearing loss - often not directly perceived - and a usually deep ringing or roaring in the ear. A Ménière's attack can occur out of complete well-being - even when lying down - and last from 20 minutes to many hours.

If a vertigo attack lasts less than 1 minutes, it is either a special form of Tumarkin drop (▶ Sect. 4.2) or, for example, benign paroxysmal positional vertigo, otolith vertigo or a brief migraine attack (◘ Table 5.1).

- **Documentation in the acute vertigo attack**

As very few Meniere's attacks occur in a doctor's office or in hospital it is not easy to get to the doctor's "during the attack." As a result, many ENT physicians often don't see their patients during an attack. But after the attack a nystagmus can't be seen any more. Thanks to modern mobile phones, the situation has now improved considerably. Most of them have a camera function. In addition, a "hearing test app" can usually be installed. This makes it possible to document eye movements in a Meniere's attack "live" and to record hearing loss during or shortly after the attack.

- **The following procedure is recommended**

Preparatory steps:

1. In the time without an attack, you, or someone close to you, try to get familiar with the camera function in the mobile phone, and rehearse the normal sequence until you can recall it without thinking. During your attempts look toward the camera but direct your view beyond the top of the camera.

Attention:

- The eye movements are to be filmed, not the movements of the eyelashes.
- Normally, the eyes do not move involuntarily.
- Normally, your eyes do not move involuntarily.

2. Install a hearing app on your mobile phone.

   Take a hearing test at your doctor's or acoustician's office during times without vertigo, and then take a hearing test with your hearing app. This will give you an idea of how exactly the hearing App can measure.
3. Save this hearing test as a starting point and rehearse using the mobile phone app until you can use it safely.

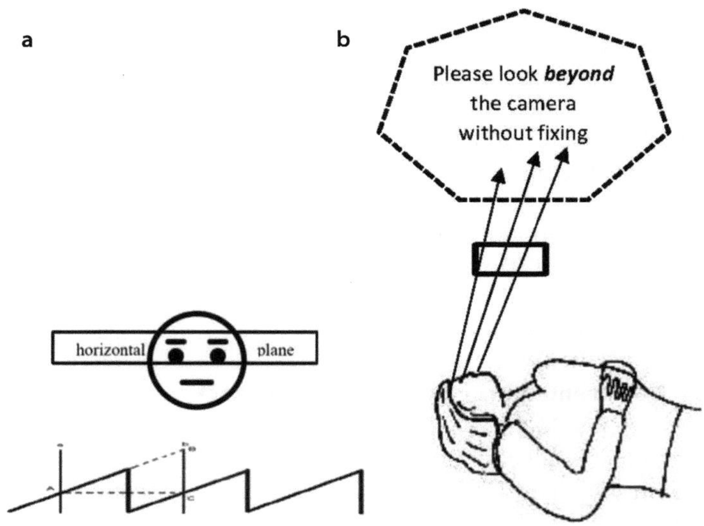

Fig. 6.1 **a** An involuntary eye tremor with predominantly horizontal direction - from "ear to ear" - is typical for a Meniere's attack. A slow phase alternate with a fast (reset) phase. **b** Look toward the camera but direct your view upward beyond the camera

During an acute attack of vertigo or dizziness

1. Activate the camera function in your mobile phone on your own or with the help of someone close to you.
2. Look in the direction of the camera. Please keep your eyes open, even if your dizziness may become stronger.
3. Please look "unintentionally behind" the camera - without focussing on any certain object. Menière disease is a peripheral disturbance of the balance system, so it is possible to suppress or reduce the nystagmus by fixating objects like the camera. This would make it difficult to evaluate the recorded video.
4. Look to one side first - and then to the other side.
5. **The involuntary eye movements (nystagmus) should be filmed, not the movements of your eyelashes.**
6. **As soon as possible after the attack, do a hearing test using a mobile phone app.**
7. **Save the video recordings and the hearing test, e.g. on a USB stick or a CD, and make it available to your doctor** (Fig. 6.1).

Preliminary cautious interpretation

Involuntary eye movements (nystagmus) in a Meniere's attack usually show a horizontal direction (eye tremor in the plane of the ears). The frequency of the eye movements increases - as a rule - when looking to one side and decreases to the other side. This is an important indication for the affected side.

Other eye movements, e.g. vertical (from the chin to the forehead) or rotating, usually do not fit to a Meniere's disease, but rather to a vestibular migraine.

Of course, one's own description also often may help if it can accurately reflect the experiences.

I am very interested in the first vertigo event. I beg the patient to described to me in detail.

Then I ask them to show me, which they feel is no longer possible and which they have avoided since then the latest in the case of long-term illnesses, it is necessary to take a comprehensive psychosomatic medical history. Realistically, this usually exceeds the time frame in ENT practice, unlike in psychosomatic clinics, special outpatient clinics or with psychotherapists.

6.2 Balance Examination (Vestibular Examination)

Even without apparatuses, you can get a good and at least orienting impression of the balance situation and the interaction of the individual balance components.

6.2.1 Standing and Walking Examination

Standing (apparently easily) on both legs with eyes closed (Romberg test) and then standing on one leg - first with eyes open and then with eyes closed - may give an indication of damage to the vestibular organ. As a specification, patients can be asked to raise both arms during this examination.

■ "Tougher" Romberg test

In the "Tougher "Romberg test, one foot is placed close behind the other in the so-called "tandem position" so that the toes of the rear foot touch the heel of the front foot. Patients with unilateral hypofunction of a vestibular organ tilt to the side of the damage and make an evasive movement.

■ Unterberger's test

When walking on the spot with closed eyes, unilateral damage of the vestibular organs leads to a deviation to the damaged side (◘ Fig. 6.2).

It is useful to repeat these tests to check the reliability of the body's responses. If abnormal muscle tension, overexertion or coordination difficulties are found, a neurological examination is advised. This includes an orientational exami-

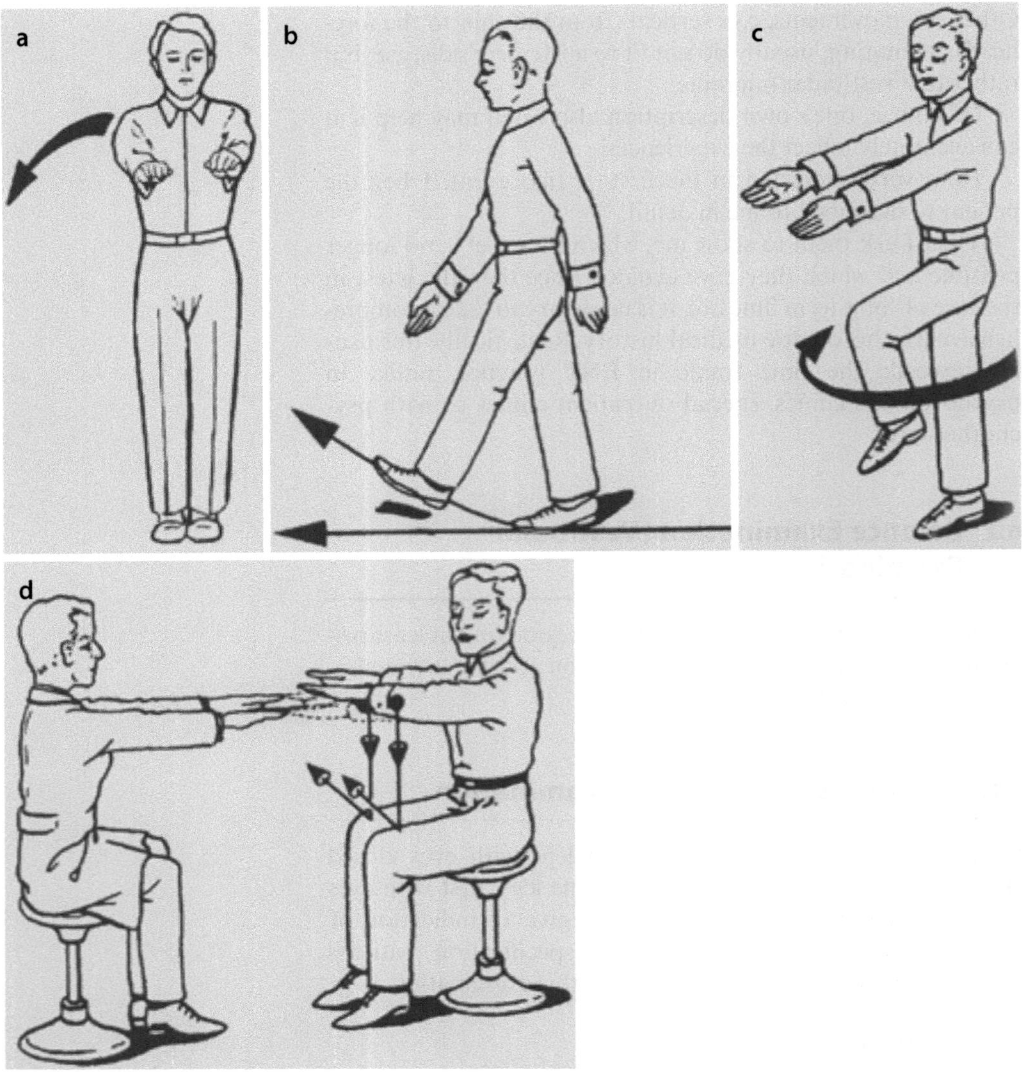

Fig. 6.2 Deviation reactions (to the right). **a** Romberg test, **b** gait deviation, **c** pedaling test according to Unterberger, **d** pointing test. (From Boenninghaus 1990)

nation of strength, coordination and tensile strength as well as reflexes (Bronstein and Lempert 2017).

- **Gait unsteadiness is to be distinguished from vertigo from the inner ear**

Gait unsteadiness can occur in many diseases. However, they are rarely associated with vertigo, eye tremor or hearing impairment and are rarely found in diseases of a vestibular organ (Bronstein and Lempert 2017).

▪ Sensitivity to vibration in the shin

A tuning fork can be used to check the sensitivity to touch and vibration in the shins and ankles. This is limited early in polyneuropathy, which is often found in diabetes and alcohol abuses. Then the information from the soles of the feet is missing - the gait becomes unsteady.

6.3 Examination of Eye Movement

▪ Most important source of information after medical history

The examination of the eye movement is an important source of information. It provides information about the possible involvement of structures in the central nervous systems. From a neurological point of view, the examination of eye movements in patients with vertigo is only surpassed in importance by the medical history.

Examiners should look for spontaneous, fixation and gaze evoked nystagmus as well as convergence, smooth pursuit, saccadic and vestibular eye movements, the vestibulo-ocular reflex (VOR) and its possible suppression and the optokinetic reflex.

Important questions are:

- Can you find spontaneous nystagmus?
- Can *positional nystagmus* be induced as a sign of benign paroxysmal positional vertigo?
- Do you find gaze jumps (saccadic gaze sequence) in slow following movements or too slow jumps (saccades) with fast following movements?
- Does a *gaze direction nystagmus* or a lack of suppressibility of the VOR *indicate a* disease in the central nervous system (mostly of the cerebellum)?

Peripheral diseases of a vestibular organ - as in Ménière's disease - show a nystagmus in the horizontal plane.

Large-amplitude directional nystagmus, with the inability to fix the eyes on an object, indicates brainstem or cerebellar damage on the side of the nystagmus.

In the upright patient, any nystagmus other than the horizontal-torsional nystagmus is probably of central origin and cannot - only - be due to Ménière's disease.

▪ Smooth pursuit

To investigate smooth pursuit, the patient is offered fixation targets, such as two fingers or a pen, which is moved about 30° to the right and left, and up and down, in front of the eye.

Perfect pursuit is when the velocity of the eyes matches that of the moving object. One must be sure that the patient remains attentive and, if in doubt, use new "attractive" objects or verbally encourage the patient. To many saccades in order to follow could be pathological.

Saccades

Saccades are fast refixation eye movements, with velocities up to 500 deg/sec. Their velocity is directly proportional to the size of the saccade. Some of them are "automatic" or reflexive, for instance in response to an unexpected sound or visual target, some of them are voluntary, such as saccades in the dark or in response to voluntary commands ("right", left" etc.) as tested in the clinic They are tested by having the patient alternately fixate two fingers held out, first right and left and then up and down. Two main abnormalities, inaccurate targeting and slowing could indicate central nervous system impairment.

- Too small saccades are found in cerebellar diseases, but also lesions elsewhere in the central nervous system.
- Excessive saccades usually indicate cerebellar disease; slow saccades suggest brainstem or eye muscle disease.

Caution with depressant medications

The most common reasons for non-specific abnormalities are age and centrally acting drugs. Therefore, it is always important to consider patient age, alcohol use (to be excluded if possible) and psychotropic drugs.

> Disturbances of the eye movements and saccades could indicate a central impairment. Peripheral impairments as in Ménière's disease shows inconspicuous eye movements.

6.3.1 Suppression of the VOR

In this position, the patient is rotated - for example, on a swivel chair in the office. While turning, the patient should look straight ahead at his hands. The head and hands remain in the same position. (in real life, the procedure would correspond to fixing the wristwatch while going around the corner).

The necessary suppression of the vestibulo-ocular reflex (VOR), which would otherwise start "automatically", is a central performance! This can be impeded by diseases in the central nervous system, mostly of the cerebellum.

6.3.2 Head Impulse Test – Testing von the Vestibulo-Ocular-Reflex (VOR)

Without apparatus, the function of the semicircular canals can be checked qualitatively (in the sense of yes or no). For this purpose, the examiner performs a short jerky movement of the patient's head in one plane at a time. This triggers the VOR (◘ Fig. 6.3).

The patient should fixate the nose of the examiner, for example. In healthy patients, the VOR ensures that the gaze remains stable and that no saccades are necessary.

▪ Effective function testing of the semicircular canals possible

To test the right horizontal semicircular canal, the patient's head is first turned slightly to the left and the patient is asked to fixate the tip of the examiner's nose continuously. The examiner then rapidly turns the head towards the center while the patient maintains fixation.

In case of unilateral failure of one or more semicircular canals, the patient cannot maintain fixation. Then the eyes go with the head (to the right) during the rapid rotation of the head, so that the patient after reaching the middle position of the head has to perform reset saccades in the opposite direction (to the left) in order to return the eyes to the fixation point. These reset saccades can be observed by the examiner opposite.

Experienced examiners can use the head impulse test to make separate statements for all three semicircular canals.

▪ Video-based head impulse test for all semicircular canals

With the development of video systems and glasses, an even more precise assessment can be made. The entire course from the beginning of the head movement with the reflex move-

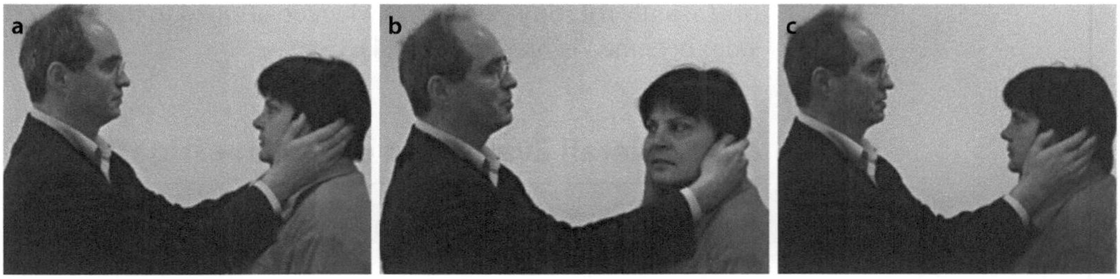

◘ Fig. 6.3 The head impulse test. To test horizontal semicircular canal, the patient **a** is asked to fixate the tip of the examiner's nose in the starting position before **b** the patient's head is first turned slightly to one side, while the patient is further asked to fixate the tip of the examiner's nose continuously; **c** the head is then turned rapidly to the center by the examiner while the patient maintains fixation

ments of the eyes to the phase after completion of the head impulse test can be documented. In this way, even reset saccades that are not visible to the "naked eye" become visible and objectifiable.

In Ménière's disease, the head impulse test (KIT) usually shows normal results for a long time, while pathological values are already seen in the cold-warm testing (caloric).

This is *an important* constellation of findings that is particularly helpful in distinguishing it from a unilateral vestibular neuritis (Plontke and Gürkov 2015). In the latter case, the head impulse test is particularly limited in the acute stage.

> An appropriate constellation of findings for Ménière's disease is a normal KIT with pathological caloric testing.

6.3.3 Positioning Maneuvers

It is essential to perform a positioning maneuver on both sides in every case of vertigo. On the one hand, benign paroxysmal positional vertigo is probably the most common organic form of vertigo, which can be detected and treated with this maneuver. On the other hand, Ménière's disease can often be confused with positional vertigo. One can perform it according to Epley or to Semont.

The following sequence of positions describes the Epley maneuver:

1. The patient begins in an upright sitting posture, with the legs fully extended and the head rotated 45 degrees toward the side in the same direction.
2. Then the patient is lowered into a supine position (on the back), with the head held approximately in a 30-degree neck extension, with the head remaining rotated to the side.

With Frenzel glasses, if positional vertigo is present, eye tremors (usually rotating nystagmus when positioned to the affected side) become visible (◘ Fig. 6.4).

6.3.4 Overall Evaluation of the Investigation

Roughly, the following distinctions can be made - with Bronstein and Lempert (2017):

- *Diseases of the vestibular organ*
  - show in the acute stage spontaneous nystagmus, which beats mainly horizontally and a little rotating in the fast phase to the healthy side,

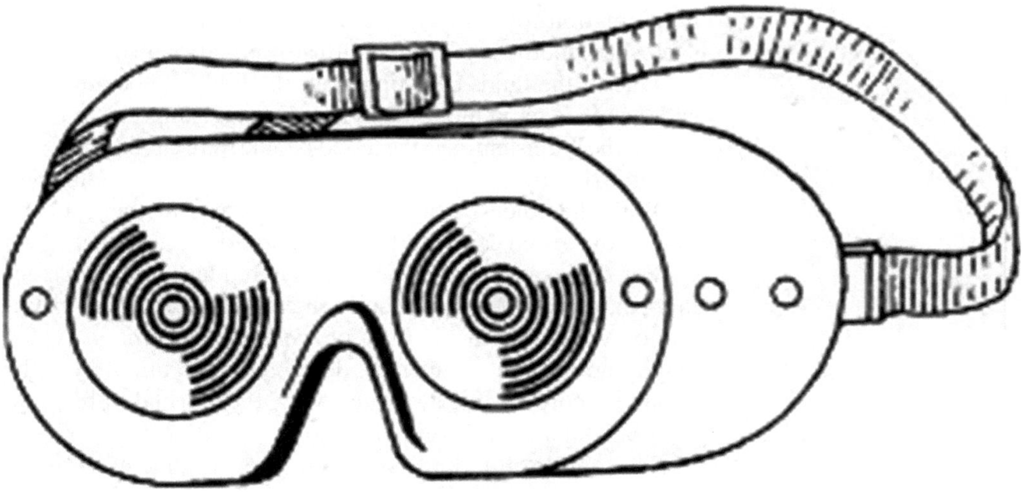

Fig. 6.4 Frenzel glasses. (From: Boenninghaus 1990)

  - show a VOR that is not fully functional.
  - *the other eye movements remain undisturbed.*
- *Central diseases* show
  - disturbed eye movements,
  - disturbed suppression of the VOR and gaze jumps (saccades).
  - in *most cases, no* VOR deviations are *found.*

"Estimated over the thumb" means for the investigator:
- A patient without brainstem symptoms and with normal eye movement is unlikely to have central disease.
- A patient with clear brainstem symptoms must be assumed to have central disease until proven otherwise.
- A patient with abnormal eye movement will have central disease even if his history sounds relatively peripheral.

6.4 Apparative Examination of the Semicircular Canals

6.4.1 Caloric (Thermal) Test

By flushing the sides with cold (30 °C) or warm water (44 °C) via the external auditory canal, the "lateral" semicircular canal of the organ of equilibrium, which lies furthest out, can be irritated. It should be noted that both vestibular organs should be examined under the same conditions. Before this, an examination of the external and middle ear is required. This is to determine that neither an earplug or a bone outgrowth nor an inflammation of the eardrum or a middle ear infection ("blocked middle ear") impairs the examination itself.

Due to the fluids deviating from the body temperature, the endolymph is set in motion and thus the same impression is created in the brainstem as if the tested people were circling horizontally in space. In response, the eyes via the VOR show nystagmus.

With the cold solution, nystagmus starts to the opposite side of the tested ear, with the warm liquid to the same side.

For this examination, the patients are placed in a horizontal position with the upper body slightly elevated on an examination couch. With the help of *video documentation* (video oculography), the number of deflections per minute can be reliably recorded and evaluated with the normal value, and especially in a lateral comparison.

The unpleasant thing about this test is that nausea can occur and one can feel maneuvered into a vertigo attack. This is not the case, however, and after a short time, this feeling subsides as soon as the excitement subsides with the draining of the water. If there is no reaction at all, the lateral semicircular canal probably no longer has function.

▪ Only lateral semicircular canal is verifiable

It should be noted here that the "cold-warm rinse" can only record the lateral semicircular canal - and the brain's response. This accounts for just 20% of the vestibular organ.

In addition, the caloric irrigation test represents "only" a very weak, low-frequency test stimulus (0.003 Hz) in relation to the dynamic width of the VOR (5–7 Hz in the head impulse test).

> In Ménière's disease, partial ranges are often impaired. Thus, the low-frequency range tends to be impaired, while the high-frequency range still shows normal test results (for a long time) (Walther et al. 2012).

6.4.2 Rotational Testing: Examination in a Swivel Chair

▪ Real-life incentives

Much more physiological than caloric irrigation are fast rotary movements. For the lateral semicircular canals this can already be done "qualitatively" in a simple office chair, following the eye movements during the movements of the chair. For exact, evaluable statements one needs a swivel chair and a video oculography. This is an expensive piece of equipment and requires, in addition to the expensive purchase, anchoring in the floor that can withstand the rotational forces.

In a swivel chair, the bilateral functionality of the horizontal VOR can be tested - but only together - in a frequency-dependent manner from 0.5–1 Hz.

Differentiated testing with different, also higher frequency stimuli can be useful for specific questions (such as corresponding inquiries about the functional capacity of the vestibular system and questions about occupational activity). Testing also provides good information about compensation after a loss of balance.

6.5 Examination of the Otolith Organs

In the meantime, the possibilities for examining the otolith organs, that is, the sacculus and the utricle, have improved considerably.

6.5.1 Examination of the Sacculus

- **Bridge between equilibrium and hearing part**

> Vestibular-evoked myogenic potentials (VEMP) derived from the cervical muscle (c-VEMP)

When testing the saccule (that detects upward and downward movements and anatomically forms the bridge between the vestibular and auditory components), one can take advantage of the fact that the saccule has both: vestibular functions and -evolutionarily- auditory functions for low-frequent sounds. Thus, low-frequent tones can be presented via headphones as "clicks" in an examination arrangement (Fig. 6.5a, b). These have a minimal but measurable influence on the large neck muscle via a reflex arc. The reflex arc leads from the saccule via the vestibular nerve, the vestibular nuclei, the interneurons and motoneurons to the cervical muscles at the sternocleidomastoid muscle.

- **High muscle tone necessary**

The changes in the neck muscle (sternocleidomastoid muscle) can be derived with a special device suitable for this purpose, as with an ECG. In a healthy person, there is first a positive wave on the tested side, then a negative wave after 21 ms. A sufficiently high muscle tone must be achieved in order to obtain a good potential derivation. For example, the patient should press his own hand with his head.

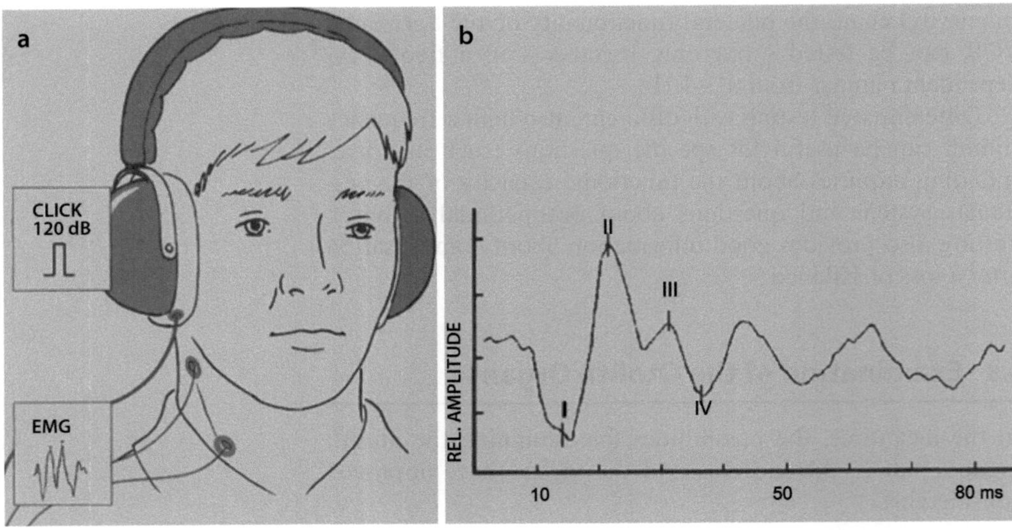

Fig. 6.5 **a** Examination arrangement in the sitting position, **b** Typical vestibular evoked myogenic potential. Potentials I and II represent the part evoked by the saccule, potentials III and IV the part evoked by the cochlea. (From: Hamann and Haarfeldt 2006)

The prerequisite for the test is an intact middle ear function. The hearing function of the cochlea does not have to be preserved so that the test can also be performed on deaf persons.

The size of wave II is measured and compared with that of the opposite side. The absence of waves as well as a clear amplitude reduction of 50% compared to the opposite side are considered conspicuous. A time-delayed course of the waves (latency change) cannot (yet) be assigned any significance (Fig. 6.6a, b).

With the c-VEMPs it is possible to assess side-separated functions of the saccule. Due to the fact that the lower part of the vestibular nerve is only supplied with impulses from the saccule and not from the utricle, it is also possible to examine whether the complete vestibular nerve is affected or "only" the lower branch in the case of a vestibular failure (Hamann and Haarfeldt 2006; Walther et al. 2010).

- **Sacculus involvement in Ménière's disease**

In Ménière's disease, the derivation of the VEMP gives the possibility to determine if the saccule is involved.

In Ménière's disease, three response patterns of the VEMP can be found:

- In the symptom-free interval, one can expect laterally normal potentials as long as the sacculus is not affected by the disease process.

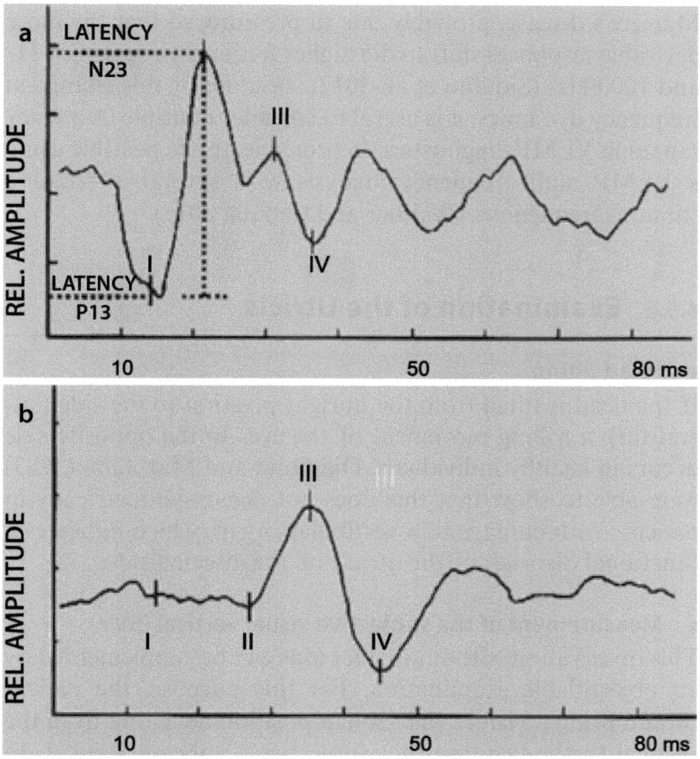

Fig. 6.6 Evaluation parameters of the VEMP. **a** Representation of the determination of latency and amplitude, **b** Missing potential complex P13–N23 with N34–P44 obtained

If the sacculus is still functional but already bulges towards the middle ear, significantly larger VEMP can be derived on the impaired side. This finding can be explained by the fact that the Endolymph hydrops, the endolymph membrane is pressed closer to the oval window, thus improving the transmission of sound pressure. The enlargement of the VEMP on the diseased side is therefore to be interpreted as an expression of an endolymph hydrops (Hamann and Haarfeldt 2006).

With increasing loss of function, it is also no longer possible to derive potentials.

Thus, the VEMPs can be evaluated so far rather in the course and sometimes show strong, not always evaluable fluctuations. In advanced stages with permanent damage to the saccule, the potential amplitudes of the VEMP are absent or significantly reduced. The optimal frequency of 500 Hz for derivation of the VEMP may change depending on age and during the course of Ménière's disease. As in the semicircular-canals the sensory cells for the lower frequencies seem to become more restricted in otolith organs in the course of

Ménière's disease, probably due to pressure, so that the more derivable responses shift to the higher frequency range (750 Hz and 1000 Hz) (Sandhu et al. 2012). Because of this change in frequency dynamics, it is useful to consider multiple frequency ranges in VEMP diagnostics. In principle, this is possible using a VEMP multi-frequency analysis with several alternating stimulus frequencies (Walther and Cebulla 2015).

6.5.2 Examination of the Utricle

▪ **Head tilting**

If the head is tilted from the upright position to the side (lateral tilt), a rolling movement of the eyes to the opposite side occurs in healthy individuals. Diamond and Markham (1983) were able to show that this does not occur symmetrically in patients with damage to a vestibular organ, which indicates a functional disorder of the utricle on the affected side.

▪ **Measurement of the subjective visual vertical (SVV)**

This observation without further aids can be supplemented by an objectifiable examination. For this purpose, the patient should bring a visible, line from a position deviating from the vertical to the position that subjectively appears vertical. In the meantime, this can be done with an additional function of the video-oculo-graphy.

Healthy persons can adjust the SVV with a precision of 0 +/– 2.5°. After the unilateral impairment of a vestibular organ, a misjudgment to the affected side of up to 20° can be found, but this returns to normal after weeks.

In the meantime, a much simpler experimental setup is clinically sufficient. So, a self-made translucent "bucket" with a solder attached to the end can provide useful results.

▪ **"Turning "during the caloric test**

For the investigation of the utricle, which registers the horizontal directions (to the left and the right) during upright gait, one can take advantage of the fact that the evolutionarily old utricle determines the reaction of the semicircular ducts, which were added later - evolutionarily - and thus also the direction of nystagmus.

▪ **Nystagmus direction turns**

Westhofen established an experimental set-up in which the patient is turned from the elevated supine position onto the abdomen in a head hanging position at the time of maximum nystagmus movement during cold-warm irrigation. In healthy subjects, the direction of nystagmus changes after the turn (Düwel et al. 2005).

If this change in direction of the eye movements does not occur, Westhofen concludes that there is damage to the utricle, but "only" in the sense that there is a functional restriction or not. One cannot draw any conclusions as to how great the damage is.

In the practical procedure, the patient is first subjected to a warm rinse at 44 °C, as in the normal caloric test.

▪ From the back to the belly

In the second step, instead of the usual 30 °C, a colder stimulus of 20 °C is used. The aim of this is to make the maximum eye tremor movements easier to detect. In addition, after the maximum eye movements have been reached, the patient is moved from the supine to the prone position. The slight bending of the head "forward" towards the abdomen of 30° is maintained (◘ Fig. 6.7b). This results in a 180° change in the position of the horizontal semicircular canal relative to the earth's gravitational pull.

In order to be able to reposition the patient safely, a lounger with a movable head section that can be lowered is desirable. Reversal of nystagmus direction occurs with a short delay after repositioning (◘ Fig. 6.7c).

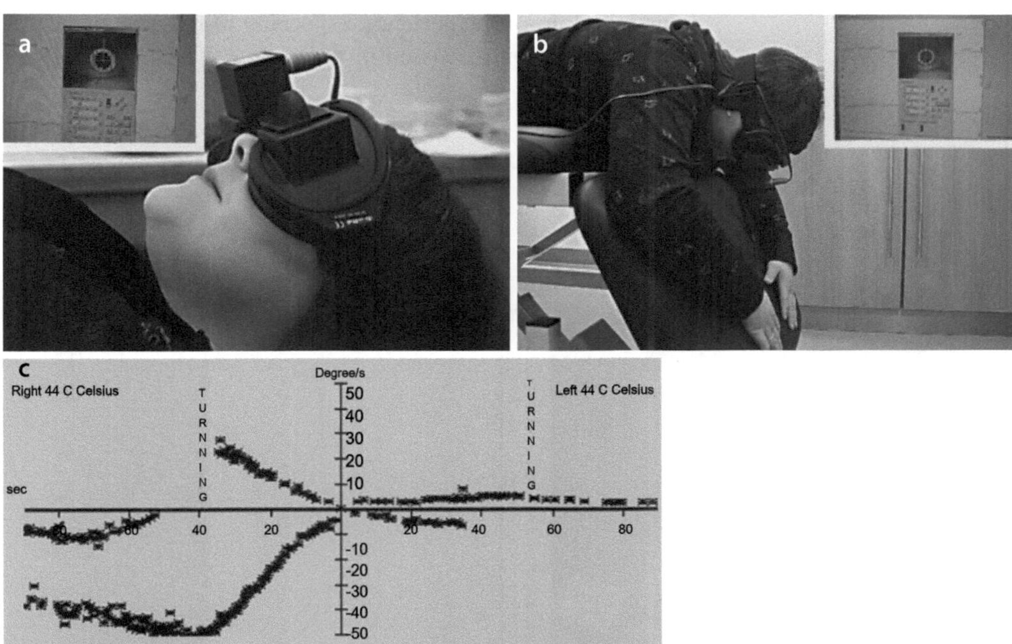

◘ **Fig. 6.7** Thermal test. **a** In the elevated head position (pronation), **b** reversed in the prone position (supination) **c** Evaluation: The velocities of the slow nystagmus phases are plotted, with the time axis starting in the middle in each case and continuing outward. After reaching the culmination phase during cold irrigation (arrow), the patient is brought from the prone to the supine position. (From: Walther 2007)

> Vestibular evoked myogenic potentials (VEMP) - derived from the eye muscles (o-VEMP)

▪ Side separated utricle information

In a similar examination setup to the examination of the sacculus, side-separated information can be obtained about the utricle. Again, low-pitched tones, as "clicks", are offered via headphones. These minimally influence the tense lower eye muscles of the opposite side via a reflex arc. The eyes should look upwards with the strain (◘ Fig. 6.8).

However, this small change can be measured with a special device suitable for this purpose, as with an ECG. The "n10 component" is measured after approximately 10.5 ms and the "p15 component" after approximately 16.5 ms on the right. Then the size of wave II is compared with that of the opposite side.

With the o-VEMPs, it is possible to assess laterally separated functions of the utricle. However, since the saccule also sends a small part of its nerve impulses via the same nerve part as the utricle, it is still unclear to what extent changes in the saccule also have an effect (Walther et al. 2010).

As with the c-VEMPs (see above), the absolute VEMP amplitudes vary greatly during the course of Ménière's disease. However, the o-VEMPS are *an* important clue in the course and, in our experience, especially in the case of gentamicin elimination discussed in ► Chap. 7. Thus, especially in

a b

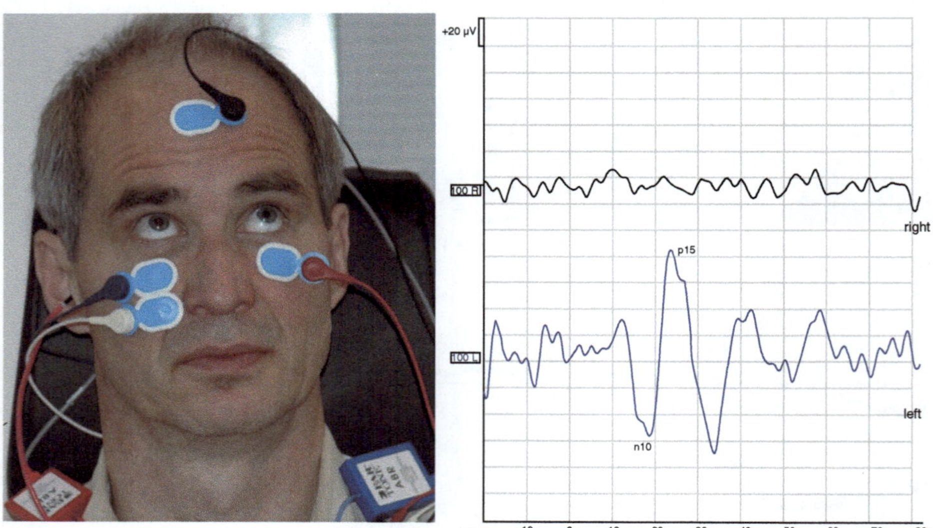

◘ **Fig. 6.8** Ocularly derived vestibular evoked potentials (o-VEMPs), **a** derived from the inferior eye muscles during upward gaze. **b** The left side shows a normal potential pattern with responses after approximately 10 ms (n 10) and 15 ms (p15), while in comparison - for the right side, which was switched off with gentamycin - no potentials can be derived

the case of Tumarkin drops (► Chap. 4), it may also be a question, beyond the clinical evaluation, whether the elimination could already be sufficient.

▪ Dynamic subjective vertical (SVV)

If one wants to know more about the function of the otolith organs, the patients - fixed on a rotating chair - have to be rotated in different directions of the room like on a centrifuge with constant speed. The reactions of the eye movements are again derived.

For a side-separated examination of the utricle, the seat is shifted by about 3.5 cm during the rotation around the horizontal axis at a rotational speed of, for example, 300°/s, so that one labyrinth at a time lies exactly in the axis of rotation. This ensures that only the "outer" labyrinth is stimulated (unilateral centrifugation), which corresponds to a tilting of the vector by 11°. In a healthy person, a tilt sensation is triggered towards the irritated, that is, the outer side.

This tilting, perceived by the patient, must now be made visible to the examiner, which is possible with the aid of a "subjective vertical". The angle between the body axis and the line of light serves as the measured variable. In healthy persons, this angle corresponds approximately to the real tilt angle up to about 30° (Helling 2008).

Determination of SVV and video documentation of eye counter roll using videoculography allows quantitative and nearly unilateral functional testing of the utricle during this minimally eccentric rotation (Clarke et al. 2001).

▪ Eccentric rotation

However, the equipment required for this "eccentric rotation" in the swivel chair is currently only available in very few centers.

> In the end, all findings must be evaluated together and coherently in relation to each other - also considering the partially limited statements and in respect of the preliminary state of our knowledge. No finding alone represents a diagnosis and probably no computer program, no matter how differentiated, can replace the clinical decision that is necessary in the end.

▪ Posturography

Useful for documentation.

Posture and postural changes can be documented and recorded with posturography (recording of posture). The basic concept is the measurement of foot pressure while standing upright on

Table 6.1 Dynamic aspects of vestibular function tests

Caloric test	Rotatory test and eye movement examination, VEMPs	head-shaking	Head Impulse Test	Vibration
0.003 Hz	0.5–1 Hz	2 Hz	5–7 Hz	10–150 Hz

a plate specially designed for this purpose, which involves the construction of several scales. Body fluctuations are recorded in an optically reproducible manner: A deviation reaction or a tendency to fall to the disturbed side can then be seen.

First, the patient stands with open eyes on a firm plate, then with closed eyes on a soft surface. The degrees of difficulty can be extended and varied in many ways.

Disturbances in the interaction between the proprioceptors, the eyes and the vestibular organ as well as the muscular responses to deviations can be detected. It is problematic that many factors play a role, including the form of the day. Thus, ultimately, only clues can be obtained. However, posturography is suitable for recording part of the course of balance therapy and thus making the success visible.

Inexpensive for documentation

Table 6.1 shows the dynamic aspects of vestibular function tests.

6.6 Hearing Tests

6.6.1 Pure Tone Audiogram

Air duct

Hearing tests are necessary - at the latest - if the dizziness is accompanied by hearing changes or aural fullness. In Ménière's disease, there is typically a flat, but a mostly trough-shaped hearing loss in the low-frequency range and, to varying degrees, also in the mid-frequency range.

During the hearing test, 7–10 frequencies that are important for the human hearing are given to the patient via headphones. The sound reaches to inner ear (cochlea) through the air into the outer ear and the middle ear. In technical jargon, this part of the hearing test is called the "air conduction".

▪ Zero line as the mean value

The baseline volume corresponds to the average hearing ability of healthy adolescents and is referred to as the "zero line". The zero line is therefore not an absolute zero or even silence, but an average value. Consequently, there are "minus values" if the patients hear even better at certain frequencies than adolescents.

Starting from this, the volume of each frequency is successively increased in steps (by 5 dB each) until the sound is heard. This is recorded in a pure tone audiogram.

In ◘ Fig. 6.8a, the transverse row shows the individual frequencies with the designation Hertz (Hz): on the left are the low tones (125–2000 Hz), in the middle tones (2000–4000 Hz) and on the right the high tones (4000–8000 Hz). The vertical row indicates the individual volumes expressed in decibels (dB). The scale ranges from –10 to +100 dB (◘ Fig. 6.9).

> In a healthy ear, the curve lies between 10 dB and 20 dB depending on age; in a damaged ear, the curve deviates significantly downwards. An important reference point is the 60-dB line. This is the volume at which people normally speak to each other at a distance of 1 m.

▪ Bone conduction

In the next test patients have to hold a sound-emitting tone button against the bone behind the ear, the mastoid. The sound does not reach the inner ear through the air, but through the skull bone. This bypasses the outer and middle ear.

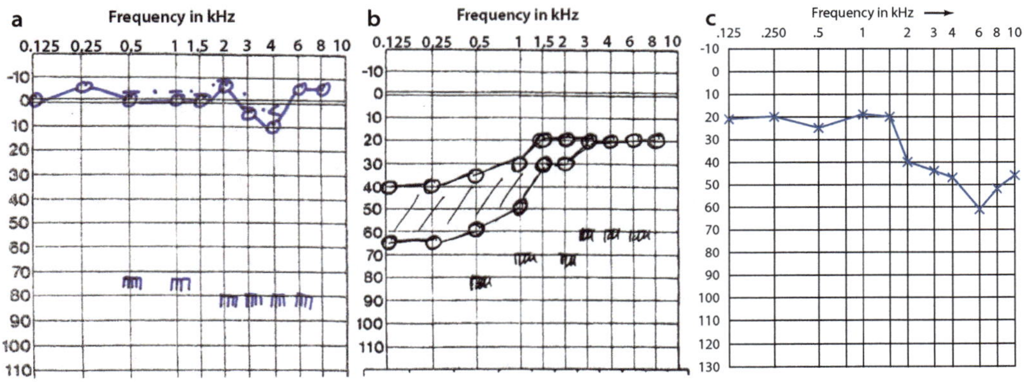

◘ **Fig. 6.9** Pure tone audiometry: **a** "Normal" hearing as in an adolescent, **b** Low frequency hearing loss as in Meniere's diseases, **c** High frequency hearing loss as after noise exposure

Otherwise, the procedure is the same as for the hearing test via the headphones and "the air". The "bone conduction" achieved in this way is also recorded in the audiogram.

The values are calibrated in such a way that the results of the air and bone measurements are almost identical.

It is possible with the help of the joint evaluation of "air" and "bone" conduction, to determine

- Severity,
- Art,
- Place and
- Possible cause of hearing impairment

Obstructions in the middle ear

This makes it possible to distinguish whether the sound was able to reach the inner ear unhindered at all. If there are problems in the outer ear (earplug) and/or in the middle ear, for example, in the case of otosclerosis (ossicular calcification), there is a sound conduction disorder. This means that the sound cannot be conducted well into the inner ear. In this case you can see that better results achieved over the bone threshold than over the air threshold. The reason for this is that the obstacle in the middle and outer ear was bypassed by going over the bone.

However, if the sound has reached the inner ear unhindered, but could not be received and transmitted properly, a so-called sound perception disorder is present. In this case, the inner ear is affected, typically in the case of noise damage or hearing loss.

In Ménière's disease (◘ Fig. 6.8b), the hearing test reveals a usually trough-shaped hearing loss in the low-frequency range and - to varying degrees - also in the mid-frequency range. In chronic cases, the hearing loss may also extend to the high-frequency range.

Ménière's patients may have a sound conduction component - an "air-bone gap" - especially in the low frequency range - without an obstruction in the middle ear being the cause. This probably occurs in about 14–30% of Meniere's patients (Lee et al. 2014). Lee et al. 2014 attributes this phenomenon to the effects of endolymphatic hydrops on sound transmission.

Discomfort threshold

With each hearing test, it is also checked at what point sounds are no longer tolerable well. For this purpose, at each test frequency, the sound is slowly increased until the patient - according to his or her perception - says: Stop, from now on it becomes uncomfortable. This is documented in the audiogram as the discomfort threshold for each frequency.

■ **Internal practice standard necessary**
To determine the discomfort threshold, we ask patients to press the button (stop button) when the sound is perceived as just too loud or uncomfortable. Care should be taken to maintain a consistent standard within the practice that provides a means of comparison over time.

6.6.2 Speech Audiogram

The hearing test with simple tones is an important basis. However, hearing and understanding speech are crucial for our ability to listen. If the pure tone audiogram shows that there is a significant hearing loss for tones, this is followed by a test of speech comprehension.

■ **Word and number sequences**
In the speech audiogram - via the headphones - first individual words and then number are played. One begins with a volume that is adapted to the results from the air and bone conduction and increases this from test series to test series. Then standardized fixed series of monosyllabic words are played through the headphones. The percentage of numbers or words understood at the different volumes is counted.
This examination is essential in determining whether a hearing aid can improve the hearing situation.

6.7 Tinnitus Determination

To determine the tinnitus, we ask the patient to pick out a tone that corresponds to his tinnitus or comes as close as possible. This is usually easier in higher tone in frequencies between 4000 and 8000 Hz. In Ménière's patients, the low-frequency sound is often perceived as rather roaring, so that a sound mixture may also have to be offered.

Once the patient has decided on a tone, the tone is raised louder and louder in 5 dB steps until the patient can indicate that the tone appears louder than the tinnitus from the outside. This is noticed as tinnitus concealability.

▪ Tinnitus loudness between 5 and 15 dB

The tinnitus loudness is calculated from the tinnitus concealability minus the hearing loss at this point. The result is usually a tinnitus loudness between 5 and 15 dB above the hearing threshold, even in Ménière's patients.

6.8 Otoacoustic Emission and Distortion Products

▪ Sound waves from the ear

As described in ► Chap. 2, we distinguish between inner and outer hair cells in the inner ear. The outer hair cells move permanently. These movements can themselves generate sound waves and thus tones. These very quiet sounds from the inner ear can be measured and evaluated with the aid of the finest microphones and the increasingly extensive use of computer technology.

However, the outer hair cells can also be sonicated in a very differentiated way and their reactions can be measured. In order to be able to measure these minute effects, one needs excellent technology, a highly complex computer program and specialists. Under these conditions, we learn a lot about the functional state and the reactivity of the outer hair cells in the cochlea.

The method reaches its limit when the hearing loss exceeds 40 dB, which is often the case with Ménière's disease in the low-frequency range.

6.9 Electrocochleography

▪ Typical changes in endolymphatic congestion

Hints of endolymphatic congestion - in the auditory (!) part - can be obtained by electrocochleography (ECochG). In most cases, a fine needle electrode must be placed in the middle ear through the eardrum near the round window niche, a summation potential of the basilar membrane and a summation action potential of the auditory nerve can be distinguished. The ratio of negative summation potential (SP) in the inner ear to the action potential of the auditory nerve (CAP) provides a characteristic picture in endolymphatic hydrops.

This is shown by a relative increase of the SP amplitude compared to the CAP amplitude. It is assumed that the SP amplitude is increased by the hydrops because the elasticity of the basilar membrane is changed, and it is displaced basally towards the scala tympani. However, an increased SP-AP quotient also occurs in perilymph fistulas and dehiscence of the superior arcade (Plontke and Gürkov 2015).

Nevertheless, we "only" get statements about the proportion in the hearing duct.

6.10 Brain-Evoked-Response Audiometry (BERA)

- **Tumor exclusion**

In this "objective hearing test", the path of the auditory impulses is followed from the inner ear to the auditory center. For this purpose, defined sounds are played with headphones. The resulting brain waves are recorded at the head as in an EEG. In this way, it can be determined - without radiation exposure - whether there is an obstacle on the way from the inner ear to the brain. This could be a tumor, which is fortunately very rarely the cause of hearing disorders. Nevertheless, this possibility must be ruled out. Therefore, this procedure is often used.

However, for hearing loss above 50 dB, it loses its significance. Then other methods, such as the computer tomogram, must be used.

6.11 Glycerol Load Test (Klockhoff Test)

Hints for an endolymphatic event in the auditory area (!) can bring the glycerol load test. For this test, patients must drink a well-filled glass of very sweet liquid. Quickly absorbed through the gastric mucosa, the concentration of the ingredients in the blood increases. In order to dilute them again, fluid - also from the endolymph tubes in the ear - is drawn out of the body.

This means that an endolymphatic hydrops - if present - becomes smaller and the hearing test better. The result is considered positive (in the sense of confirming the diagnosis) if an increase of at least 10–15 dB is detectable in three adjacent frequencies in the pure tone audiogram. Although only (!) 70%

of all Ménière's patients show a positive result, if it occurs, this is an almost certain indication of an endolymphatic event – in the hearing duct!

- **Strain on taste and circulation**

This test is very unpleasant. The same effect can also be achieved in a less stressful way with diuretics. Thus, in view of significantly improved diagnostic possibilities, the formerly useful tool belongs in my opinion in the museum, especially since also here no distinction can be made between Menière disease and endolymphatic congestion only in the hearing part.

6.12 Manual Examination of the Vertebral Segments

Manual therapists examine the function and mobility in each vertebral segment. Considering the biomechanical possibilities, the range of motion and the quality of movement of the individual sections are then assessed. The findings determined on this basis, for example, whether a joint has excessive or limited mobility, are assigned to the disorders and pain reported by the patients. After comprehensive safety tests for the cervical spine, manual therapists try to contribute to a balanced function of the individual vertebral joints by stretching and lengthening (Hülse et al. 2005).

- **Neck stiffness and tension**

In Ménière's disease, some neck stiffnesses and tensions can also be found, which, however, have mostly developed reactively in the course of the disease. These can benefit from good manual therapy and break the cycle of tension, pain and more tension. They have no influence on the inner ear-related vertigo intensity.

6.13 Imaging Techniques

A significant advance in the diagnosis of Ménière's disease is the visualization of endolymphatic hydrops with MRI (magnetic resonance imaging), even though this examination cannot be used as a standard procedure in suspected Ménière's disease for reasons capacity and cost.

For this purpose, the contrast agent gadolinium is administered either into the vein or into the tympanic cavity. The advantage of the intratympanic application is the relatively rapid accumulation of the contrast agent in the inner ear. In the MRI a semi-quantitative "three-dimensional" image can be created.

Hydrops - as it also occurs in Ménière's disease - is indirectly detectable in MRI if the contrast agent gadolinium accumulates in the perilymphatic space but not in the endolymphatic space of the inner ear. In the meantime, changes in size can certainly be detected, and one can get a - calculated - three-dimensional impression. It is also possible to follow the course of the disease on the basis of the development of the hydrops (Gürkov et al. 2012, 2015).

Gürkov et al. (2016) suggest that an increase in endolymph volume of 33% to 50% indicates "mild" endolymphatic congestion.

If the endolymph volume expands to more than 50% of normal, they assume a significant endolymphatic congestion (hydrops).

Nevertheless, even this procedure cannot provide definitive certainty for the diagnosis of Meniere's disease.

Endolymph hydrops in the saccule is also found on imaging in 10% of healthy individuals and in 40% of patients with significant hearing loss without vertigo (Attye et al. 2018).

In addition, endolymph hydrops can also be detected in other vertigo syndromes such as vestibular migraine (Gürkov et al. 2015).

■ It is not the outer form that is decisive

Above all, it must not be forgotten that it is the external shape that is calculated in these examinations. However, the actual damage is usually not in the external form, but at the cellular level.

Either way, therapy is based on the clinical picture, not the image calculated from an MRI.

"Daring" - and from my point of view not very helpful for the patient - is the idea that one can make a prediction for the course of a possible disease from the detection of endolymphatic congestion.

6.14 Psychological-Psychosomatic Diagnostics

■ Psychological assessment of medical history

A psychological and psychosomatic diagnosis first of all consists of listening and asking questions, which, despite all openness, is quite structured. In the foreground is the question of what constitutes, has produced, maintains or intensifies the illness. Thus, psychotherapists and psychosomatics - with the patients (!) - look beyond the organic findings for the consequences and the meanings of the illness for the respective individual and unique person. The therapist:

- ask to describe their suffering with their words and their feelings;
- ask what impact this has on them and their environment;
- want to know for what specific goals they want his help;
- point out that they probably cannot deal with Meniere disease as such, but the suffering from it;
- ask about the factors that could have caused the suffering from Ménière's disease, with different weighting;
- ask about influences that perpetuate the suffering from Ménière's disease;
- ask about the personal perception of the disease and its course.

Dizziness as a diagnostic tool

If the therapist then experiences dizziness himself, this may be due to the intuitive grasp of the situation with his patient (countertransference feeling). Consequently, this is an additional diagnostic criterion. It is also possible that the therapist is unsure whether he can work safely with the patient.

On the relational level, dizziness can also be perceived as an appeal to enable the patient to hold on. Thus, the therapist also needs a clear, secure, firm idea of what is coming. Otherwise, he is in danger of becoming dizzy with the patient himself. Then the patient as well as the therapist can and must decide whether they are suited to each other for coping with the dizziness.

Visual analogue scale

The intensity of the dizziness can be assessed, for example, using a scale between 0 and 100. The intensity scale ranges from 0 = no dizziness to 10 = mild dizziness to 100 = most severe dizziness.

Recording the evaluation and consequences

I ask the persons to check whether the symptomatology occurs more frequently in dependence on certain situations, and ask them to write down:

- What are the immediate consequences of your vertigo or dizziness?
- What do you do during vertigo?
- What do you avoid avoiding dizziness?
- What is the "cost" of avoidance?
- How does the environment react to your vertigo?
- Is that helpful?

Diary

I ask patients to record the frequency of occurrence, duration over time, and varying intensity of their balance situation, for example, on a full-page printout as in ◘ Table 6.2.

Until the final diagnosis is made and, if necessary, also for recording the course and success of therapy, a diary for recording frequency and duration can be helpful. The disadvantage of the diary is sometimes that it can increase the attention for vertigo sensations that were otherwise not perceived as pathological.

Diary rubrics are:

Has there been any triggers? For example, head movement, change of head position, standing up, special situation (e.g. shopping, narrow spaces), over-exertion, rest...

◘ Table 6.2 Diary

Date/Day	Time	Duration in minutes	Character of the dizziness/vertigo (in your own words)	Perceived strength (0–100)	Perceived triggers	Accompanying circumstances	What happened after that?	Other

- *Have you experienced any other symptoms?* For example, headache, hearing or visual disturbance, nausea/vomiting, sensitivity to light or sound, flickering before the eyes, unsteadiness in standing or walking, rapid heartbeat, shortness of breath, sweating, anxiety.
- *Have any therapies been given?* For example, positioning maneuvers, analgesics, anti-nausea medication, blood pressure or blood sugar levels.

6.15 Psychological Questionnaires/Test Diagnostics

Psychological questionnaires and tests cannot replace the taking of the medical history and in particular the differentiation between organically triggered vertigo and reactive psychogenic dizziness. However, they can give an initial hint of the extent of psychological impairment. Prerequisites for this are that

- they fit to the symptom,
- the examiner has a clear idea of what he wants to know and does not treat the result as just another laboratory value and check it off,
- the patient is able and willing to cooperate.

Then psychological questionnaires make it possible to record the usually significant psychological component (above all anxiety disorders, depression and somatization disorders) of vertigo in about 2/3 of patients suffering from vertigo for a long time.

6.15.1 Dizziness Handicap Inventory (DHI)

The DHI is a questionnaire for the assessment of "self-perceived incapacity" related to dizziness.

The questionnaire combines questions aimed at organic causes of dizziness such as circulatory problems and positional vertigo with questions about psychological effects and anxious or depressive feelings.

Examples:

- Do you have difficulty reading because of your problems?
- Do your problems increase with more demanding activities, for example, sports, dancing or household chores?
- Are you afraid to leave the house because of your problems?

- **Perceived dizziness**

The DHI contains a total of 25 questions, 7 of which are about the physical limitation of performance due to the perceived dizziness symptoms, another 9 questions about associated functional limitations, and finally 9 questions about emotional involvement. The total score is between 0 and 100.

6.15.2 Hospitality Anxiety and Depression Score (HADS)

- **Anxious and depressive symptoms**

The Hospitality Anxiety and Depression Score, HADS, is a short and well-accepted self-report measure with seven alternating anxiety and seven alternating depression items. It measures the severity of anxious and depressive symptoms during the previous week (Herrmann and Buss 1994).

Examples:

- I feel tense or overstimulated: most of the time - often - from time to time - not at all
- I feel slowed down in my activities: almost always - very often - sometimes - not at all

The assessment is made by forming sum scores of the subscales. The two scales comprise the following dimensions (for orientation purposes, values greater than or equal to eleven per subscale are considered conspicuous).

6.15.3 Patient Health Questionnaire (PHQ-D)

The Health Questionnaire for Patients by Löwe et al. (2002) measures anxiety, somatoform and depressive disorders. Using scale sum values, severity levels can be formed, for example, for the areas of depressiveness and anxiety.

For depression assessment, the PHQ-D can provide directional insights with just two questions. It asks:

- How have you felt affected by the loss of interest and pleasure over the last two weeks?
- How often have you felt affected by dejection, melancholy, or hopelessness?

The possible answers are
- "not at all" (0 points)
- "on some days" (1 point)
- "on more than half of the days" (2 points)
- "almost every day" (3 points)

The scores for both questions are added together, resulting in scores from 0 to 6. A score of 3 or more is likely to indicate significant depression.

The assessment of anxiety disorders can - as an orientation - also be carried out based on two questions:
- During the last two weeks, how often did you feel affected by the following complaints:
  - Nervousness, anxiety or tension?
  - Not being able to stop or control worry?

The answer choices are:
- "not at all"
- "on some days"
- "more than half the days"
- "almost every day"

Again, the numerical values from 0 to 3 are assigned accordingly. With a value of 3 or more, a debilitating anxiety disorder is likely.

6.15.4 University Research

Interdisciplinary diagnostics

Psychosomatic-psychometric diagnostics ideally and for scientific investigation necessarily consist of clinical diagnostics, for example, according to operationalized psychodynamic diagnostics (OPD II), structured diagnostics (SKID I) according to ICD-10 and - depending on the underlying disease - the application of various psychometric instruments. This includes anamnesis as well as family and couple diagnostics. In the case of very complex and chronic diseases, it is advisable to start with a diagnostic admission to an appropriately specialized clinic that can perform differentiated interdisciplinary diagnostics (Eckhardt-Henn, Tschan, Best and Dieterich 2009).

As screening questionnaires Eckhardt-Henn, Tschan, Best and Dieterich (2009) recommend the use of the symptom checklist SCL 90, the HADS, the AVK (questionnaire on body-related fears, cognitions and avoidance) and as specific questionnaires on vertigo the VHS (Vertigo Handicap Scale) as well as the VSS (Vertigo Symptom Scale).

Conclusion

Questionnaires alone are not enough. In the end, the problem remains, which cannot be solved by questionnaires alone, that Ménière's disease cannot be detected by audiometric and neurotological examinations alone. Information on the frequency and length of attack can often only be determined with uncertainty, since keeping a "dizziness diary", for example, is only rarely recommended and is probably even more rarely adhered to. The determination of the individual disposition and psychological impairment is even less precise. In this case, the decision on therapy should be determined by the patient's level of suffering. Here, a symptom- and disease-specific questionnaire could help to make a therapy decision on an expanded basis, if the results are understood and not just filed away like another laboratory value.

6.16 The Most Important Thing at the End: Evaluating and Assigning

In the end, all findings - the organic and the psychological - must be evaluated and discussed together and put coherently in relation to each other.

No finding alone constitutes a diagnosis

Even though we have more and more detailed knowledge, the details only make sense in connection with the other components of the balance system. Probably no computer program, no matter how differentiated, can replace the clinical decision that is necessary in the end.

In Ménière's disease, the puzzle of hearing and balance findings changes in the course of the disease. If one adds the balance findings to the staging presented by Jahnke (1994) (▶ Chap. 3), which was primarily based on the severity of the hearing loss, the following constellations will probably be found - in most cases (◘ Table 6.3).

Table 6.3 Stages of Ménière's disease with possible associated hearing and balance findings

Stages of Ménière's disease (according to Jahnke 1994)	Clinic	Hearing results	Balance Findings
Stage 1	Attack vertigo between 20 minutes and several hours Fluctuating hearing Low-frequency tinnitus	Hearing may completely normalize after an attack of vertigo	Caloric testing conspicuous, C-VEMPS possibly conspicuous, possibly shifted to higher frequencies. KIT incon-spicuous " O-VEMPs rather inconspicuous
Stage 2	Vertigo, dizziness and fluctuating hearing	Hearing still improves after an attack, but does not return to normal.	Caloric test conspicuous, C-VEMPS probably conspicuous KIT mostly inconspicuous O-VEMPs rather inconspicuous
Stage 3:	Significant hearing loss, still dizziness, but it is usually weaker and less frequent	No or hardly any fluctuation, hearing loss with increasing expansion to the mid- and high-frequency range	Caloric test conspicuous, C-VEMPS probably conspicuous KIT becomes conspicuous O-VEMPs conspicuous Swivel chair asymmetrical
Stage 4	"Burnt out" Ménière's disease Hardly any or no vertigo attacks, sometimes Tumarkin drops.	Moderate to severe hearing loss	Caloric test abnormal, C-VEMPS abnormal KIT impaired O-VEMPs conspicuous Swivel chair asymmetrical

Literature

Attye A, Eliezer M, Medici M (2018) In vivo imaging of saccular hydrops in humans reflects sensorineural hearing loss rather than Meniere‘s disease symptoms. Eur Radiol 28:2916–2922

Boenninghaus HG (1990) Hals-Nasen-Ohrenheilkunde. Springer, Berlin Heidelberg New York

Brandt T, Dieterich M, Strupp M (2012) Vertigo. Leitsymptom Schwindel. 2. Aufl. Steinkopff, Darmstadt

Bronstein A, Lempert T (2017) Dizziness. A practical approach to diagnosis and management. Cambridge University Press, Cambridge

Clarke AH, Schönfeld U, Hamann C, Scherer H (2001) Measuring unilateral otolith function via the otolith-ocular response and the subjective visual vertical. Acta Otolaryngol Suppl 545:457–464

Diamond SG, Markham CH (1983) Ocular counterrolling as an indicator of vestibular otolith function. Neurology 33:1460–1469

Düwel P, Walther LE, Sanders M, Ilgner J, Westhofen M (2005) Otolithenfunktionstests – Ein differenziertes, qualitätsgesichertes Screeningsystem. Laryngorhinootologie 84:653–659

Eckhardt-Henn A, Tschan R, Best C, Dieterich M (2009) Somatoforme Schwindelsyndrome. Nervenarzt 80:909–917

Gürkov R, Flatz W, Louza J, Strupp M, Ertl-Wagner B, Krause E (2012) In-vivo visualized endolymphatic hydrops and inner ear functions in patients with electrocochleographically confirmed Menière's disease. Otol Neurotol 33(6):1040–1045

Gürkov R, Berman A, Dietrich O (2015) MR volumetric assessment of endolymphatic hydrops. Eur Radiol 25:585–595

Gürkov R, Pyyko I, Zou J, Kentala E (2016) What is Menière's disease? A contemporary re-evaluation of endolymphatic hydrops. J Neurol 263(Suppl 1):71–81

Hamann KF, Haarfeld R (2006) Vestibulär evozierte myogene Potenziale. HNO 54:415–428

Helling K (2008) Otolithenfunktionsstörungen und Therapieoptionen HNO 56: 996–1002

Herrmann Ch, Buss U (1994) Vorstellung und Validierung einer deutschen Version der Hospital Anxiety and Depression Scale (HAD-Skala), ein Fragebogen zur Erfassung des psychischen Befindens bei Patienten mit körperlichen Beschwerden. Diagnostica 40:143–154

Hülse M, Neuhuber W, Wolff HD (Hrsg) (2005) Die obere Halswirbelsäule, Pathophysiologie und Klinik. Springer, Heidelberg

Jahnke K (1994) Stadiengerechte Therapie der Menièreschen Krankheit. Dtsch Arztebl 91:428–434

Lee HJ, Jeon JH, Park S, Kim BG, Lee WS, Kim SH (2014) Prevalence and clinical significance of spontaneous low-frequency airbone gaps in Meniere's disease. Otol Neurotol 35(3):489–494

Lopez-Escamez JA, Carey J, Chung WH, Goebel JA, Magnusson M, Mandalà M, Newman-Toker DE, Strupp M, Suzuki M, Trabalzini F, Bisdorff A (2015) Diagnostic criteria for Menière's disease. J Vestib Res 25(1):1–7. https://doi.org/10.3233/VES-150549

Löwe B, Spitzer RL, Zipfel S, Herzog W (2002) PHQ-D Gesundheitsbogen für Patienten. Manual Komplettversion und Kurzform, 2. Aufl. Pfizer, Karlsruhe

Patel M, Agarwal K, Arshad Q, Hariri M, Rea P, Seemungal BM, Golding JF, Harcourt, JP, Bronstein AM (2016) Intratympanic methylprednisolone versus gentamicin in patients with unilateral Ménière's disease: a randomised, double-blind, comparative eff ectiveness trial. Lancet 388:2753–2762

Plontke SK, Gürkov R (2015) Morbus Menière. Facharztwissen HNO LRO 94:530–554

Sandhu JS, Low RH, Rea PA, Saunders NC (2012) Altered frequency dynamics of cervical and ocular vestibular evoked myogenic potentials in patients with Ménière's disease. Otol Neurotol 33:444–449

Walther LE (2007) Diagnostik und Therapie vestibulärer Störungen. In: Biesinger E, Iro H (eds) Schwindel. HNO Praxis heute, vol 27. Springer, https://doi.org/10.1007/978-3-540-47448-7_6

Walther LE, Cebulla M (2015) Frequenzdynamische Analyse der Otolithenfunktion mittels vestibulär evozierter myogener Potenziale (VEMP). Laryngo-Rhino-Otol 94:153–155

Walther LE, Hörmann K, Pfaar O (2010) Die Ableitung zervikaler und okulärer vestibulär evozierter myogener Potentiale. Teil 1. HNO:1031–1045

Walther LE, Hörmann K, Blochin M, Blödow A (2012) Rezeptorfunktion der Bogengänge Teil 1: Anatomie, Physiologie, Diagnostik und Normalbefunde. HNO 60:75–88

Therapy of Ménière's Disease

How to Deal with the Disease?

Contents

7.1 Enlightenment and Counselling – 182
7.1.1 Attention: Interactions Between Patient and Doctor – The Doctor–Patient Relationship – 183

7.2 Acute Therapy – 187
7.2.1 Emergency Medical Assistance: First and Second Vertigo Attack – 187
7.2.2 Own Emergency Preparation – 189

7.3 Therapy Between Vertigo Attacks – 192
7.3.1 How Can Therapeutic Success Be Determined? – 192
7.3.2 Proven Therapies – 195
7.3.3 Non-proven Conservative Therapies – 213
7.3.4 Surgical Interventions – without Proven Effect – 221

7.4 Basic Outline of Psychosomatic Treatment – 226
7.4.1 Relaxation Techniques – 226
7.4.2 Psychotherapy – 227
7.4.3 Psychodynamic Psychotherapy – 228
7.4.4 Behavioral Therapy Approaches – 229
7.4.5 Systematic Desensitization – 229
7.4.6 Psychotropic Drugs – 238
7.4.7 Inpatient Psychosomatic Treatment – 240

7.5 Alternatives/Outsiders: Opportunities and Threats – 242
7.5.1 Homeopathy – 243
7.5.2 Acupuncture – 243

Literature – 244

H. Schaaf, *Ménière's Disease*, https://doi.org/10.1007/978-3-662-63610-7_7

▪ The Wise Men and the Elephant

Once upon a time, there were five wise but blind scholars. They were sent on a journey by their king to find out what an elephant was. So they set out on a journey to India. There they were led to an elephant. The five scholars stood in a circle around the animal and tried to get an idea of the elephant by feeling it.

The first sage had stood by the animal's head and palpated the elephant's trunk. Returning to their king, he reported, "An elephant certainly resembles a water pipe."

The second scholar had felt the elephant's ear and objected, "No, an elephant is rather like a large fan."

The third replied, "But no, an elephant is like a thick pillar." He had touched the elephant's leg.

The fourth sage said, "It is like this: an elephant is like a short rope with fringes at the end," for he had only felt the tail of the elephant.

The fifth sage reported to his king, "An elephant is like a kind of king's throne." That scholar had touched the back of the animal.

Each examines a different part of the body (but each only one part), such as the flank or a tusk. Then they compare their experiences with each other and find that each individual experience leads to its own completely different conclusion. It takes an overview to be able to put the individual aspects together into a more complete picture.

In the case of Ménière's disease, it can be difficult to keep an overview of the "labyrinth" of dizzying and hearing-restricting events, even if every expert – in his or her field and with his or her knowledge – certainly does his or her best. It makes a difference, who looks at whom in which course of the disease (acute or chronic). Also it makes a difference, if one looks primarily at the disease or the ill person. Likewise, the perspective is influenced from the fact, whether one is more conservatively or surgically oriented, or one is specialized in neurootology or neurology or in "psyche", or is more research-oriented. At least, not at last, it matters, if one is or was affected with Menière's disease himself or herself.

▪ Who can help in times of need?

In principle, Ménière's disease falls within the scope of the ENT specialist. The recognition of many possible differential diagnoses (▶ Chap. 5), especially migraine, is in the responsibility of neurologists. The first contact person and usually also the companion during the disease will usually be the general practitioner. Psychotherapists and psychosomatics are usually the last to see the person suffering from Ménière's disease if essential aspects in the maintenance of vertigo cannot coped.

- **Changing expertise**

Thus, the Ménière's patient may meet with different specialists at different stages of his disease, each of whom may be more or less familiar with the disease. It is a sign of competence on the part of the therapists to recognize and address their own gaps in this rare but highly complex clinical picture. This opens up the possibility of either becoming more competent – together with the patient – and/or referring the patient to the right authorities. Sometimes a coordinated team can be found in the few clinics that regularly work with Ménière's patients.

It is favorable,

- *when medical professionals:*
  - know about the course and the changeability of the clinical picture,
  - take into account the fact that a Ménière's patient does not always suffer from Ménière's vertigo, but may develop benign paroxysmal positional vertigo more than other people, often have a (reactive) psychogenic dizziness component or perhaps suffer from migraine;
  - perceive the psychological side, respect it and, if necessary, be able to set a professional course. What usually exceeds the possibilities of the general practitioner by far, are the time-intensive intermediate steps and a professional – psychotherapeutic – processing of the distress of the affected persons;
- *when psychotherapists:*
  - organically – at least roughly – know or be informed,
  - not interpret every dizziness and vertigo as psychogenic;
- *when patients themselves:*
  - despite dizziness and despair, have the motivation and the will to work on the changeable parts and to deal with the unchangeable parts.

- **Assistance possible**

Although there is no cure in the classical sense, medicine – despite all its limitations – has a lot to offer in the case of Ménière's disease and can lay the foundations for:

- Recognition (diagnosis) of the disease and the increasingly better differentiation from similar appearing diseases
- Enlightenment and counselling
- Effective attenuation of the acute vertigo attack
- Increasingly better technical compensation aids for hearing loss
- Reduction and elimination of the function of the vestibular organ, if the vertigo attacks become excessive.

Possibly – if not likely – it could be that expiring time has the largest (most significant) share of all the "conservative" measures.

Stahle described that after an average of 9 years, Ménière's disease seems to "burn out" in 75% of untreated and non-surgically treated (!) patients, that is, the vertigo attacks tend to get weaker or disappear completely (Stahle et al. in: Huang 1991), accompanied by a unilateral, serve hearing loss.

In the process the function of both parts labyrinth is (usually) damaged step by step – with its expression in vertigo attacks. This damage reduces subsequently the basis for further functioning. But it also ensures that the next attacks of vertigo – as a tendency – become weaker and occur less frequently. In the end, the loss of function is accompanied by freedom from attacks.

The passing of the organ can be dramatically exacerbated by Tumarkin drops (→ ► Chap. 4).

Accordingly, any therapeutic measure that is not aimed at reducing function (gentamicin administration, neurectomy) will show more "success" the later it is applied.

Perhaps everything that does not harm helps to get over the time better.

7.1 Enlightenment and Counselling

The course and management of the disease can be favorably influenced by a comprehensible explanation. Perhaps even more than with other diseases with physical and mental components, organic understanding – in the sense of understanding and knowledge – is necessary with Ménière's disease.

> Ménière's disease is not a diagnosis of death or destruction. It refers to a disease of the inner ear and not a disease of the central nervous system such as a "stroke".

Understanding reduces uncertainty

The better the disease can be understood and the uncertainty can be reduced, the more possibilities of dealing with the dizziness will become apparent. Then also the subsequent problems become smaller. This is especially true for the phenomena of reactive psychogenic dizziness and of the escalation of anxiety components.

The physician should meet the patient's need for knowledge and distress with as much understanding as possible. At the same time, it is important to explore what is still possible and also to point out the limits of what is feasible in order to avoid disappointment in the patient. On this basis, (comprehensible) explanations and instructions, including self-help guides, help to reduce the anxiety and anxiety behavior. (Yardley and Kirby 2006).

7.1.1 Attention: Interactions Between Patient and Doctor – The Doctor–Patient Relationship

▪ Reflections on a difficult balancing act

There are diseases where the relationship between doctor and patient is less complicated. This is the case when, even after a difficult diagnosis, therapy can be initiated that promises a cure or at least a lasting improvement. In the case of Ménière's disease – as described in detail in ▶ Chap. 5 – even the diagnosis can be difficult. If the organic (!) part of Ménière's disease appears to be confirmed, there still remains – to put it mildly – a greater degree of therapeutic uncertainty in the course of treatment.

Even the non-psychosomatically trained family doctor or ENT specialist can feel the often great distress and deep despair of the Ménière's sufferer. However, this "does not fall within his area of expertise".

At the same time, the – understandable – expectation of the person suffering from vertigo to get back the lost security from the doctor can trigger feelings of uncertainty and dizziness in the practitioner himself. This phenomenon is well known as "Countertransference of feelings" in psychotherapy. It is defined as redirection of a psychotherapist‘s feelings toward a client – or, more generally, as a therapist's emotional entanglement with a client.

As "sympathetic" as this may seem from the patient's point of view, it is nevertheless "unsettling" for the practitioner – and usually does not exactly bring about what the patient had wished in terms of support and security from the doctor.

Thus, in an encounter, there are always (at least) two actors. Between a patient and the doctor, many things are predetermined. In the case of Ménière's disease, two people meet in a hierarchical relationship that is characterized by distress and vertigo on the one hand and a (hoped-for) special competence on the other.

On the factual level, the patient seeks clarification, advice and the most effective therapy possible. The doctor offers the diagnostics – necessary from his point of view or available to him – and makes suggestions within the scope of his profession.

On the mostly unspoken emotional and expectation level (selection: please tick as appropriate) the patient
- hopes for,
- requests,
- expects,
- claims
- desperate,
- plaintively,
- demanding,

that the doctor
- heal him,
- allows him to control his balance and
- gives him back his diminished, lost security.

> A relationship between patient and doctor, which is dominated by vertigo, dizziness or swindle, often puts each other to a stress test.

It is already difficult for a doctor to endure not being able to be "healing". Together with an unbearable expectation of the patient, the physician *may be* tempted to give "something anyway", even if this "something" is not useful. This explains why the belief in betahistines is still passed on, even though they are – now proven (Adrion et al. 2016) – no more effective than placebo in Ménière's disease.

In yielding to this pressure (to the patient's risk), the doctor risks illusory security on thin ice, which can collapse with the next vertigo. Thus, in the disillusionment and the dizziness – perhaps now beyond measure – the reliability delegated to him also dwindles. Thus, disappointed hopes are also a serious side effect.

If, on the other hand, the doctor keeps his recommendations and measures closer to reality, this increases the truthfulness of his statement, but often disappoints expectations and hopes. This dilemma often leads to a true odyssey of the patient to right, truthful, less suitable or often even swindling experts.

On the other hand and at the same time, however, unpleasant wishes and reflexes can be triggered in the practitioner against the dizziness and insecurity brought to him. Thus, the practitioner can also understandably respond with:
- "With the dizziness (one) can't help you anymore either."
- "Go (but) somewhere else, to a specialist or a psychotherapist."
- "It's not organic (not Ménière's), it must be different vertigo altogether."
- "You must be fibbing."

This can serve the understandable self-protection but is unfavorable for the patient.

▪ **What might help in the patient-doctor relationship?**

Therapy literally means accompaniment. This also means that the encounter between patient and doctor (therapist) can be oriented towards repetition. It is not always necessary to do "something". Sometimes it is enough to find out what is possible and what is not.

It is advantageous for the patient -and the doctor, if the patient – as well as the dizziness allows – is prepared. Thus the patient should

- think about the questions that are important to him in advance and, if possible, write them down, so that he does not forget the most important ones at the end or only asks the most important ones at the end, when time is pressing or has run out,
- bring the available findings,
- keep a balance diary,
- list the previous medications,
- maybe even bring someone (partner, friend) with him and ask the doctor if they can be there,
- himself repeat what he understood and what could be the next step,
- ?

For the patient, too, it is favorable not to expect more from the doctor than he can achieve – even with the best will in the world. So it is good for both sides if the doctor can be freed from his – perhaps hoped for – role as healer and "away-maker".

It is beneficial for Ménière's patients when physicians

- understand and confirm and, if possible, the credibility of the complaints,
- know about the changeable course and the changeability of the clinical picture,
- can offer explanations understandable to the patient, both for the organic part and for the possible development of a psychogenic part,
- reconsider and act appropriately, if the quality of vertigo changes (e.g. in the case of an added positional vertigo and a (reactive) psychogenic dizziness component),
- encourage appropriate active balance activities (sports, exercises, etc.),
- avoid questionable or rather unsafe interventions,
- perceive and respect the psychological side and, if necessary, set a professional course,

- have the patient summarize what they understand, so that any information bias can be corrected,
- make appointments for follow-ups (rather than saying the patient may not come back until "with vertigo"),
- involve self-help groups.

In this context, it is supportive and appreciative, if not even decisive, if the patient can be seen as a person with an illness, despite all the uncertainties of the illness and time limitations. Then one can also hope for the power of words.

Thus, the feeling of being able to influence the experience and the course and, in the best case, to get the dizziness under control, depends both on the experience with the doctor or "the medicine", which is experienced as helpful or unhelpful, and on the patient's possibilities of coping.

In the first phase, the struggle (with oneself and others) for acceptance is as necessary as it is understandable that there is still further research into solutions and alternatives. The better the condition can be understood and the uncertainty reduced, the more options for dealing with vertigo become apparent. In the further course, it is often a matter of understanding the phenomena of reactive psychogenic dizziness and the possible extension of the anxiety component. Then the secondary problems also become smaller. ◘ Table 7.1 gives an overview of the stage-appropriate relationship management in Ménière's disease.

It is favorable for Ménière's patient if *he* can feel "in good hands" with his doctor and therapist. Then he can implement what is feasible because he does not expect the impossible, which can make his counterpart despair.

At the same time, a reference by the doctor to the fact that he has reached the limits of his own competence in certain questions can be just as truthful as it can build trust, especially if it can be combined with a reference to another competence center.

Prospectively, it is a question of help for self-help, which also includes the commitment of those affected in self-help groups. These can be the "Meniere's Society in England.

The following will demonstrate:

- what the therapy is like in an acute vertigo attack,
- which therapies are effective in reducing or eliminating vertigo events,
- which therapies are offered in addition,
- how a psychosomatically oriented, inpatient Ménière's therapy can look like.

Table 7.1 Stage-appropriate relationship management in Ménière's disease

Stage-specific treatment	Favorable for Ménière's patients	Rather unfavorable
At the time of diagnosis	Diagnosis on the most reliable basis possible, taking into account the differential diagnoses (especially migraine) and the use of special neurotological diagnostics	Make tentative diagnoses without sufficient certainty
In the beginning after diagnosis	Comprehensible enlightenment Reference to literature and self-help groups	"There's nothing *you* can do about it."
In the course of the disease	With all realism a piece of justified hope and above all appropriate accompaniment Trial with intratympanic cortisone	Predicting a fateful path to deafness and bilateral loss of balance
In case of widening of the hearing loss	Hearing aids, also to preserve directional hearing	Waiting "until stable hearing threshold"
If the fear component is extended	Enlightenment, the involvement of psychotherapeutic support, antidepressants	"Not my responsibility."
In case of extension of the vertigo component	Possibility of safe elimination (intratympanic gentamycin) Neurectomy of the vestibular nerve	Ineffective surgical interventions with repeatedly dashed hopes

7.2 Acute Therapy

7.2.1 Emergency Medical Assistance: First and Second Vertigo Attack

At the first Ménière's attack and in the case of very severe attacks, an emergency doctor is usually called. If the attack is recognized as such or if the patient can give decisive indications, it helps against vertigo if an antiemetic agent is slowly injected via access to the vein or given via an infusion, or is used as a suppository itself.

- **Antiemetics**

Dizziness is usually reduced by 100 – 150 mg of dimenhydrinate or 5–10 mg of diazepam. This may or may not be followed by hospitalization with bed rest.

Furthermore, ENT physicians will consider infusion therapy with different additives, mostly with cortisone over days, as long as the diagnosis of Ménière's disease is not certain. As a rule, 500 ml infusions with different additives, mostly with cortisone, are administered over several hours per day. Withdrawal from a stressful environment is just as useful as supportive medical education. Additional benefits are provided by relaxation techniques such as Jacobson's Progressive Muscle Relaxation, with detailed instructions usually provided on CD.

- **Cortisone**

Since inflammatory reactions at the endolymphatic sac have been discussed as a component of Ménière's disease (Rask-Andersen et al. 1991), cortisone has been used repeatedly in the treatment of Ménière's disease. According to the study by Patel et al. (2016), the earlier administration of cortisone into the middle ear will become more important (see also ► Sect. 7.3.2).

Plontke and Gürkov (2015) discuss in detail the possible mechanisms of action. They weigh up how possibly the production of the endolymphatic fluid could be influenced, whether via a "stabilization of the vascular barrier" or, for example, via an effect on the hormone vasopressin. Studies on cell cultures of human cells from the utricle taken during surgery on a neurinoma of the vestibular nerve show evidence that glucocorticoids may act via aquaporin 3 in regulating endolymph volume (Nevoux et al. 2015).

The hope is that this may also affect the function of the endolymphatic sac so that it could once again provide better resorption performance.

- **Cortisone for large hearing changes**

We give – if there are no other concerns, such as diabetes – 250 mg in the morning for 3 days. If success is achieved, we give Decortin as a tablet 16 mg in the morning for 1–2 weeks.

Symptomatically, we additionally recommend the implementation of a relaxation procedure (guided by CD) such as Progressive Muscle Relaxation according to Jakobsen.

- **Cortisone into the middle ear (intratympanic cortisone administration)**

In the meantime, it is increasingly being tested whether the administration of cortisone directly in front of the inner ear could have positive effects with regard to the frequency and severity of vertigo attacks. The advantage is that cortisone should not have any side effects outside the ear (Novoa et al. 2014).

In the Tinnitus Clinic Dr. Hesse, we give – in the case of – first-time – major hearing loss and in the case of an identified Ménière's disease after local anesthesia with 2% Xylocaine (15–20 minutes with Gelitta on the eardrum and then suction) Dexamethasone 4 mg (0.4 ml) / Hyaluronic acid (0.1 ml) = 0.5 ml or Fortecortin Inject 100 mg 0.4 ml / Hylo-COMOD 0.1 ml = 0.5 ml every second to the third day.

We carry out a maximum of 5 to 7 applications.

- **"Steal effect"**

Not useful and rather unfavorable are "blood liquefying" drugs.

In the past, "blood liquefying" agents, especially pentoxifylline, were added to the infusions and later as tablets. The "liquefaction" of the blood was intended to make it easier for the red blood cells, the erythrocytes, to wriggle through even the narrowest end sections of the blood vessels.

Low-molecular dextran or levulose, sorbitol, starch solutions (hydroxyethyl starch, HES) and other "blood substitutes" can indeed influence the flow properties (viscosity = viscosity) of the blood and achieve an increase in blood flow to the inner ear. It is a cause for concern that areas with a good blood supply are better supplied with blood than areas with a poor blood supply, so that – despite an overall increase in blood flow – there can be an undesirable distribution which puts the deficient areas at an even greater disadvantage. This is called the "steal effect".

In addition, approaches that promote blood circulation are not plausible in the case of known Ménière's disease.

Morgenstern (1994) summarizes:

> Even if an increase in blood flow was achieved, it is difficult to imagine an influence on the actual pathological substrate (the diseased structure), the endolymphatic hydrops.

Therefore, in the treatment of Ménière's disease, "circulatory agents" should be avoided as well as "hyperbaric oxygen therapy" in a hyperbaric chamber.

7.2.2 Own Emergency Preparation

If the Ménière's patients themselves know about the diagnosis and have already undergone one or the other acute treatment, it makes sense and is effective to prepare oneself for an attack – without an emergency doctor.

To do this, you will need the items listed below.

▪ Pre-care: suppositories and tablets against nausea

Take vestibular suppressants always with you

For precaution and your own sense of security take vestibular suppressants such as 2–3 *Vomex A* (dimenhydrinate, *diazepam* or *dimenhydrinate* as suppositories in your pocket.

The suppositories are safer in an emergency, when you are on your own because unlike tablets, they cannot be vomited. Although the effect is slower than with an injection into the vein, this is usually much faster than any emergency doctor can be called and come.

Also, make sure you have suitable packaging (e.g. a tin) so that the suppositories do not melt! It is also useful to have an ampoule of an antiemetic medication at home (prescribed by a doctor you trust!) so that a doctor who is called in has something to hand immediately. *Vomex A, for* example, is not a standard item in the emergency kit!

If diarrhea also occurs, talk to your doctor about lorazepam melting tablets that are dissolved over the tongue (Expidet form). The big problem, however, is that multiple doses of lorazepam can become addictive very quickly, so this drug should only be used to treat the vertigo attack!

The Ménière's patient should know that the vertigo attack is not stopped by the medication, but is dampened "centrally" – and in the process also the centers of alertness and attention.

I have had a good experience with the drug "dimenhydrinate" for central nausea, both as a patient and as a practitioner. For this pharmacologically a central reduction of the excitability of the equilibrium and the vomiting center has been described as the main effect. With diazepam and related drugs as well as neuroleptics, the antiemetic effect is only one, in this case, desirable side effect.

▪ What to look out for during pregnancy?

During pregnancy, of course, special caution is required, especially if a more frequent use. As a rule, the package inserts are of little help here. These always advise, as a precaution, to take the drug during pregnancy only after consulting a doctor, then the responsibility is shifted. In the German standard work on drug side effects and interactions published by Ammon, the following is found for the above drugs presented for emergency use: In the case of diphenhydramine, a degradation product of dimenhydrinate, "there is a suspicion of a connection between ingestion and damage such as cardiac malformations and mongolism" (Ammon 1991, p. 215).

"With regard to teratogenicity (teratogenic: producing malformations in the embryo), there is only speculations in the case of the benzodiazepines (such as diazepam). The possible teratogenic potency is too low to be statistically proven so far" (Ammon 1991, p. 215). With regard to diazepam, prospective studies would give no indications of teratogenicity. Nevertheless, it is recommended that diazepam should not be taken during the first 3 months of pregnancy.

■ No absolute security

Although single doses are certainly far less dangerous than continuous doses, there is no absolute safety for any drug. From what I have read, taking diazepam, which has now been on the market for a very long time and is not known to have any serious side-effects, seems to me to be the least dangerous for the control of Ménière's attacks.

■ Bag

It is a good idea to carry a bag with you in case vomiting occurs despite carrying medication with you.

■ Mobile phone – with video function

In order to leave as much room for movement as possible and still be able to request help, even when running in the woods, a mobile communication aid such as a mobile phone is recommended.

■ Record eye movements!

If the mobile phone also has the option of video recording, the eye movements during a seizure can be recorded – if necessary, by people nearby or by an accompanying person. This helps enormously to determine afterwards whether the seizure was organic or psychogenic.

See also detailed instructions under 6.1 – and be prepared!

If you do not want to be admitted to hospital – for example from home – and want to release the doctor from his responsibility, it is advisable to have a letter reads as follows:

Statement of the Ménière's sufferer

I suffer from Ménière's disease (right/left)/with hearing loss right/left. In an acute Ménière's attack with nystagmus, nausea, vomiting and possibly shock-like sweating, therapy with dimenhydrinate supp. and, if necessary, with dimenhydrinate i.v. is the treatment of the first choice. However, the administration of diazepam (5–10 mg i.v.) is also possible.

- I was given dimenhydrinate in ampoules to take home. In addition, I am known to have the following diseases, such as:
  - Heart failure
  - Angina pectoris
  - Pulmonary
  - ...

- (Please mark with a cross where applicable and delete where not applicable)

- If the diagnosis "Ménière's attack" (leading symptom nystagmus) seems clear and there are no signs of another illness requiring hospitalization (heart attack or stroke), I would like to and can be treated at home with, for example, dimenhydrinate in an infusion.

- Venous access can be removed by myself or by the family doctor. Thus, in the event of a Ménière's attack, I would also like to receive emergency medical care at home and I take responsibility for this.

7.3 Therapy Between Vertigo Attacks

7.3.1 How Can Therapeutic Success Be Determined?

When the first, second and perhaps third attacks are over and the hearing loss is possibly perceived as more limiting, the question arises as to what – in the case of a – confirmed – Ménière's disease can reduce the frequency and severity of the vertigo attacks, better prevent them and perhaps also bring back the hearing and possibly reduce the ringing in the ears.

In the area of tension between expectations of the expert and the desire to give the patient something that might even help, there is no lack of offers, that promise relief or even healing. But one can also do "bad business" with the desperation of people. In the case of Ménière's disease, there is a wide field and a large number of more or less sensible treatment proposals.

The following applies to most attempts at therapy for Ménière's disease: Relatively independent of what was done, according to the investigators, about two-thirds of the patients benefited. In the meantime, it can be said very clearly that this was due to two reasons:

- Thus, it is still difficult – even for many investigator groups – to clearly diagnose Ménière's disease. A clear distinction between inner ear-related and psychogenic vertigo attacks is unlikely to have been observed.

- On the other hand, the criteria for assessing success usually proved to be extremely fuzzy. Who wants to say whether the observed successes are related to the respective measure or fall into a symptom-free interval, or, if the vertigo is assessed, exclude that Ménière's disease has "burned out" in the meantime.

■ Feedback to practitioners important

All procedures show that patients often change practitioners when they are dissatisfied with the results. This is understandable, but without feedback, it makes it difficult to monitor the results of the treatment. Therefore, I would like to encourage everyone to tell the practitioners what the results of the procedure performed were. This can also be done in writing and at least increases the possibility of learning more. In spite of all the shortcomings, one has to respect the vast majority of those who do research on Ménière's disease and grant them that they work on symptomatology, that is rare and shows "natural changes" over many years. t. Their work – except for the drug studies – is hardly rewarded.

■ Success Criteria of the Committee on Hearing and Equilib rium

While five major professional societies agreed in 2015 to narrow down the diagnosis of Ménière's disease (► Sect. 7.1.1), the 1995 revised version of the American Committee on Hearing and Equilibrium still applies to the assessment of the course of therapy.

■ Success of therapy by controlling the rate of vertigo attacks

$$n = \frac{Average\ number\ of\ vertigo\ attacks\ per\ month, 24\ months\ after\ therapy}{Average\ number\ of\ vertigo\ attacks\ per\ month, 6\ months\ before\ therapy} \times 100$$

■ Disability

- Grade 1: No disability
- Grade 2: Minor disability (intermittent or persistent vertigo or dizziness that precludes employment in a hazardous job).
- Grade 3: Moderate disability (intermittent or persistent vertigo or dizziness requiring sedentary behavior).
- Grade 4: Severe disability (severe symptoms that make the person unable to work)

Most publications report success when grade 2 is reached. This is certainly often a considerable success compared to the previous situation. However, it is important to understand what is meant by the rather friendly term "low disability" or "moderate disability" before expectations become too high.

Unfortunately, it is to be assumed that the different vertigo experiences in their organic and psychogenic parts were "not always" kept apart.

Before all the time factor must be taken into account. The later an intervention – no matter which one – takes place in the course of Ménière's disease, the greater the chances that these measures will be accompanied by a reduction in vertigo attacks (frequency and intensity). This may even be statistically noticeable.

■ Very strict: success criteria of the Cochrane Collaboration

Improving the scientific basis

The Cochrane Collaboration is an international network of scientists guided by the principles of evidence-based medicine. The central aim of the Cochrane Collaboration is to improve the scientific basis for decisions in the health care system. This goal is achieved primarily through the production, updating and dissemination of systematic reviews for the evaluation of therapies. These are published online in the Cochrane Library database.

The Cochrane Collaboration only considers good and, above all, objectifiable and evaluable studies and assesses them with regard to effectiveness.

Studies are not included if there is reason to suspect that the patient selection, as well as the choice of methodology and the analysis itself, might not stand up to critical scrutiny or comparable studies.

Now, there is certainly no need for an evidence-based review of whether it is necessary to jump out of a plane with a parachute. However, the Cochrane Collaboration provides a pleasant counterpoint to the sometimes wave-like therapy fads and, not least, against the statements of opinion makers, often couched by "interested" providers.

For Ménière's disease, the Cochrane Collaboration has reviewed the following therapies: Intratympanic gentamicin, intratympanic cortisone, saccotomy, betahistine, diuretics and balance therapy.

7.3.2 Proven Therapies

■ Balance exercises

It is helpful – until proven otherwise – to carry out a graduated balance training. In order to "get back on track" from the state of vertigo, it makes sense to intensively promote and challenge the entire balance system. This should promote body awareness and training, especially of proprioceptors (mechanosensory neurons located within muscles, tendons, and joints) and the eyes, but also confidence in the further possible ability to balance.

The aim is to strengthen confidence in physical ability to function and to work on different triggers for vertigo. This is more likely to succeed under the guidance and in a group than alone.

■ Balance Diary

The main purpose of a balance diary is to record progress and development. The assignment as "balance diary" has – differently accentuated than the "dizziness calendar" – not the problem, but more the goal in mind. Thus, the balance diary is a good basis for one's own work and for monitoring progress. At the same time, it can be one (1) building block for psychotherapeutic support, which may become necessary.

Although the vestibular system usually recovers "on its own" after an acute Ménière's attack, functional losses of the affected organ occur after repeated attacks. Balance and movement training helps to repair the deficits in the vestibular network that are frequently observed in the course of Ménière's disease and – after any necessary surgery on the vestibular apparatus – to shorten the compensation period (Gottshall et al. 2005).

■ Offset by compensation

It is also important here to work with a positive basic attitude and a realistic assessment of the available possibilities. Thus, even larger failures can be compensated by a central compensation. In addition, the experience of one's own abilities helps against an otherwise expanding fear, which in turn restricts the balance behavior.

Smaller weaknesses may remain, for example, if one organ of equilibrium has completely failed. The functional restriction can be compensated for as far as possible via the opposite side, except for (then too fast) movements to the diseased side. Here, the handling of this particularity must and can be trained. This is now also explicitly recommended for Meniere's patients – during the vertigo-free period (Basura et al. 2020).

Possible fall prophylaxis

If additional problems are present, such as a sensitivity disorder under the feet (e.g. in the case of polyneuropathy), visual disorders or other neurological diseases (central vascular diseases, degenerative diseases), this complicates the success. Thus, if necessary, one must still work on prevention of falling.

The most significant factor in the lack of success is physical rest and avoidance of even the activities; that would be feasible with little problem. Reasons for this are often lack of clarification, lack of encouragement and fear. Unfavorable are often added calming medications, which are sometimes recommended *instead of* balance training.

Increase stability, increase self-confidence

Until proven otherwise, balance exercises – performed – help to increase stability, improve mobility and increase self-confidence. This also applies to reactive "psychogenic" dizziness! This could be evaluated – evidence-based in 27 studies evaluated by the Cochrane Collaboration with 1668 participants as "safe and effective for unilateral loss of balance" (Hillier and McDonnell 2011).

No significant difference was found between the methods. The most important thing is that it is done.

In the following, I would like to present the "classic" exercise sequence of Cawthorne and Friedmann (1969) and Cooksey (1946). Ultimately, most balance exercises are based on this.

Cawthorne Cooksey Exercises

In bed

- Eye movements – first slowly, then faster (at least 5 times):
  - Up and down
  - From left to right
  - Fix one finger and move the finger back and forth
- Head movements – first slowly, then faster, later with eyes closed:
  - Move the head forward and backward
  - Move the head from left to right

Sitting

- Eye movements – first slowly, then faster:
  - Up and down

  - From left to right
  - Fix one finger, and move the finger back and forth
- Head movements – first slowly, then faster, later with eyes closed:
  - Move the head forward and backward
  - Move the head from left to right
- Move shoulder up and down and circle
- Bring the whole body forward and pick up an object

Standing
- Eye movements first slowly, then faster:
  - Up and down
  - From left to right
  - Fix one finger, move the finger back and forth
- Head movements – first slowly, then faster, later with eyes closed:
  - Move the head forward and backward
  - Move the head from left to right
- Move shoulder up and down and circle
- Bring the whole body forward and pick up an object
- Raise from sitting to standing position with eyes open and closed
- Throwing a small ball from one hand to the other at eye level
- Throw a small ball under the knee from one hand to the other hand
- Come back from sitting to standing and turn around once, one after the other in one direction and then in the other direction.

With the group
- One person stands in a circle, throws the ball to a person and the person throws the ball back
- Walk through the room with eyes closed and open
- Walking up and down a slope or inclined plane with eyes open and closed
- Walking up and down a staircase with eyes open and closed
- Any game with walking and stopping movements such as bowling and all ball games.

▪ Feldenkrais Method

Learning of a special kind

The Feldenkrais Method is a special kind of learning because it reveals almost infinite possibilities of the body in movement. The idea that self-realization and happiness can be found through body experience and body awareness is one of the guiding principles of Moshé Feldenkrais, the founder of this body method. Showing what is physically possible through mental actions characterizes many of his exercises.

I came across Feldenkrais after treating my inner ear with gentamycin. What appealed to me was that neither gymnastic nor athletic performance was required. Instead, it's about small, gentle movements and certain attention to the small differences and quality in movement. This then sets in almost by itself.

In principle, the Feldenkrais exercises can be learned without an expert, so that I still practice regularly, at the latest when I feel stiff, clumsy and/or unsteady on my legs again.

▪ Tai Chi

Sensorimotor balance

We work in the clinic, in addition to individually tailored, special balance training, with Tai Chi Chuan exercises. These exercises are well suited in the group and also without a Far Eastern worldview to promote the conscious perception of body sensations and sensory stimuli as well as to regain or rediscover sensomotoric balance. The disadvantage is that they require guidance – at least in the beginning. This in turn can lead to the fact that one meets other people in the group who join in the practice and support the progress together.

From experience, people will participate more in any type of balance training with others.

▪ Neurofeedback procedures

Expansion through additional stimuli

Balance therapy has been significantly expanded through the use of neuro(bio)feedback techniques. In this process, the patient receives an additional stimulus while performing balance exercises, either in the form of an auditory signal, a (galvanic) stimulus on the tongue or via vibration. They signal deviations from the body's normal position to the patients so that they can perform a corrective movement (Basta and Ernst 2008).

This can be particularly useful for patients who – for example, in the case of bilateral loss of balance – show limitations in sensory perception and then receive more noticeable and thus usable feedback for them in this way.

▪ Hearing aids to support the hearing function

Hearing loss is an important component of Ménière's disease and can lead to social isolation. Although unilateral hearing loss can usually be compensated for roughly, it usually leads to loss of directional hearing, as directional hearing is only possible on both sides. It also leads to reduced perception, which can also affect thinking, since speech and thinking performance are largely coupled.

■ Diminishing Tinnitus

If tinnitus is present, the hearing impaired are more likely to notice it because the masking external sounds are missing. For this reason, a hearing aid can often work wonders for patients with tinnitus, not only in compensating for hearing loss but also in masking tinnitus (■ Fig. 7.1).

In Ménière's patients whose hearing loss has affected the speech area, hearing aid should be used.

■ Patient must be able to use the hearing aid

A prerequisite is that the patient can use a hearing aid.

A common objection to hearing aid fitting in Ménière's patients is the possibility that the hearing threshold may shift more often. This is one of the particularities to be considered, which requires a special effort of time, knowledge and cooperation from the patient, the doctor and the acoustician. Thus, the hearing aid may need to be readjusted from time to time and a new device may need to be fitted.

Various environment-adapted programs help to perceive speech, especially in noisy environments.

■ Hearing Training

Of course, it is necessary to adjust hearing aids in accordance with the fluctuating hearing threshold. Often, special hearing training is also necessary. Especially the constant fluctuations

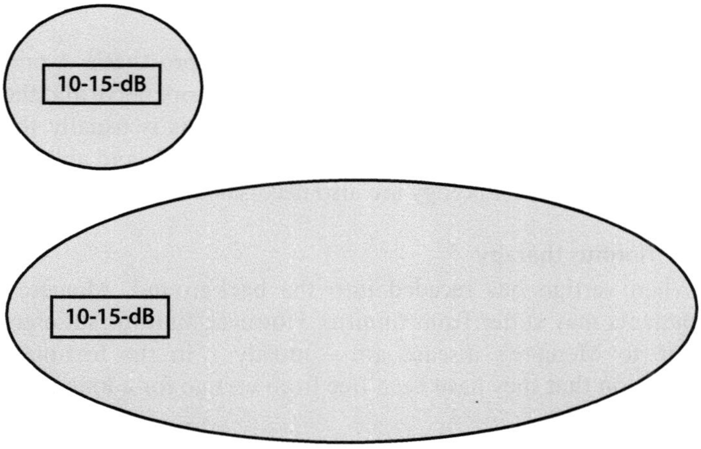

■ **Fig. 7.1** **a** The tinnitus, which is usually determined 10–15 dB above the hearing threshold even in Ménière's patients, accounts for up to 90% of the hearing reality in the affected ear in the case of hearing loss, **b** a hearing aid can help to reduce the tinnitus, to 10% of the perception by expanding the acoustic perception, in which voices, birdsongs or snow crunching can be heard again

of the hearing threshold (fluctuation) require a high degree of knowledge on the part of the patient. Adequate training includes listening strategies and experiencing different listening situations.

▪ CROS devices for unilateral deafness

If the course of the disease and/or treatment has led to unilateral deafness, spatial hearing is no longer possible. In order to compensate for this, so-called CROS devices (contralateral-routing-of-signals) were constructed. These essentially consist of a microphone unit behind the deafened ear, which is connected wireless on the other side of the ear.

▪ Directional Hearing

This helps especially against one-sidedness in social communication. So it is possible again to talk to people on the right and on the left instead of being de facto cut off from one half in a company. It is also useful in traffic to hear vehicles from both sides before they get too close.

▪ Cochlear implant ("CI")

In most patients with Meniere's disease, the hearing loss is limited to one side. In this case, the hearing loss can usually be reduced with the help of hearing aids. However, if this is only insufficiently possible, a so-called cochlear implant ("CI") can become useful – even on one side.

In this way, above all, directional hearing can be preserved and speech comprehension improved. Both are good prerequisites for maintaining the quality of life.

A cochlear implant is an electronic inner ear prosthesis. A prerequisite for the use of the cis is that the auditory nerve and the central auditory pathway remain intact. This is usually the case in Meniere's disease patients. Sufficient skills and abilities to operate the technology are also necessary.

▪ Tinnitus therapy

When vertigo has receded into the background, Ménière's patients may suffer from tinnitus. However, tinnitus sufferers due to Ménière's disease are – mostly – in the fortunate situation that they have been free from vertigo for a long time.

For Ménière's patients without significant impairment due to vertigo, we work along with a neurotological step therapy as with other tinnitus sufferers. This is based on four pillars:

- Serious and medically sound information, which the patient can understand for himself, supported by comprehensive neurotological diagnostics

- Hearing Therapy for Habituation
- Psychotherapeutic treatment of the tinnitus condition

In Ménière's patients, special attention should be paid to the fact that, that ringing in the ears may actually become louder at times. This can have the meaning (in the sense of information) that a vertigo attack is imminent.

■ Use tinnitus with meaning

Here it is important to learn to distinguish between insignificant and significant tinnitus. The insignificant tinnitus, always the same, usually perceived as deep background noise, without information character, is treated like other types of tinnitus. The tinnitus with meaning can announce a possible attack and therefore, as terrible as it is, can be used to prepare for the attack. Much is already gained here if both can be distinguished.

■ Cortisone into the middle ear (intratympanic cortisone administration)

In late 2016, a double-blind study of 30 patients each over 2 years was published (Patel et al. 2016). These were identified between 2009 and 2013 from a total of 256 patients eligible for elimination with gentamycin 40 mg/ml or, alternatively, intratympanic administration of methylprednisolone (62.5 mg/ml). Cortisone, unlike gentamycin, is not expected to cause additional hearing deterioration. These 60 patients were assigned in a double-blind fashion to one of the two procedures. Thus, neither the patients nor the practitioners knew which drug they were administering – planned twice with one-week intervals – through the eardrum into the middle ear.

Also surprising for the investigators, both methods showed the same effect. In both groups, the number of vertigo attacks were reduced very early after the injections and remained stable for 2 years.

Both groups – again surprisingly – did not differ significantly with regard to hearing loss. One can speculate whether this was due to the progression of the disease. Credit may also be given to the fact that – as is increasingly common – only a little gentamycin was used.

The only thing missing is a comparison group with a placebo or an obvious wait-and-see group, then the study would be even more meaningful. Nevertheless, the comparison with an established method (intratympanic gentamycin) that has been sufficiently studied against placebo is meaningful (see below).

If you're looking for where "the rub might be," it's allowed to ask,

- what happened to the 196 patients who were not eligible for treatment
- if the support of the English self-help organization "Meniere Society" influenced the patient composition
- if the – in comparison to the English health care system – rather high support effort plays a (positive) role for both good results
- why an intravenous administration of cortisone – in contrast to gentamycin – apparently does not show any recognizable permanent effects.

In the end, empirically – despite all the astonishment and the questions about the unknown mechanism of action – a good result remains for the methylprednisolone.

Thus, the comparison with an established method (intratympanic gentamycin), which has been sufficiently studied against placebo (Postema et al. 2008), is so meaningful that in the end a good result remains for the use of cortisone. Therefore, we offer intratympanal cortisone in our clinic, if there is sufficient suspicion of a Menière's disease and the patients want this approach.

- **Our approach in the clinic Dr. Hesse in Arolsen**

Because patients with methylprednisolone report a painful sensation in the middle ear for several hours, we use the more tolerable Dexamethasone 4 mg (0.4 ml) / hyaluronic acid (0.1 ml) = 0.5 ml or Fortecortin® Inject 100 mg 0, 4 ml / Hylo-COMOD® 0.1 ml = 0, 5 ml.

According to Espinosa-Sanchez and Lopez-Escamez (2016), despite the lower concentration in endo- and perilymph compared to methylprednisolone, dexamethasone might nevertheless be more effective because it is more rapidly taken up by endocytosis into the stria vascularis and surrounding soft tissue, where it acts intracellularly.

This means that although the concentration in the fluid portions of the vestibular organ is lower, it gets there faster, from where dexamethasone it should be effective.

In the follow-up published in 2019, it is reported that the presented results were very stable even after 5 years of follow-up. For example, in terms of dizziness reduction, there was still no significant difference between the gentamycin group and the cortisone group (Harcourt et al. 2019).

However, there was a significantly higher need for follow-up injections in the cortisone group.

Again, it should be kept in mind that the "natural" course of Meniere's disease may have led to increasing convergence in both groups regardless of intervention.

Taking into account the now proven ineffectiveness of betahistine, one will certainly be allowed to advise intratympanic cortisone administration in a step-by-step plan. This would – theoretically – lead to much better management of a disease that limits the quality of life and the psychological state, especially due to the unpredictable vertigo attacks.

■ Chemical reduction of the vestibular function, destruction of the labyrinth

Gentamycin into the tympanic cavity: intratympanic gentamicin administration

If the organically caused Ménière's vertigo occurs to frequently, an effective method is the administration of gentamycin – toxic (poisonous) for the inner ear – into the middle ear. This can reduce the frequency and severity of Ménière's attacks and (depending on the frequency of use) eliminate them. What is endangered here – as by the progression of Ménière's disease itself – is the hearing part.

It is probable that most Ménière's sufferers have already tried some of the measures discussed later, before they have to face this procedure. Nevertheless, I have deliberately put these methods first, as it is one of the most effective procedures in terms of what it is intended to do. Numerous studies are available, including two double-blind peer-reviewed studies accepted by the Cochrane Collaboration.

■ Clarification before surgery is essential

Before this intervention – which reduces the function of the vestibular organ and involves the hearing part – it must be clarified before:

- Is it really Ménière's disease (and not vestibular migraine or perilymph fistula or a dehiscence of the upper semicircular canal?
- Are the vertigo events inner ear-related attacks or a predominantly reactive psychogenic event, perhaps complicated by additional, but eliminable paroxysmal positional vertigo or the "objective" experience of the unilateral loss of function during very fast movements?
- What is known about the compensation possibilities in the balance system of the affected person, what about vision, stability and possibly improved coordination?
- What is the influence of depressant substances or addictive substances, medicinal or self-inflicted?
- What is "often"?

- **History**

Aminoglycosides, the name of the substance class to which gentamycin and streptomycin belong, "suppress" (damage) the sensory cells in the inner ear. The effect thus corresponds to radical surgical methods. However, gentamycin specifically damages the vestibular organ of balance more than the hearing part (cochlea).

The ear-damaging effect of aminoglycosides was discovered in the treatment of tuberculosis. In addition to the main effect, the repressed infection, the long-term treatment showed a hearing loss, double vision and eye tremor; this suggested damage to the vestibular organs. For conscious vestibular elimination, streptomycin was first used in intravenous form by Fowler (1948) and via direct access to the middle ear by Schuknecht (1957). Since practically all patients became deaf, the procedure was abandoned.

In 1997, Lange (1977) took up the method and refined it by using gentamycin, which is less toxic to hearing.

- **By diffusion into the inner ear**

Gentamycin enters the inner ear fluids by diffusion across the membranes of the tympanic membranes, mainly via the round window (◘ Fig. 7.2). Vascular connections between the middle ear mucosa and the labyrinth presumably also play a role in transport. Because aminoglycosides are highly water-soluble, they accumulate and distribute in the inner ear fluids. They do not cross the blood-brain barrier.

After gentamycin elimination, clear differences in saccule and utricle damage can be detected (Helling 2008). Thus, the determination of the VEMP showed for all patients showed a complete loss of sacculus function. In contrast, the utricle remained intact in one third.

- **Cautious administration**

Delayed effect

Initially, intratympanic gentamycin elimination was used only for very poor hearing (stage 3). In the course of increasing experience with this method, it has become apparent that gentamycin is both absorbed into the inner ear with a delay and degraded only slowly (Magnusson et al. 1991). This has led to the fact that nowadays significantly smaller amounts of the active substance are used and – due to the delayed effect – a longer waiting period is required for the therapeutic success, that is, the absence of vertigo. Partial elimination of the vestibular organ also seems to be sufficient to improve the symptoms (Magnusson et al. 1991). As a result, fewer and fewer side effects were observed.

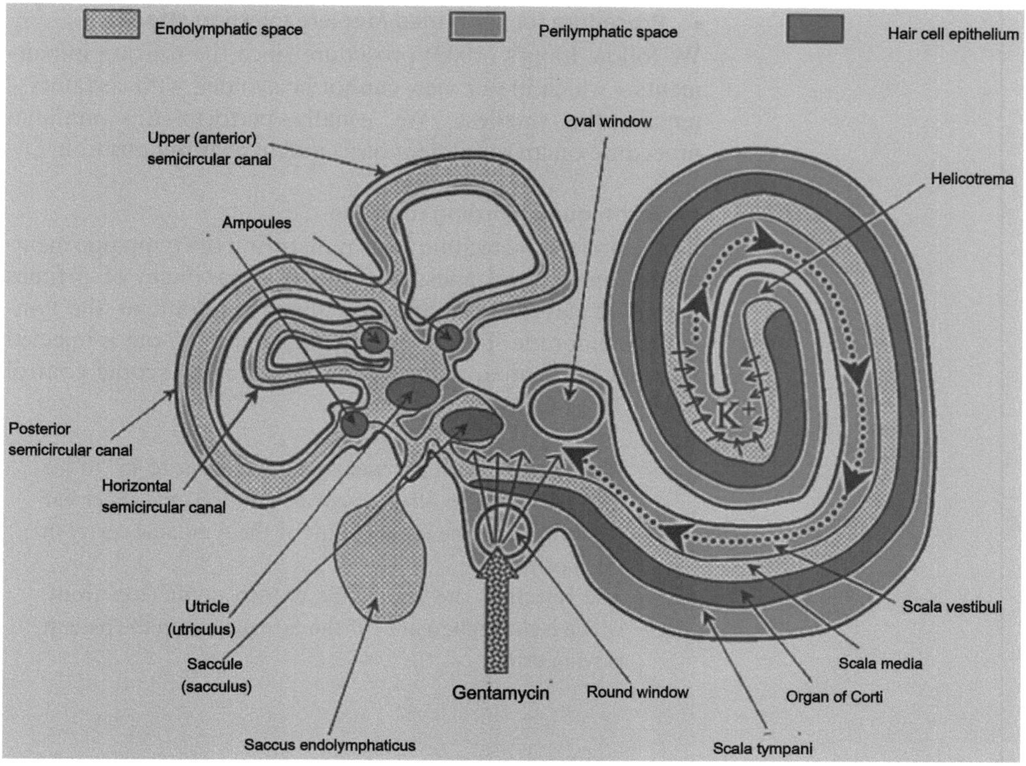

Fig. 7.2 Positional relationship of cochlear and vestibular endolymph and perilymph spaces, highly schematized. Short thin arrows: K+ enters the scala vestibuli from the endolymph of the scala media in the apical region of the cochlea due to increased permeability or rupture of the Reissner membrane. Dotted line (in the direction of the large arrowheads) K+ has invaded the perilymph, enters the vestibular area in the scala vestibuli, and may lead to activation of vestibular afferents there. Large marbled arrow + long thin arrows: Pathway of gentamycin after intratympanic application through the round window into the perilymph of the scala tympani, into the basal cochlear area, and the vestibule. (From Gleich et al. 2008)

Lang (2003) was one of the first to observe, after almost 30 years of personal experience with the method, that hearing did not deteriorate significantly with only a few gentamicin applications, but sometimes even recovered somewhat.

An important aspect with regard to hearing concerns the uptake and distribution of gentamycin in the inner ear after administration into the middle ear. Here, Plontke et al. (2007) was able to show that gentamycin accumulates predominantly in the base of the cochlea and from there reaches the endolymph of the vestibular portion (see also Gleich et al. 2008, Fig. 7.2).

However, since it has been found that with this method.

- vertigo can be safely suppressed, and
- hearing does not exactly improve, but usually does not have to deteriorate significantly, the method was already recommended for stage 2b (Jahnke 1994) if more than two attacks of vertigo occur per week (Morgenstern 1994).

▪ Procedure for confirmed Ménière's vertigo attack

We follow Lang's (2003) procedure since the hearing impairments – which in our view cannot be avoided with certainty – remain the smallest. We usually perform this minimal procedure on an outpatient basis and in a sitting position.

▪ Technique according to Lange

Lange prefers the technique of puncturing the tympanic membrane (under local anesthesia up to a maximum of 3 times within 15 days) in the anterior upper quadrant of the tympanic membrane. Then 0.3 ml gentamycin = 12 mg is injected through the tympanic membrane under microscopic control (see → ◘ Fig. 7.3).

- The patient lies on his back and turns his head 45° to the healthy side. The affected ear lies on top; the inner ear windows form the lowest point of the tympanic cavity in this position.
- The injection site should be chosen at the top front, which is the highest area of the eardrum when the patient is lying down.

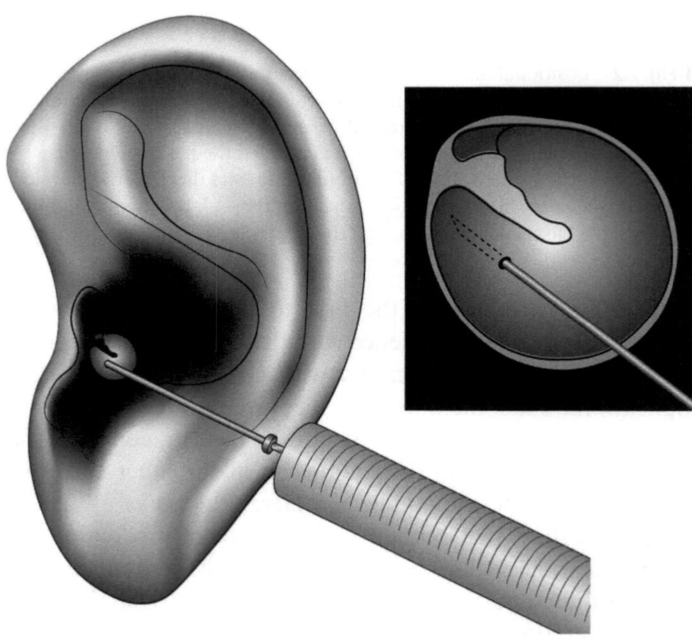

◘ **Fig. 7.3** Injection of gentamycin into the anterior tympanic quadrants under local anesthesia. (After Lange 1998) (Drawing: Michaela von Aichberger)

- The gentamycin thus inevitably accumulates in the niches of the inner ear windows. After the injection, the patient remains lying with his head turned to the opposite side for at least 30 minutes. The gentamycin thus remains concentrated in the window niches.
- In the described head position, the eustachian tube opens into the tympanic cavity at the very top. The liquid gentamycin can therefore not flow off prematurely or be transported away.
- On day 1, 0.3 ml gentamycin is applied into the middle ear.

  53% (n = 30) of Lange's 57 patients (2003) required only one gentamicin dose.
- On the eighth day, the injection is repeated if there are still no reactions (nystagmus or vertigo).

  This was the case in 27 of Lange's patients (2003).
- If no inner ear symptoms are present on day 15

  (about 1/4 of patients at Lange), treatment is given for the last time.
- Then wait for at least 2–3 months until a new therapy.

Quaglieri et al. (2014) studied 174 patients over a period of 7 years. In 41%, one administration of gentamicin was sufficient, in 44% two to nine administrations were required. Only 4% did not have a satisfactory outcome and underwent transection of the vestibular nerve (neurectomy, see below). In 13% of the patients, after several years of freedom from symptoms, vertigo recurred, which could be eliminated by a further gentamicin administration.

The access is stopped at the latest when dizziness occurs. This is the sign that the labyrinth functions fail and the basis for the attack-vertigo is removed. What remains is a – decreasing – nausea and a trembling of the eyes towards the healthy side, which accompanies the destruction of the labyrinth (failure nystagmus). It ceases when the central nervous system has become accustomed to the new situation with only one functioning vestibular organ.

With the above-described procedure according to Lang (2003), the absence vertigo is no more severe than vertigo already experienced.

Because the aim is not the elimination but the reduction of the function of the vestibular organ, it is possible that after a longer period of time dizziness or vertigo may again become noticeable. This is then not a failure of the method, but an indication that gentamycin – with the same idea – should be injected again.

Studies in guinea pigs showed that regeneration of hair cells in the vestibular organ can occur as early as 24 weeks after gentamicin application (Wang and Wang 1997). This is another reason why gentamycin may have to be given again. However, a regeneration of the cochlear hair cells could not be found (Forge et al. 1998).

▪ Regeneration of the vestibular cells conceivable

Lang's (2003) optimism went so far as to recommend the use of low-dose gentamycin treatment at a very early stage in cases of repeated severe Ménière's attacks.

Also, Lang (2003) would not hesitate to treat the opposite side after successful unilateral therapy.

▪ High success rates

The success rates of intratympanic gentamicin application are – measured by the elimination of inner ear-related attack vertigo – high.

For the Cochrane Collaboration, among a large number of studies, Pullens and van Benthem (2011) evaluated those by Postema et al. (2008) and Stokroos and Kingma (2004) as prospective, double-blind, and placebo-controlled. Both found a significant reduction in vertigo symptoms in the gentamycin group. Stokroos and Kingma (2004) reported hearing loss, Postema et al. (2008) – unexpectedly – even saw slight hearing improvements, averaging around 8 dB.

Based on these results, the procedure is considered effective for the treatment of vertigo in Ménière's disease – coupled with the risk of hearing loss. However, no significantly increased rate of hearing loss was found with low-dose gentamycin therapy. These results are broadly consistent with data from a meta-analysis by Huon et al. (2012).

A quantitative meta-analysis (Salt et al. 2008) confirmed that single injections with possibly necessary repetitions at longer intervals (usually several weeks) until the absence or significant reduction in the number or severity of vertigo attacks are the safest with regard to observed hearing loss (Plontke and Gürkov 2015).

▪ Outputs and side effects

Until the balance system has compensated the (partially) switched offside, there remains an eye tremor to the healthy side (failure nystagmus). This depends on the total amount of gentamycin that has become necessary. The less is necessary, the less is also the dizzy time afterwards.

In the case of a prolonged course of Ménière's disease with many attacks, the absence of vertigo after gentamicin elimination will usually be slight, whereas it may be more pronounced at the beginning of Ménière's disease with only a few attacks.

- **Missing effects**

Diffusion barriers for gentamycin

Failure to achieve therapeutic success can occur in 10% to one-third of cases (Plontke and Gürkov 2015). This may be due to anatomical peculiarities of the inner ear windows, for example, due to mucosal membranes, etc. (Crane et al. 2009; Rah et al. 2014). In this case, tympanoscopy (opening or dislocation of the tympanic membrane to view the middle ear) and, if necessary, removal of the "false membranes" and direct entry of gentamycin can help (Plontke 2011).

- **What is so "often" that you can decide to do the procedure?**

Individual conditions

The decision to eliminate the inner ear is as difficult as it is individual. No one likes to destroy a sensory organ. ENT doctors in particular are rightly hesitant to induced or accepted restriction of hearing.

Morgenstern (1994) mentions twice a week as a criterion, referring to organically induced attacks. This may be too much for a person who could lose his job. One vertigo attack a month can be too much if the ability to drive is endangered and the uncertainty regarding the question: "Will the vertigo come today or will it go" leads to endangerment of the ability to work. Two episodes of vertigo a week can be tolerated if the attacks are weak and the person concerned is retired. However, two attacks can also be too much for a pensioner if this increases the risk of falling and one does not want to spend the last few years in the room withdrawing with fear.

Ultimately, therefore, must be evaluated individually. But then there is much to be said for reducing unnecessary dizziness.

I myself have benefited greatly from the termination of my Ménière's disease by a gentamicin administration. This is another reason why I have a very positive attitude towards the procedure.

I would also not wait until – unilaterally – the hearing has decreased by itself, if by then possibly an occupational disability, invalidity or massive depressive reactions had set in.

▪ Clarification on gentamycin elimination

If one considers the possible side effects and risks of gentamycin elimination, one must think of the following side effects, most of which are very rare:

- During local anesthesia to numb the eardrum, there may be minimal bleeding in the external auditory canal or irritation of a small nerve.
- During the puncture (with a millimeter small puncture of the eardrum under local anesthesia), there may be minimal bleeding and irritation or injury to the underlying structures.

The administration of gentamycin into the middle ear causes the gentamycin to enter the inner ear and also the auditory part, so that hearing deterioration may occur. These hearing impairments are very small if the dose is low enough. Sometimes the hearing even recovers to the original hearing level before the gentamicin was administered. Nevertheless, it cannot be ruled out, that a significant hearing loss may occur, which in rare cases may lead to deafness.

- An intended side effect of gentamicin administration is the elimination or at least the reduction of the vestibular part in the inner ear. This usually results in dizziness, which in most cases only lasts for a short time (about one day). Spinning vertigo-like in Ménière's attack can also occur, but typically in the other direction, that is, the eye movement does not go in the direction of the affected ear, but points to the opposite side as dropout nystagmus.
- Depending on the amount of gentamycin and the functioning of the vestibular organ, this dizziness can either last only a few hours up to a day. Feeling of insecurity and dizziness can remain for a day, in a few cases up to several days, which however gets better bit by bit and above all with increasing practice.
- As in the case of Ménière's disease itself, driving incapacity must be assumed after gentamicin administration until the dizziness symptoms have reliably disappeared – for at least 1 month. – Also sufficient compensatory mechanisms (e.g. no compensatory nystagmus after rapid head-turning movement, no deviation to one side when stepping on the spot) must have developed.

▪ Cutting of the vestibular nerve: neurectomy

If the dizziness originating in the inner ear cannot be adequately controlled, it seems obvious to cut the nerve connections between the peripheral sensory organ and the central balance center.

If it is possible during the operation to spare the auditory nerve, which lies close to the vestibular nerve and joins it in a common main nerve, the vertigo should be controlled and the remaining hearing preserved. Performed by experienced surgeons, good long-term results with a low risk of complications have been reported (Helms 1985; Hillman et al. 2004; Schlegel et al. 2012; ▣ Fig. 7.4).

- **Transection of the vestibular nerve**

Nevertheless, neurectomy does not "protect" against fluctuating hearing disorders due to persisting endolymphatic hydrops with further fluctuating hearing.

The prerequisite for this measure is a neurosurgical intervention. Like any intervention, this has its specific risks, which rarely occur with experienced surgeons. Nevertheless, Moller

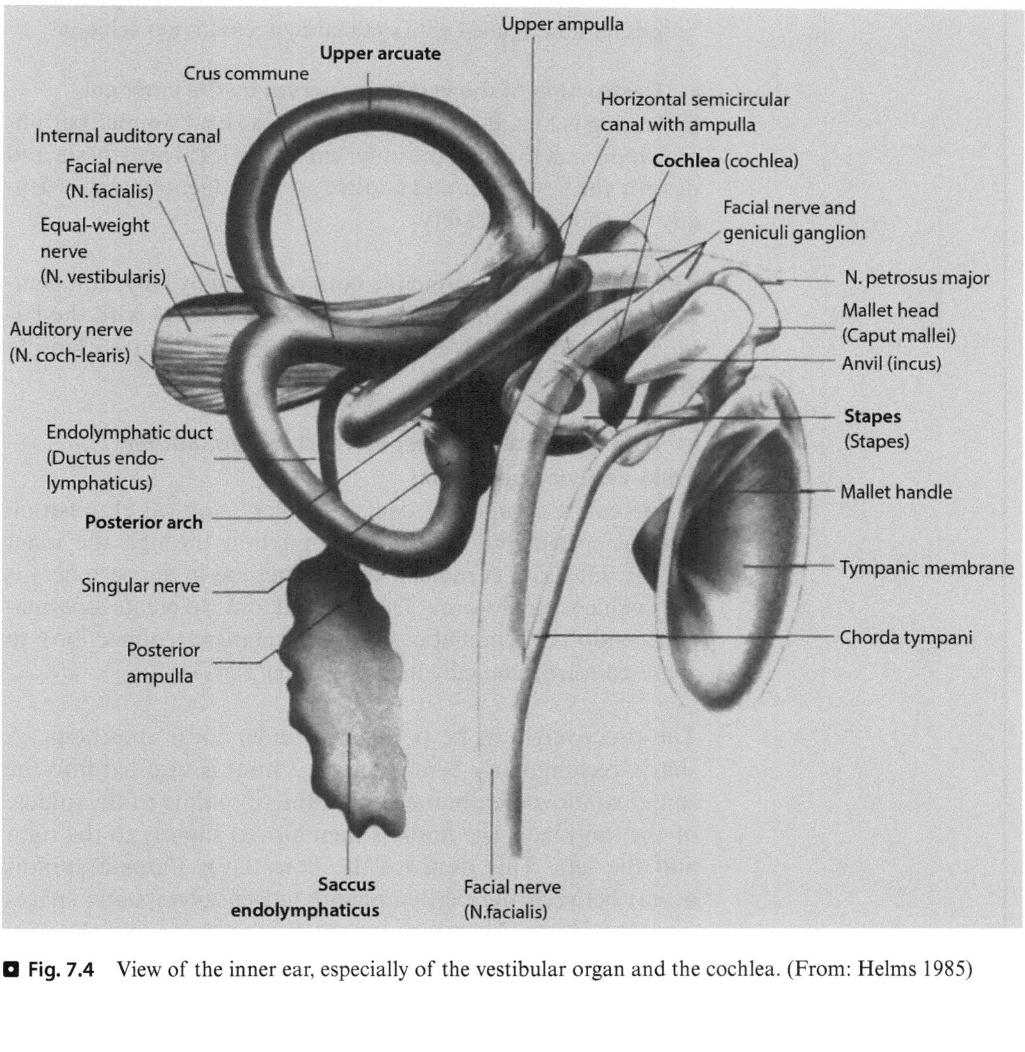

▣ **Fig. 7.4** View of the inner ear, especially of the vestibular organ and the cochlea. (From: Helms 1985)

et al. (2009) reported on 18 patients in a hospital specializing in this procedure that good results were achieved in terms of vertigo elimination. However, facial nerve palsy occurred once and cerebrospinal fluid flow (the fluid around the central nervous system) occurred twice after surgery.

▪ Finding the vestibular nerve through the temporal bone

The worse the hearing ability is, the simpler the surgical technique can be and the more certain is the success. For example, if the hearing is still present, the procedure is performed through the temporal bone ("transtemporal") and the vestibular nerve, which is still separate from the auditory nerve, is located and cut. With the help of microsurgical techniques and differentiated approaches, and the closely adjacent auditory and facial nerves can be spared as far as possible.

> The condition after neurectomy corresponds to that of a unilateral loss of balance. Therefore, balance training methods must be applied until optimal compensation is achieved.

▪ Destruction of the vestibular nerves by the inner ear

If hearing is lost, it is also sufficient to seek a "simple" peripheral approach through the inner ear under local anesthesia and destroy the vestibular and auditory nerves. Gentamycin is usually also added for safety.

This measure has in principle been replaced by labyrinth elimination with gentamycin, as described above. As with the latter, surgical labyrinth elimination also initially causes lapsing vertigo.

▪ Destruction of the inner ear: cochleosacculotomy

Endo-perilymphatic shunt

If the ear is completely deaf, "simpler" surgical elimination options (peripheral labyrinth elimination through the inner ear) are effective. A radical surgical method in the periphery is the cochleosacculotomy. This method aims to create a permanent endo-perilymphatic shunt (permanent connection) to avoid endolymphatic hydrops (Walther 2005).

The procedure can be performed under local anesthesia. A sharp, rectangularly bent hook (2–3 mm) is inserted into the round window membrane so that the tip points to the middle of the footplate. The hook is then moved slightly to the right and the left. This destroys the bony layer (lamina spiralis ossea) between the perilymphatic and endolymphatic spaces (cochlear duct). The procedure is then repeated and the window is closed with connective tissue (Walther 2005).

The method is more widespread in America than in Europe. Long-term success in eliminating vertigo ranges from 82% to 89% (Montandon et al. 1985). Because of the high percentage of subsequent hearing loss, the method is only indicated for patients with severe hearing loss. Often cochleo-sacculotomy is performed as a "second-line surgical therapy" after a lack of response to function-preserving procedures (Westhofen 2013). Since it leads to complete loss of labyrinth and cochlear function, patients are simultaneously offered cochlear implantation to improve their hearing.

Caution: If implantation of a cochlear implant is later considered on the affected side, this procedure may jeopardize the basis for this.

- **Summary: A possible step-by-step plan**

The following approach seems to be useful in the course of the disease:

If the organic vertigo increases, the administration of cortisone into the middle ear seems to be helpful – at least for a large part of the affected persons.

If (after that) the – inner ear related! – vertigo – continues to occur more often than can be tolerated and if the hearing in the speech area has failed, also deactivating measures come into consideration. These include the administration of gentamycin into the middle ear or the severing (neurectomy) of the vestibular nerve.

If the psychogenic vertigo or emotional distress takes over, experts, who can recognize from the outside what is causing the Meniere's patient to lose balance, maybe helpful. These experts are usually psychotherapists.

7.3.3 Non-proven Conservative Therapies

The following selection from A-Z is the opinion of "experts" (from the medical field).

- **Aciclovir and valaciclovir**

There is probably hardly anyone who has not come into contact with a herpes virus in the course of growing up. Thus, herpes viruses are also considered when hearing loss and balance disorders cannot be explained otherwise. This could be preceded by a weakening of the immune system, which allowed the viruses, which had been defended against until then, to become harmful.

Nevertheless, it is unlikely that herpes viruses – in the sense of Ménière's disease – repeatedly trigger vertigo and hearing loss. Thus, Gacek (2015) is scientifically very much alone with his opinion on the antiviral treatment of Ménière's disease (Helling 2015). He undertook long-term treatment (1 year and longer!) with acyclovir or valacyclovir, which is fraught with side effects, and reported hearing improvement in 12 of 31 patients. For 19 patients without therapeutic hearing improvement, he speaks of control of vertigo in 9 patients during this time. The others could not be helped with continuous antiviral therapy.

▪ Arlevert

Arlevert is a combination medication of the sedative dimenhydrinate (40 milligrams) and the calcium antagonist cinnarizine (20 milligrams).

The sedative component is supposed to dampen dizziness, but – according to the experts, recruited for the "Handbook of Dizziness" (created by the pharmaceutical company) – in this combination, it is not supposed to impair attention (vigilance) and reaction time.

▪ Mechanism of action nebulous

The calcium antagonist cinnarizine, tested on a hair cell model (!) of a guinea pig, is supposed to inhibit "non-physiological" impulses from the vestibular organ. Why cinnarizine should succeed in inhibiting only non-physiological impulses from the vestibular organ and not the physiological ones (e.g. in the healthy vestibular organ on the opposite side) probably remains as nebulous as the extension of the field of application to almost all types of vertigo – from loss of equilibrium to psychogenic vertigo to motion sickness.

All experience indicates that the vestibular system – except in the acute phase – does not benefit from its attenuation and thus reduction of its abilities but from promotion and challenge. It is true that without balance function there is no dizziness, but there is also no coordination ability and safety in movement. (Also note on taking dimenhydrinate during pregnancy above).

▪ Betahistine

Until now, hardly anyone with fluctuating hearing or a suspected case of Ménière's disease could avoid the prescription of a drug from the group of betahistines. Now a well-conducted study by betahistine propagators has found that betahistines work no better than placebo, whether they were dosed low or high.

If one has thought or hoped that the betahistine discussion is over, one must find oneself disappointed.

▪ A seemingly endless story

Betahistines or betahistine dimesilate are related to histamine. These are tissue hormones that can dilate but also constrict blood vessels. In 1972, betahistine was shown under experimental conditions in animals to increase blood flow within the cochlea (Martinez 1972). This had raised hopes – among therapists and patients – that betahistine could also intervene in the still complex and largely unclear process that can lead to Ménière's disease. Nevertheless, in humans, no really confirmed success in terms of frequency and severity of seizures has been recorded. Thus, a review of the seven studies accepted by the Cochrane Review Group shows no evidence that betahistine helps (James and Burton 2011).

As early as 1991, Paparella stated, "It is extremely doubtful that any so-called vasodilator drug in the labyrinth significantly affects blood flow in the inner ear." Morgenstern (1994) commented, "Even if an increase in blood flow could be achieved, it would be difficult to imagine an influence on endolymphatic hydrops."

> *Rationally, this is true for all drugs that are supposed to influence Ménière's disease by improving blood flow.*

Nevertheless, betahistine remained very popular among those who prescribe it. Thus, many practitioners are glad to be able to put in the hands of the desperate patient a drug that at least does not seem to show serious harm. This is understandable, but not rational.

The highlight of the story so far – with some friendly support – is that despite – to put it mildly – "uncertain data" betahistine is designated as "indicated" in a guideline "Vertigo" (2008) "based on an open observational study":

This also meant that too many publications had to refer to the "presumed effect" of betahistines in order for the article to be accepted "on a scientific basis". However, a large number of hardly substantiated, but "friendly" approving studies were published.

▪ Again no evidence of efficacy

If, on the other hand, a good study (Gürkov et al. 2013) finds that betahistine does not affect hydrops, then perhaps the dose was too low, or the study instrument (MRI) too poor.

Under the leadership of the group around Strupp, the aim was to find out whether (or actually that) a higher and longer administration of betahistine reduces the frequency of vertigo in Ménière's disease, after a fierce propagation of "more betahistine". The study design was on a basis that could have shown a more benign result:

- Thus, confirming the diagnosis was associated with some uncertainties.
- Only patients who had not previously responded to the low dosage, that is, were already at a significantly later stage of the course of the disease, were studied, which is very likely to have an influence on the reduction of vertigo attacks.
- The "management" of the study by many, often changing "investigators" at different sites makes a uniform assessment "problematic".
- The evaluation based on patient diaries cannot reliably distinguish between a reduction in Ménière's attacks and the – at least frequently occurring – psychogenic dizziness or, for example, benign paroxysmal positional vertigo with subsequent unsteadiness.

▪ Neither high nor low dose more effective than placebo

The study then found – methodically clean – that placebos for the treatment of Ménière's disease are just as "effective" as the previous standard dosage of betahistine and also as the high-dose therapy with betahistine.

> » Long term prophylactic treatment with betahistine dihydrochloride (at daily doses 2×24 mg or 3×48 mg) does not change the time course of vertigo episodes related to Ménière's disease compared with placebo. Placebo intervention, as well as betahistine treatment, showed the same reduction of attack rates over the study's nine-month treatment period. (Adrion et al. 2016)

The latest attempt to establish betahistine in Meniere's patients with the realization (after more the 50 years!), that betahistine has a high "first-pass effect" (approx. 99%). So Betahistine taken as a tablet is largely broken down by an enzyme called monoamine oxidase (MAO). Accordingly, only a minimal amount enters the blood. This late observation, however, raises the question of the value of publications that have published "proofs of efficacy" of betahistine, i.e. of a drug that has not reached further than the liver.

In order to prevent the degradation of betahistine, a drug can be given which – irreversibly – reduces this degradation. These are the so-called MAO inhibitors. These are given in the symptomatic co-treatment of Parkinson's disease in order to allow the medication required for this to take effect in a sufficient form. This results in irreversible inhibition of the enzyme monoaminooxidase B (MAO-B) and inhibition of dopamine degradation.

Thus, the price for better betahistine uptake – not for its efficacy, which no one has yet validly verified – is the acceptance of the possible side effects of the MAO inhibitor.

These are:

Dry mouth, loss of appetite, dizziness, sleep disturbances, confusion, anxiety, hallucinations.

Transaminase increase, orthostatic hypotension, and cardiac arrhythmias.

There may be an increase in the effects and side effects of sympathomimetics, psychostimulants, nasal drops, antihypertensives, antihypertensives, sedatives, and ethanol.

Simultaneous use of selegiline and antidepressants (especially SSRIs) may lead to serious reactions, such as flushing, hyperthermia, seizures, cardiovascular disorders, mental disorders (confusion, hallucinations) and even coma.

> Combination with dimenhydrate (e.g., Vomex) for dizziness attenuation in acute attacks also appears to be problematic according to the package insert of the drug.

However, many patients with Parkinson's disease seem to tolerate MAO inhibitors well.

But interactions need to be considered, which may be less practiced in an ENT setting.

So it takes a lot of conviction to bring out what we consider to be heavy guns in a disease that, for all its vertigo potency, has a markedly different severity of disability and limitations than in Parkinson's disease with progressive degeneration in the brain.

The evidence from studies to date provides no basis for this belief. Except in one animal experiment, no really convincing effect has been shown so far, and this was not about M. Meniere, but about blood flow in the cochlea.

The multiple "approximate" results without a control group are invalidated by the large-scale study performed by Adrion et al. (2016).

■ What remains?

It is more than understandable for patients to take what has certainly been a trial with few side effects so far, in order not to leave out anything that might help or that has been heard to help.

Understandably, many practitioners are happy to be able to give a desperate patient a drug with a great deal of certainty that at least does not seem to show any serious harm.

However, this option is eliminated when an MAO inhibitor is added.

The current state of affairs is that there is no evidence of organically explainable efficacy (Devantier et al. 2020), nor can there be if the betahistine is already metabolized before it can reach the desired target.

For Ménière's patients, it would of course still be desirable if there were a simple and above all curative solution for Ménière's disease. As long as this cannot exist, placebos should at least be known as such to the doctor. Dashed hopes are also a serious side effect.

- **Diuretics**

Diuretics are dehydrating drugs and are intended to achieve in a fast procedure that even the endolymph hydrops can only carry little water if the "person surrounding the hydrops" only offers little. That is why this measure is mainly used during the time of the attack.

- **No long-term effect**

Although this may seem plausible at first sight, no prolonged success can be ascertained. The mechanism by which hydrops develops is different and the electrolyte balance of the inner ear cannot be permanently influenced by such factors, otherwise, a normal hearing would not be stable. Thus, the Cochrane Collaboration states that no effect can be proven for this measure (Burgess and Kundu 2006).

- **Reduction of stimulants**

Alcohol can cause spinning dizziness

Nicotine constricts the blood vessels and thus also hinders the supply of important nutrients. Smokers will understand that this is not helpful.

Not infrequently, the stimulant alcohol is used to escape from misery. But alcohol is a very effective "balance poison". It has a specific effect on the inner ear and can – in the right dose – even cause spinning dizziness. In addition, alcohol has a direct effect on perception and the balance centers in the brainstem. Therefore, alcohol should really only be consumed for and with pleasure.

Coffee and tea are in principle weak neurotoxins. As long as they still have a stimulating effect, they can help to ensure that the coordination and control centers in the brainstem are activated by a higher level of alertness. Even after an extensive literature review, caffeine has no demonstrable negative effect on the symptoms of Ménière's disease (Trinidade et al. 2014).

▪ Restricted sodium, high potassium diet

Without lasting influence

A similar idea to diuretics exists when recommending a low-salt diet. The total amount of fluid in humans is closely coupled with their sodium (salt) content. Potassium is the "antagonist" of sodium in electrolyte balance. Also here no longer success can be found and regulation processes compensate mostly again fast possible effects. Thus, Plester already briefly summarized in 1979: "Dietary sodium deprivation cannot influence the regulatory disturbance of the endolymph."

The (probably seriously meant) study of 18 patients by Naganuma et al. (2006) must be regarded as almost contrary to this. They headline their work on a defined fluid intake with: "Water could cure patients with Ménière's disease". Indeed, they found improvements in vertigo (as in the non-treated group) and improved hearing in the "water" group.

At the very least, it is clear that externally restricted or increased fluid intake may have little to do with the course of Ménière's disease.

▪ Picrotoxin

Picrotoxin is found naturally mainly in the seeds of the Asian climbing plants Anamirta paniculata and Anamirta cocculus, which are called "Cocculus indicus". Picrotoxin acts pharmacologically as an antagonist (opponent) at the GABA receptor, a switching point for messages between two nerves (neurotransmitters). GABA (gammaaminobutyric acid) has a reinforcing effect in the peripheral-vestibular system and an inhibitory effect in central-vestibular pathways. Among other things, it stimulates respiratory activity, but also the tendency to epileptic seizures.

Ehrenberger in Vienna recommends a picrotoxin dosage of 3 times 1 mg/week as a suppository for long-term therapy of Ménière's disease. Weikert et al. (2008) treated 18 patients with picrotoxin suppositories at a dose of 3 times 1 mg weekly and compared them with patients taking betahistine at the standard dose. The patients surveyed reported a decrease in vertigo sensations within 12 months. However, statistically valid data on this are not available.

However, certainly, picrotoxin cannot have a causal effect on Ménière's disease. It is questionable whether permanent prophylaxis with as yet unexplained side effects is in a justifiable relationship to the real frequency of attacks.

The drug has been withdrawn from the German market because of its side effects in emergency medicine.

▪ Avoidance of allergens

Since immunological and allergic factors have been discussed in the development of Ménière's disease, the list of questionably involved allergy-causing substances has become longer and longer. On it are chocolate, potatoes, oranges, milk, tomatoes, coffee, meat and more.

▪ Omission diet

If there is a chain of effects, this is certainly very individual, that is, you have to find out for yourself which component is harmful, that is, specifically worsens the disease. This component can be determined, for example, with an omission diet. After a few days of fasting with unsuspicious liquids, the components of the normal food are gradually added and it is observed whether one of the substances aggravates the disease. This should then, of course, be omitted. It is advisable not to abandon medical supervision because of the side effects of diet (deficiency of proteins or vitamins).

▪ Vertigoheel

In homeopathic medicine "Vertigoheel" is used as a globule ("cocculus") for the treatment of dizziness, nervousness, nausea, kinetosis.

▪ Vitamins

Vitamin A, E and B

Vitamins A and E in particular are considered important, as they both play a significant role in the metabolism of sensory cells in the inner ear as well (Löhle 1980).

Vitamin B is recommended for all nerve damage. To supply the body with sufficient vitamins, however, a trip to the pharmacy is not absolutely necessary. A balanced diet with plenty of vegetable components, fruit and fresh raw vegetables, now and then sauerkraut, provide more vitamins than the body can use.

Vitamin A is found, for example, in vegetable oils, kale, spinach, cheese, eggs, butter, soy and white beans, fennel and corn.

Vitamin E is concentrated in nuts, berries, avocado, savoy cabbage, eggs and butter, all vegetable oils – especially sunflower oil – corn and buckwheat.

Vitamin B is found in barley, rice, soybeans, broccoli and kale, for example.

> To consider:

> If nothing – surgical is done: On average after 9 years, Ménière's disease seems to "burn out" in 75% of untreated

and non-surgically treated (!) patients, that is, the vertigo attacks become weaker or disappear completely (Stahle et al. and Kitahara in Huang 1991).

7.3.4 Surgical Interventions – without Proven Effect

The following selection is also based on the opinion of "experts".

- **Tympanostomy tube into the middle ear (pressure reduction)**

Tympanostomy tubes for ventilation problems
By inserting a so-called tympanic tube into the eardrum, the ventilation of the middle ear is improved. Tube dysfunction with ventilation problems can occur in about 1/3 of all patients. In this case, the symptoms can be similar to those of Ménière's disease (Westhofen 2008). Thus, there is always speculations that fluctuations in middle ear pressure may influence the course of Ménière's disease (Park et al. 2013). In this case, the insertion of a tympanostomy tube as a simple measure is already helpful in many cases. Westhofen sees the indication for tympanostomy tube treatment when a value of 50 daPa and more is found in impedance audiometry.

It is important to note that this does not address Ménière's disease "in the common definition", but rather a middle ear problem. But this is certainly more of an academic problem for the patient if the symptoms are reduced or even eliminated.

- **Does additional "pressure pulse" help against Ménière's vertigo?**

Since a few years a "pressure pulse generator", with the name "Meniett 20" is offered. It generates a "pulsating" pressure of 12 mbar (corresponding to a 12 cm water column). After placing a tympanic tube, the pressure pulse is supposed to ensure that this pressure is propagated from the middle ear to the inner ear via the connection to the inner ear. There, the endolymphatic hydrops should be influenced.

An intermediate increase of the perilymphatic pressure should lead to a decrease of the endolymph hydrops by influencing the valve mechanism in the endolymph flow (sinus endolymphaticus). Accordingly, the alternating pressure should be applied by the patients for self-treatment 3 times a day.

Now it is difficult to explain why pressure changes in the middle ear, such as those caused by swallowing and yawning, or changes in the oxygen or carbon dioxide content of the middle ear spaces, do not also cause an influence on the inner ear.

Westhofen (2008) compared the published results of pressure application using Meniett with the 34 Ménière's patients they treated who had tubal dysfunction and were treated with a tympanostomy tube – without a pressure pulse. He found similar results to the Meniett treatment. Here's how he sums it up:

▪ No additional effect

> The idea that impulsive pressure application in the middle ear enables pressure relief of the saccus endolymphaticus cannot be substantiated as a therapeutic principle for Ménière's disease against this background. (Westhofen 2008)

The Cochrane analysis sees no evidence for a confirmed effect of "pressure pulse therapy" after evaluating five conclusive studies (van Sonsbeek et al. 2015).

▪ Interventions on the endolymphatic sac (saccotomy)

With all ambiguities, the saccus endolymphaticus seems to be responsible for the fact that the endolymph cannot be discharged sufficiently. The saccotomy aims at relieving the pressure of the endolymphatic hydrops. Contrarily a recently propagated procedure separates the endolymphatic sac from the labyrinth (see below).

While the guidelines of the "German Neurological Society (2008)", classify this intervention as "obsolete", ENT physicians who perform surgery, in particular, propagate its effectiveness – probably also with the idea of not damaging hearing if the operation goes well (Ernst 2011; Baier and Ott 2008).

▪ Saccotomy in the light of the Cochrane Collaboration

In a review for the Cochrane Collaboration, Pullens et al. (2021) found insufficient evidence for the efficacy of endolymphatic sac interventions, taking into account the study criteria already mentioned:

> Two trials included in this review provide insufficient evidence of the beneficial effect of endolymphatic sac surgery in Ménière's disease. (Pullens et al. 2021)

▪ Procedure

The saccus endolymphaticus can be reached surgically behind the ear (◘ Fig. 7.4). To do this, the surgeons must first clear out the so-called mastoid process in order to get close to the labyrinth from there. The meninges are then exposed in the posterior fossa and the saccus is usually found relatively far forward. This is also the only place in the endolymphatic system, according to Meyer zum Gottesberge and Stupp (in Link et al. 1980), where an opening is possible without danger to the vestibular apparatus and the risk of injury to the meninges (dura) is small. The saccus is located a good 1 cm from the labyrinth, so that the risk of deafness due to the operation, although given, is to be regarded as low.

- **The basic idea and fundamental concerns**

The saccotomy was already introduced by Portmann in 1927. He opened the saccus and directed it into the open cell system of the mastoid process. In this way, he released the mostly shrunken organ from its scarred embrace (after inflammation or immune reactions) and ensured the drainage of the excessive fluid.

- **Successes not higher than with placebo surgery**

This basic idea has spread worldwide. However, it has been modified in many ways because it turned out that the success was quickly undone by adhesions and regrowth of the ablated bone. However, even all variations with different ablation routes and sizes as well as various ablation implants always come up with the same success rates in long-term follow-up examinations despite sophisticated approaches and explanations (e.g. Kitahara 1990, pp. 181–187; Huang et al. in Huang 1991, pp. 145–154; Radeloff et al. 2009; Westhofen 2008). These are not higher than the successes of a so-called placebo operation. In this case, only the mastoid process was removed, and here too the described improvements occurred (Thomsen et al. 1981).

This confirms all doubts about explanations of the pathophysiological basis, which Schuknecht already pointed out in 1981 (in Vosteen 1981, pp. 236–241):

- The surgical epithelial damage resulting from the opening can only further reduce the resorptive capacity (because, according to Morgenstern 1985, the saccus does not have a simple filtering function, but exhibits an active activity regulating the ionic milieu. Therefore, it is to be expected that injury or even destruction would only have to produce more negative results).
- Since the pressure in the subarachnoid space (fluid-filled space under the meninges) is greater than in the endolymphatic system, a surgically created artificial connection (drainage) between the two can actually only lead to cerebrospinal fluid entering the endolymphatic system, thus

increasing the pressure even further and not, conversely, allowing endolymphatic fluid to drain away.
- Drainage tubes (artificial connectors) are almost certainly quickly rendered inoperable by connective tissue.

In addition, Schuknecht describes the difficulty that in some cases the saccus is either so small that drainage is not possible, or it is surgically blocked by bone or connective tissue in such a way that a surgical procedure is not possible.

■ Follow-up

Since no lasting improvement has been achieved in one-third of all saccotomized patients, (Westhofen 2008), proponents of the method have given thought to how to proceed. Huang suggests that not only resurgent dizziness should be included in considerations for reoperation, but also deteriorating hearing. He assumes that hearing can be preserved by surgery (Huang et al. in Huang 1991, pp. 145–154). In addition, a revision operation offers the possibility to find out which factor has led to the renewed problems, so that the procedure can be further improved.

■ Higher failure rates

However, the second procedure, like any revision procedure, is not only more difficult but also associated with higher failure rates. Moreover, these failures occur earlier: Whereas with the first intervention, dizziness only accumulates after 2 years and more in the approximately 30–40% of patients for whom the procedure could not guarantee freedom from dizziness, with the second intervention this is already the case after half a year (Huang and Lin in: Huang 1991, pp. 131–144).

■ Conclusion: Hope dies at last

What remains is an ultimately unclear situation and the confidence that by widening the often constricted conditions, a better flow of blood and lymph in this region will be made possible, so that indirectly the resorption of lymph will also be improved (Jahnke 1994). Most otolaryngologists, such as Paparella (2006), hope that this surgery will keep other options open and that at least subjective improvements can be achieved. Perhaps less considered is that disappointed hopes are also a serious side effect.

From my point of view – but without any surgical experience – I have to say that I cannot understand this intervention. Therefore, I do not recommend a saccotomy, but to the cortisone or gentamycin treatment as described above.

The blockade of the endolymphatic duct

It is astonishing that the contrary operation, the deliberate closure of the endolymphatic duct (Saliba et al. 2015), is said to have at least the same effect as the saccotomy – without side effects: "There is significantly better control of the vertigo attacks when compared to the traditional ESD. In addition, there were no significant complications or adverse events."

After an appropriate surgical opening, the endolymphatic duct (Ductus endolymphaticus) should be blocked with clips so that no endolymph can flow. Then (as expected) a hydrops develops, but – surprisingly – *in those previously classified as Ménière's patients,* it should remain without Ménière's symptoms. After some time, the endolymph would then be better reabsorbed by other intracochlear structures.

The procedure is described as a non-destructive technique – although a functional unit previously assumed to be the end organ is interrupted. In addition, the quality of life is said to be "even better" than with saccotomy (Gabra et al. 2016).

Now, in a disease where there is no gold standard (except perhaps the time of the disease), it is difficult to find a valid comparative measure. Whether the saccotomy of all things is resilient, which is called obsolete by some and cannot really be explained in its mode of action by others, must be questioned. So far there is probably also no control investigation outside of the first descriptors themselves.

The unanswered questions remain:

- Why should no Ménière's *remain* or develop after occlusion of the endolymphatic duct and a backflow with endolymph hydrops?
- If it were anyway, why can't it be done without ligating the duct?
- Is the cause of Ménière's disease now supposed to come from the saccus endolymphaticus – in contrast to what has been assumed so far?

Temporary labyrinth anesthesia

Von Illberg propagates a temporary elimination of the labyrinth with procaine or lidocaine. Both are short-acting local anesthetics (local anesthetics) whose effect wears off after a short time.

According to von Ilberg's idea, the vegetative nervous system of the inner ear is blocked for a short time. Afterwards the pressure balance of the inner ear should stabilize again and the vertigo attacks would "calm down". This idea is neither scientifically supported nor proven. There is no disease concept coherent to it from the users. Their observation that after

("after" does not mean "through") labyrinth anesthesia the vertigo attacks become less is reported in a retrospective study in 24 (!) patients (Gstöttner and Adunka 2004).

Basis for vertigo remains

The disadvantage could be – unfortunately to be expected – disappointed hopes if it turns out that organic vertigo could not be influenced by the labyrinth anesthesia since nothing has changed in the functioning of the inner ear conditions causing vertigo.

7.4 Basic Outline of Psychosomatic Treatment

Ménière's disease can lead to the fact that the physically triggered uncertainty can also affect mental processing. Thus, support for the soul may become necessary in order to find a – possibly new – balance again and to maintain the ability to live and work.

Psychotherapeutic help can be particularly relieving when psychogenic dizziness occurs. It is important to clarify whether the "vertigo attacks" are attacks from the inner ear or psychogenic events, which can feel similar or the same for those affected.

7.4.1 Relaxation Techniques

Entry into coping

A first possibility and usually a start in coping with problem situations can be relaxation procedures. They often have a quickly noticeable effect. An effective procedure, which can also be learned from a CD itself and at home, is progressive muscle relaxation (PMR). Patients who suffer from tinnitus on top of their dizziness can add the seemingly unbelievable phrase at the beginning of the relaxation procedure: *All sounds reinforce my (1) calm.*

This will help them get into practice instead of straining to overhear the tinnitus.

Progressive muscle relaxation according to Jacobsen

Progressive muscle relaxation (PMR) was developed by Jacobsen. It works with the two poles of tension and relaxation. It seems to be easier for many sufferers to first tense the muscles in order to then achieve deep relaxation for the whole body.

As a relaxation posture, both the supine position and the sitting posture in a comfortable armchair or recliner are possible. In principle, in the beginning, you learn the tension and then the relaxation of individual muscle groups in the body.

It usually starts with the dominant hand and the forearm. Then the contraction and relaxation go over to the upper arm, the other side and over the forehead-cheek-part, neck-, chest-, abdominal muscles, thighs up to the non-dominant foot. At first, one should concentrate on the respective muscle group, but then slowly and continuously tense it. In doing so, a – individually – comfortable level of tension should be achieved. Afterwards, the muscle group is loosened and relaxed.

There are many good instructions for progressive muscle relaxation on CD.

Progressive muscle relaxation can often provide pressure relief from the feelings that often accompany the disease, if the tensing and releasing – mentally – is continued into the ears. That is why we prefer to use it with patients with endolymphatic events such as Ménière's disease.

7.4.2 Psychotherapy

Psychotherapy translated from Greek means: "accompaniment of the soul", so it is actually nothing reprehensible. Nevertheless, for many, belief in the soul begins only after death, and psychotherapy tends to be tainted with the smell of "crazy". Moreover, those whose problems are not purely organic are often assumed to have only themselves to blame. With organ damage, one may quibble with the expert; with the mental, it becomes personal. So it is no wonder that psychological help is often only accepted when nothing else – no matter how pointless and expensive – can help.

Professional psychotherapeutic support can be helpful in cases of psychogenic dizziness and when the disease leads to (reactive) changes such as depression, anxiety and vertigo because of anxiety. Then even the best medical examination or balance therapy alone may not help sufficiently.

▪ An empathetic view from the outside

Psychotherapy has as an important element the function of the empathetic view from the outside. This can help the to recognize things that are there, but cannot be perceived.

In the case of patients with vertigo, the psychotherapist should have at least enough organic knowledge to feel safer than the patient. Only in this way can he in turn credibly show his patient that he may stumble with him, but will not fall over. Above all – as a wish and as a requirement for psychological psychotherapists: not every dizziness should be interpreted as psychogenic.

It must be clear between the person affected and the psychotherapist that psychotherapy does not influence the organic part of the illness. However, there may be justified confidence that the extent of the burden can be influenced.

Together it has to work out what the presumption is about:
- Nature of the vertigo
- Normal course of the disorder
- Possible psychological influencing factors
- Type of therapy (short to medium term with a focus on vertigo etiology and treatment as well as the chances of success)

▪ Dizziness in the initiation of relationships

Not only do patients perceive a hard time with psychotherapists, but also psychotherapists with vertigo patients. These are considered rather "difficult" because of the interweaving of organic and psychogenic factors. Sometimes dizzy patients can also cause uncertainty and even vertigo in the therapist, which can also initially confuse him and make him seek distance. If this is allowed to lead to working through this too with the patient, often an important step has already been taken.

7.4.3 Psychodynamic Psychotherapy

In the large field of psychotherapeutic approaches, one usually has to deal with psychodynamic and the behavior- therapies.

> Focus on life history and its impact on the disease.

Psychodynamic psychologists understand mental illness as a consequence of current triggers or stresses on the background of previous life development, and on the background of an organic disease such as Ménière's disease. In a psychodynamic approach, there will be the assumption that a significant part of the dizziness processing can also be a consequence or expression of a not really optimal coping attempt, which could have its foundations in the previous mental development.

The aim of psychodynamic approaches can be to understand and process the psychogenic distress expressed in suffering. A part of the psychodynamic approach to perceive also the feelings and non-linguistic messages that become clear in the patient and to use them for the treatment process. In doing so, it is important to recognize and work on conflicts or possibilities for improvement – as far as they are important for the symptomatology "here and now".

Psychodynamic psychologists assume that change requires self-knowledge. In most cases, however, this alone is not enough: What has been recognized must also be "worked through" and applied or practiced. Therefore, the transformation into action, as it is illustrated in the "Systematic Desensitization", should be part of the therapy.

7.4.4 Behavioral Therapy Approaches

Behavior therapists orient themselves to the symptom as well as to the behavior reported by the patient and to the observable behavior. More directly than in the psychodynamic psychological methods, behavioral therapy aims concretely at practical improvements of the symptom.

Unfavorable settings moderate load

The "cognitively oriented" behavioral therapy is particularly concerned with the perception, assessment and evaluation of the suffering. The working basis of cognitive therapy is the assumption that unfavorable attitudes or cognitive processes moderate individual stress. They can influence the stress on different levels and counteract an improvement process. This shows great points of contact with psychodynamic psychological methods – and vice versa.

Learning processes certainly have a decisive influence on the maintenance of symptoms, such as anticipatory anxiety in vertigo.

Then it's very practically about improving by:

- Acquisition of coping skills (e.g. in balance training)
- Actively approaching the situations that have caused dizziness so far (exposures)

7.4.5 Systematic Desensitization

A pragmatic and effective approach for the active management of vertigo experience and behavior is the approach of systematic desensitization developed by Wolpe (1958). This approach can be designed in behavioral therapy terms or extended in- psychodynamic psychology terms. This has proven to be effective and can create a great deal of *experienced* security, especially in the case of reactive psychogenic forms of vertigo.

Prepared supported staged engagement

The common thread consists of a well-prepared and supported, staged confrontation with the individual situations that trigger vertigo. Along the way and through this, a gradual improvement of the balance ability and a reduction of the – mostly inappropriate – fear can be achieved.

The procedure is divided into the following stages:
1. Identify as many as possible of the important situations and events that cause dizziness.
2. Creation of a hierarchy of fear- and dizziness-inducing stimuli
3. Educational phase (preparation)
4. Learning a relaxation method, for example, progressive muscle relaxation
5. Step-by-step confrontation with fear- and dizziness-inducing stimuli under relaxation

This includes the development of a coherent "condition model" for the person concerned, which includes organic and psychological aspects. In the process, the possibilities of new and more favorable coping strategies in dealing with emotions should become apparent. In the preparation, attention must be paid to whether the Ménière's sufferer is also able to follow along step by step.

Step 1 for the therapist

> Identify as many as possible of the important situations and events that cause dizziness.

The basic work is the elaboration and practical identification of the triggers and maintaining conditions. The therapist obtains information about triggering situations and constellations from the targeted collection of medical history and during therapy, as well as from balance training, for example. In this way, factors can be included and worked on which the person affected may not even be aware of in terms of their form and consequences. This can also include – psychodynamically – associations and fantasies of the patient.

Step 1 for the person concerned

- I pay attention to when and under what circumstances my dizziness or vertigo occurs.
- I try to distinguish which is organically triggered or if rather other factors play a role.
- **Diary**
  For this purpose, I use a diary and estimate the strength of vertigo and dizziness using the "Visual Analogue Scale".

- I ask people familiar to me how they see my dizziness and vertigo and gather clues and accompanying circumstances.

- **Step 2 for the therapist**

- Creation of a hierarchy of fear- and dizziness-inducing stimuli
- The stimuli that trigger anxiety and dizziness must be classified according to severity. This can be done by description, self-assessment and external assessment and, for example, with the help of the "visual analogue scale".

- **Step 2 for the person concerned**

Ranking of dizziness triggers

I sort and write down:

- What seems most threatening to me?
- What can be tackled first?
- What's the order in between?

- **Step 3 for the therapist**

Educational phase (preparation)

In the "educational phase", a model of the development of reactive dizziness is conveyed in order to clarify and learn the connections and possibilities of new and more favorable coping strategies in dealing with vertigo or dizziness. A central assumption of the educational phase is that behavior and experience do not proceed according to an "all-or-nothing principle", but in a sequence of phases.

In this process, a distinction is made between (ideally) four phases:

1. Preparing for a possible dizziness or vertigo -inducing situation
2. Face the possible situation causing dizziness
3. Perhaps being thrown off balance by the possible vertigo-inducing situation
4. Being rewarded for dealing with the possible situation that caused the dizziness

Imparting the necessary knowledge and jointly working out the active factors of the vertigo are usually the necessary prerequisites for further action and often take up the largest part of the work with the affected person.

- **Step 3 for the person concerned**

Do I know enough?

- What did I understand about the clinical picture and the disease process, both the organic and the psychological pattern?

- Can I already distinguish organically caused dizziness and vertigo from psychogenic triggered dizziness?
- Does that model make sense to me?
- What else do I want or need to ask?

▪ **Step 4 for the therapist and the person concerned**

- Learning a relaxation method
- In order to influence the physiological tension, relaxation training is instructed, preferably progressive muscle relaxation according to Jacobson.
- This can also be done in parallel by the person concerned with the help of a CD.
- Step-by-step confrontation with fear- and dizziness-inducing stimuli under relaxation.

▪ **Step 5a for the therapist**

Practice phase

In the exercise phase, the aim is to convey coping options, which are then tested in the form of mental images. On the level of recognition and understanding, in Ménière's disease, the content must be the practice of the recognition pattern of psychogenic versus inner ear-related dizziness.

In the practice phase, the "not yet sure of their balance" should learn more and more ways of coping, which are also tested in the form of mental images.

For example, exemplary situations can be worked through according to the ABC scheme introduced into cognitive behavioral therapy by Albert Ellis (◘ Fig. 7.5).

The ABC scheme describes how thoughts influence feelings:

- A – activating events: the triggering event
- B – beliefs: the evaluative thoughts about the event
- C – consequences: consequences that follow as a reaction to the thoughts (feelings and behavior)

Later Ellis added aspects D and E to the Scheme.

- D – disputation: a confrontation with irrational thoughts
- E – effect: Replacing irrational thoughts with rational thoughts

This provides an opportunity to identify important components in the development or maintenance of vertigo and – as far as possible – to change them.

a: (Situation)	
b: (Thoughts)	**d**: (Changed thoughts)
c: (Feeling)	**e**: (Changed feelings)

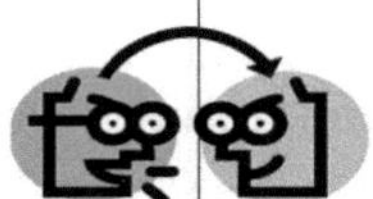

Fig. 7.5 Worksheet for mental images along with the ABC scheme with the possibility of change in thought and action

▪ Thoughts influence feelings

An important Part of the work is on "D", working on the changeable thoughts that can lead to "E" = changed feelings and reactions.

(A) I want to go shopping and experience (C) dizziness. (B) could be: I probably won't make it, I'm sure I'll get dizzy again. As (D) could be worked out that the second step can succeed if the first is taken, which can lead to (E) a more successful attempt.

▪ Thoughts can increase dizziness

Wirth (2000) has been able to collect from his patients with vertigo a variety of thoughts that "reinforce vertigo" and anxiety, such as:

- "What will people think of me if I falter like this?"
- "I may have to die now!"

- "I feel like something's broken in my head!"
- "I'm sure I'll fall and hurt myself!"
- "I can't take it anymore with these vertigo attacks!"
- "The dizziness never stops!"
- "I can't get through this dizzy spell!"
- "I'm being thrown off track!"
- "The rug is pulled out from under me!"
- "I'm losing my grip on the world!"

In addition, there can be the usually increasing recognition and then also the processing of influencing factors, which may not even be conscious for the person suffering from vertigo.

▪ Thoughts can improve balance

Recognizing these thoughts and the structure of thoughts and actions based on them leads to an understanding of the always individual concerns and needs of the patient. It also makes it possible to check them against reality and to "work through" the resulting possibilities for action and consequences.

For this purpose – based on the respective pattern of the individual affected person – "more helpful thoughts on the possibility of improved equilibrium " can usually be worked out, such as:
- "I'm sure the dizziness will stop soon!"
- "If I fix my eyes on a specific point, I can make vertigo (in certain types of vertigo) stop!"
- "I'm trying to be really calm and focus on my breath!"
- "It's "just" my vertigo, otherwise I'm fine!"

▪ Plan for difficult situations

With Ménière's disease, it is also a matter of taking precautionary measures in order to be able to move from fear and helplessness to self-determined and, if necessary, supported action and to have "a plan" for difficult situations. As already mentioned, it is important to learn to distinguish between Ménière's vertigo and anxiety vertigo.

▪ Step 5a for the person concerned

- Replaying the situations in your mind
- Collecting fears, seemingly difficult to understand and possible alternatives

▪ Step 5b for the therapist

Application phase

The application phase is focused on the step-by-step confrontation with the situation that triggers dizziness while relaxing. As a rule, one should start with the lower degrees of severity in order to be able to make positive experiences, no matter how small they may be, especially at the beginning.

- **Hands-on experience**

The gradually learned forms of coping must then be increasingly tried out – even in otherwise "dizzying" situations.

This can be approached as "self-directed" (Hoffmann 2008) or within the framework of a therapy session. Video documentation for individual follow-up helps to accelerate the learning behavior significantly.

The implementation of a self-directed vertigo exposure is associated with

- the challenge of looking as closely as possible at the threatening scene (to see as closely as possible what is happening), despite vertigo and the fear of it;
- the therapist's offer to talk about it in detail in the following lesson (to understand what is behind it);
- the possibility, at least in the imagination, to take the therapist into the situation.

- **Everyday situations are included**

In the process, the application of the relaxation learned in the meantime should be able to be used against the anxiety and the feeling of dizziness. In the course, other everyday situations with higher degrees of difficulty are then included.

- **Step 5b for the person concerned**

- *What can I actively address?*
- What do I learn from trying it out?
- What support do I need?
- What can I do myself?
- Does progressive muscle relaxation (PMR) help?
- *What can be done better – where is the problem?*
- What's next, what can I practice?
- What do I need help for?
- What do I need patience or more effort for?
- What is realistic?
- What do I learn from the situation?
- What goes better, where do I have to repeat?
- Do I see my goal as realistic and achievable?
- If applicable: what do I need for this? How can I determine and experience my success?

The therapeutic process should not end before important, very concrete situations have been successfully tried out. This is the only way to learn to cope with the situations that had caused dizziness.

It is favorable if the former dizzy person is allowed to become his own therapist at the end. Then he can also call up previous companions inwardly, but no longer has to call them. Psychodynamic psychological therapies also strive to work on triggering conscious and unconscious associations as well as possibly causing conflicts and deficits.

The concept of systematic desensitization, which has been well evaluated in terms of its effectiveness, can apparently be modified in its details and arrangement without compromising its effectiveness (Reinecker 2012).

▪ For the hurried and the brave

Confrontation until dizziness subsides

If the sufferer and therapist both feel good about each other and the outcome of the attempt, this process can also be addressed more quickly in a confrontation, high-level challenge.

Confrontation means the selection of a situation feared by the patient, in this case, associated with "dizziness", whereby the focus is primarily on the generally unpleasant avoidance behavior. The most important technical rule is that the patient should remain in a stressful situation until there is a clear reduction in fear and anxiety – and also in the experience of dizziness. This can take up to 100–120 minutes.

The patient, who must have a high degree of motivation and resilience, will experience that the feared expectations do not occur, whether under the guidance of the therapist or with a self-management to be learned by then.

I have had a good experience with the described procedure of "systematic desensitization", whereby this was mainly carried out in an inpatient setting. With all the modifications that are certainly possible, it seems important that

- Avoidance is processed,
- Fear is at least reduced,
- circling thoughts are stopped and
- new, helpful experiences can be made in practice.

> Important elements of all psychotherapeutic procedures are understanding and confidence.

All psychotherapeutic workers look at the whole tangle of problems with the help of their possibilities. The difference lies in the approach. Figuratively this could mean: They pick up different threads from the problem (symptom) tangle, especially at the beginning, which they then follow – together with the patient.

Three things are really important here:

1. Patients need to be understood by the therapist, and the therapist needs to understand them – usually through understanding their history (biographies).
2. Patients need to gain confidence that the therapist can be a competent partner in solving their problem, and the therapist needs to be competent.
3. Patients must have the motivation and will to get better, and the therapist must have an interest in progress.

Relationship: therapist – affected person

The motivation for change is – understandably – often only given in deep distress. Otherwise, what is the point of changing anything? In the end, the people affected have to enable and implement the solutions themselves. Therapists should – like mountain guides – professionally "accompany" the uninformed hiker.

Trial sessions useful

When looking for a suitable therapist, it makes sense to visit more than one psychotherapist and then decide after a trial session. It can also be helpful to get advice from friends or acquaintances. This may reveal that many more people have sought psychotherapeutic help than you thought.

Assistance possible

I only came to psychotherapy when I couldn't help it and was so shaken by my vertigo attacks and my dizziness that I thought I wouldn't be able to get up at all. During psychotherapy, I not only received a lot of help and learned a lot about myself anew, but it also saved my life in situations where I really didn't know what it was all about anymore.

So it is no wonder that I subjectively come to a positive assessment here. This cannot be generalized, and certainly, psychotherapy as a highly effective method also has side effects. One of them is that one has gained a different approach to oneself through the therapeutic accompaniment and cannot simply carry on as before. This can be painful, because the familiar, even if it is associated with unpleasantness, often still has something homely familiar, which one does not want to give up so quickly and usually cannot immediately.

From my, in the meantime also "professional" psychotherapeutic point of view, psychotherapeutic support becomes necessary when problems of coping with illness occur and the ability to live, love and work are endangered. It is particularly necessary when a psychogenic dizziness take part. Then experts are needed and often successful, and these experts are called medical or psychological psychotherapists.

7.4.6 Psychotropic Drugs

▪ Devil stuff or help?

The possibility of being able to influence mental problems with medication, psychotropic drugs, is often beneficial and at the same time seductive.

Without doubt, psychiatric drugs can help to endure the misery and suppress the symptoms. This is what many patients also expect. What is not appropriate is, that too much anxiety is tackled with diazepam-like agents.

Without brain no dizziness – but also no safe orientation, that is one consequence, the other that too many slowly but surely stumble in the direction of addiction. So caution is advisable especially with "sleeping pills and tranquilizers".

Unfortunately, the fear of addiction that rightly exists with diazepam medications make it difficult to use even the psychiatric drugs that can be quite helpful and not addictive.

▪ Support with antidepressants or neuroleptics

Antidepressant medications make one somewhat more thick-skinned in the face of psychological vulnerabilities and provide more support on the outside. Neuroleptics can favorably influence agonizing symptoms of persecutory anxiety, mental-motor excitations, hallucinations and, to a certain extent, disorders in psychoses of the schizophrenic type.

▪ Sometimes necessary or helpful

If depression develops or comes to the fore in or due to Ménière's disease, antidepressant or neuroleptic medication – as support – can be quite useful. Sometimes they are even necessary in order to be able to come into therapeutic contact in the first place, and then we also use them. In the best case, they can initiate a turnaround in the course of the disease, even if they do not cure the disease itself. Consequently, they have a similar function as crutches for a broken leg: they are usually temporary help.

The Psychiatrist Staab (2012) has found that anxiety may be a significant factor in long-lasting dizziness. As outlined in ► Chap. 3, connections of the fear circuit in the limbic system with central processing pathways allow the threshold for impulses from the vestibular organs to increase (Balaban et al. 2011). This means that there may be a reduction in the flow of information from the affected vestibular organ due to the fear response. The neurotransmitters effective in this process appear to be primarily serotonin or its counterparts, which are "neurotransmitters" known from anxiety development. For this reason, it may be useful to think of antidepressants to reduce this inhibitory component (Staab 2012).

Popkirov et al. (2018) stated:

> A positive response seems not to depend on the presence of psychiatric symptoms as treatment may help patients with PPPD but without psychiatric comorbidity. As expected, comorbid symptoms of depression and anxiety, where present, also improved. Dosing needs to start slowly and effects are usually seen with doses in the lower half of the ranges recommended for depression. As in many functional disorders, patients may be particularly sensitive to side effects, which led to one in five patients stopping during trials. (…)

Clinical response is usually seen after 8–12 weeks, and, if effective, medication should be continued for at least 1 year.

- **Antidepressants for the balance inhibiting anxiety component?**

However, this should not be the first measure and certainly not the only one. First and foremost, after appropriate explanation, should be active balance training, unless the person suffering from vertigo is so depressed that he needs appropriate antidepressant medication because of it.

Irrespective of vertigo, it has also been shown that the effectiveness of antidepressants depends to a large extent on the patient's education and cooperation, which often has to be obtained first (Kocsis et al. 2009).

- **Psychotropic drugs alone are no solution**

Thus psychotropic drugs have their justification, as a transitional regulation and as a support of other measures. However, psychotropic drugs should under no circumstances be used against the organically caused vertigo or the fear of vertigo. This prevents therapeutic changes. To ensure that psychotropic drugs are used professionally, a specialist in psychotherapy, psychiatry or a doctor with the additional competence of psychotherapy should also be consulted. A reflexive prescribing is rarely helpful.

7.4.7 Inpatient Psychosomatic Treatment

Inpatient treatment may become necessary if the treatment options for outpatients have been exhausted and/or the individual options are too limited or insufficient.

Inpatient treatment should include the following elements:

- **Therapy coordination**

Precise diagnostics: A good neuro-otological and psychosomatic diagnosis is required for clarification. Both sides need to clarify whether the vertigo attacks are attacks from the inner ear or psychogenic forms of dizziness and/or accompanying or reactive depressive crises.

- Information tailored to the patient, which is also understood by the person concerned in such a way that he or she can recognize causes and possible developments and influence them at least in part.
- *Professional psychotherapeutic support* must be able to address the psychological components in particular and facilitate changes in the way of (experiencing) life.
- Individually tailored *balance training* is designed to compensate for and help build up the delicate balance situation.
- If there is a hearing loss, with or without tinnitus, hearing aid provision should be possible. This should be supported by specific training.

The group around Eckhardt-Henn has derived a step-by-step plan (Tschan et al. 2012), which has unfortunately already ended again,

Stages for renewed stability

1. Physical exercises (needed for everyday fitness)
2. Balance training, in the simplest case on a "seesaw board" and/or along the exercise sequence (described below) of Cawthorne and Friedmann (1969) and Cooksey (1946).
3. Relaxation training (PMR)
4. Diary work
5. Exposure exercise
6. Cognitive restructuring of the thoughts reinforcing the dizziness
7. Activation of resources to improve the quality of life
8. Critical examination of the function of vertigo, also with the parts that are unconscious for the patient
9. Motivation for outpatient psychotherapy

The patient's task here is to take up recognizable and comprehensible possibilities for action and to try new steps.

■ Own investigations (I)

For the first time, we examined a total of 96 Ménière's disease patients admitted as inpatients for 6–8 weeks between 1994 and 1997 (Schaaf et al. 2000).

We found:

- 41% (n = 39) well-compensated patients with sufficient management of vertigo for them. They suffered more from hearing loss and/or tinnitus condition.
- 59% (n = 57) with reactive psychogenic dizziness components that dominated the clinical picture.

In 1998, we interviewed all 96 patients with standardized and structured questionnaires about the further course and invited them to a follow-up examination. Of these, 60% (n = 58) responded. Of these patients, 21 came for clinical follow-up.

■ A reduction in vertigo – even a persistent one – is achiev able

There was a statistically significant [$t(20) = 5.28$, $p < 0.001$] reduction in vertigo attacks from an average of 4 attacks per month before treatment ($M = 3.95$, $SD = 2.87$) to less than 1 attack per month after treatment ($M = 0.52$, $SD = 0.93$).

■ Own investigations (II)

Results of a follow-up investigation

Inspired by the discussions about the basics of "chronic subjective vertigo", we looked up the vertigo patients we treated at the Tinnitus Clinic, Dr. Hesse. We wanted to know whether our inpatient neurotological and psychotherapeutic treatment, which also focuses on vestibular disorders, helps to cope with vertigo in the long term (Schaaf u. Hesse 2015).

In 4 years, we treated 96 patients who had already returned home 1 year or more after treatment at the time of the follow-up examination. These patients were admitted – except for six – with clinical pictures from the ENT area after the originally organic dizziness problem had lasted longer. This clearly distinguishes our patient group from "psychosomatic clinics", where the psychological component is usually the sole or predominant focus.

At the time of follow-up, at least 1 year (mean 32.5 months; SD = 15.39) after discharge, 18 of 23 patients (78%) reported a sustained reduction in their vertigo symptoms. This was largely consistent with the results of the test diagnostic (HADS-D) for anxiety and depression development. Four patients reported unchanged vertigo sensations the same, *one* patient who became vertigo free during the stay suffered again from the for him intangible vertigo months after discharge – under the same circumstances that brought him to us.

This shows that – under the optimal conditions of a clinic designed for this purpose – stable improvements are possible in the long term, at least for this group of patients, even in the case of persistent vertigo complaints. This result differs from the rather sobering results of some meta-analyses, in which psychotherapeutic measures showed improvements during treatment, but which usually did not remain stable in the longer term (Holmberg et al. 2007; Schmid et al. 2011).

A comprehensive body and psyche diagnosis as well as a clarification certainly contributed to the pleasing result. The focus of the therapy was not so much on the residual handicap, but rather on the healthy person who was still present and able to function. Great importance was attached to repeated medical education, which most of the patients considered to be an important element even afterwards.

Psychotherapeutically and in balance therapy, the emphasis was placed above all on the cognitive processes and the implementation in direct experience. The often existing functionalization were at least thematized.

If anxiety and/or depression or psychiatric illnesses requiring treatment were found to be significant comorbidity, these were also treated with medication in half of those affected.

Certainly critical to the continued success is that 12 of the 18 (66%) persistently improved patients continued the learned therapies at home. For most, this meant continuing psychotherapy as outpatients as well.

7.5 Alternatives/Outsiders: Opportunities and Threats

After the description of medical and psychological approaches, some "alternative approaches" will now be briefly presented. This seems necessary, as conventional medicine leaves many questions unanswered in the case of chronic diseases such as Ménière's disease. Therefore, it is understandable that one looks for alternative methods of treatment which offer them the prospect of help, but which often also cost them "dearly".

▪ Help or dependence?

Alternative therapies" can also have their meaning, if it is about holding on, also about hoping or if they are meant as bridging with the idea "You will manage to go through life again with your own strength". They are dangerous and worsen the situation when the phrase is, "You're going to need it or you're going to need me."

Two important approaches will be described in a little more detail: Homeopathy and acupuncture.

7.5.1 Homeopathy

Homeopathy focuses less on a specific disease, such as Ménière's disease, and more on the whole person. At the beginning of treatment, there is a longer survey of the medical history from specific points of view. Once the person is "recorded", homeopaths look for a remedy that will strengthen him. Homeopathy assumes that the body is already trying everything to become healthy and that it must be supported in these efforts. To do this, homeopathic remedies are used to increase its energies.

When choosing a homeopathic medicine, the main idea is that same is cured with the same. Thus the medicine, whether taken as globules (small balls) or as drops, ideally triggers the same symptoms as the disease itself. For example, toxic substances such as arsenic and mercury are used, but in such a diluted form that conventional doctors deny any effect – positive or negative. Homeopaths, however, call the dilutions they make "potentizations", and for them, the most effective remedy is the one that has been diluted the furthest.

7.5.2 Acupuncture

- **Energy flow is to be directed**

Acupuncture is intended to direct the energy flow of the person into healing channels. In order to detect the disturbed energy flow, acupuncture is also preceded by a detailed, again specific survey of the medical history. In the meantime, there are many explanations for the effect of acupuncture, also from orthodox medicine. Especially the "Yin and Yang concept" can be reconciled with the two parts of the autonomic nervous system. However, there is – as far as I can judge (!) – no evidence that acupuncture can organically influence Ménière's disease.

Literature

Adrion C, Fischer CS, Wagner J, Gürkov R, Mansmann U, Strupp M (2016) Efficacy and safety of betahistine treatment in patients with Menière's disease: primary results of a long term, multicentre, double blind, randomised, placebo controlled, dose defining trial (BEMED trial) BMJ 2016, 352:h6816. https://doi.org/10.1136/bmj.h6816

Ammon HPT (1991) Arzneimittelneben- und -wechselwirkungen. Wissenschaftliche Verlagsgesellschaft, Stuttgart

Baier G, Ott I (2008) Die chirurgische Therapie des M. Menière Entwicklung und heutiger Stand. HNO 56:553–566

Balaban CD, Jacob RG, Furman JM (2011) Neurologic bases for comorbidity of balance disorders, anxiety disorders and migraine: neurotherapeutic implications. Expert Rev Neurother 11(3):379–394. https://doi.org/10.1586/ern.11.19

Basta D, Ernst A (2008) Moderne Rehabilitation von Gleichgewichtsstörungen mit Hilfe von Neurofeedback-Trainingsverfahren. HNO 56:990–995

Basura GJ, Adams ME, Monfared A, Schwartz SR, Antonelli PJ, Burkard R, Bush ML, Bykowski J, Colandrea M, Derebery J, Kelly EA, Kerber KA, Koopman CF, Kuch AA, Marcolini E, McKinnon BJ, Ruckenstein MJ, Valenzuela CV, Vosooney A, Walsh SA, Nnacheta LC, Dhepyasuwan N, Buchanan EM (2020) Clinical practice guideline: Ménière's disease. Executive summary. Otolaryngol Head Neck Surg 162(4):415–434

Burgess A, Kundu S (2006) Diuretics for Menière's disease or syndrome. Cochrane Database Syst Rev (Cochrane Library) 2010(4):CD003599

Cawthorne TE, Friedmann G (1969) Head movement exercises in the therapy of disorders of the equilibrium. Schweiz Med Wochenschr 99: 156–158

Cooksey FS (1946) Rehabilitation in vestibular injuries. Proc R Soc Med 39:273–278

Crane BT, Minor LB, Della Santina CC, Carey JP (2009) Middle ear exploration in patients with Ménière's disease who have failed outpatient intratympanic gentamicin therapy. Otol Neurotol 30:619–624

Devantier L, Hougaard D, Händel MN, Liviu-Adelin Guldfred F, Schmidt JH, Djurhuus B, Callesen HE (2020) Using betahistine in the treatment of patients with Menière's disease: a meta-analysis with the current randomized-controlled evidence. Acta Otolaryngol 140(10):845–853. https://doi.org/10.1080/00016489.2020.1777326. Epub 2020 Jun 25

Ernst A (2011) Perspektiven der Gleichgewichtsdiagnostik und -therapie. Laryngo-Rhino-Otol 90(Supplement 1):35–S43

Espinosa-Sanchez JM, Lopez-Escamez JA (2016) Menière's disease. Handb Clin Neurol 137:257–277

Forge A, Li L, Nevill G (1998) Hair cell recovery in the vestibular sensory epithelia of mature Guinea pigs. J Comp Neurol 397:69–88

Fowler EP (1948) Streptomycine treatment of vertigo. Trans Am Acad Ophthalmol Otol 53:293–301

Gabra N, Asmar MH, Berbiche D, Saliba I (2016) Endolymphatic duct blockage: quality of life assessment of a novel surgical technique for Menière disease. Eur Arch. https://doi.org/10.1007/s00405-015-3890-4

Gacek RR (2015) Recovery of hearing in Meniere's disease after antiviral treatment. Am J Otolaryngol 36(3):315–323

Gleich O, Strutz J, Schmid K (2008) Endolymph-Homöostase und M. Menière Grundlagen, pathologische Veränderungen, Aminoglykoside. HNO 56:1243–1252

7

Gottshall KR, Hoffer ME, Moore RJ (2005) The role of vestibular rehabilitation in the treatment of Menière's disease. Otolaryngol Head Neck Surg 133(3):p326–p328

Gstöttner W, Adunka O (2004) Labyrinthanästhesie bei M. Menière. HNO 52:265

Gürkov R, Flatz W, Keeser D (2013) Effect of standard-dose Betahistine on endolymphatic hydrops: an MRI pilot study. Eur Arch Otorhinolaryngol 270:1231–1235

Harcourt JP, Lambert A, Wong PY, Patel M, Agarwal K, Golding JF, Bronstein AM (2019) Long-term follow-up of Intratympanic methylprednisolone versus gentamicin in patients with unilateral Menière's disease. Otol Neurotol 40:491–496

Helling K (2008) Otolithenfunktionsstörungen und Therapieoptionen. HNO 56:996–1002

Helling K (2015) HNO update. Vestibuläre Störungen. In: Iro H, Werner JA (eds) HNO Update 2015 – Handbuch HNO 2015/2016. med update, Wiesbaden

Helms J (1985) Die chirurgische Therapie des Morbus Menière. In: Verhandlungsbericht der Deutschen Gesellschaft für Hals-Nasen-Ohrenheilkunde. Arch Otorhinolaryngol Suppl 1:67–118

Hesse G (Hg) (2015) Tinnitus. 2. Aufl. Thieme, Stuttgart

Hillier SL, McDonnell, M (2011) Vestibular rehabilitation for unilateral peripheral vestibular dysfunction. Cochrane Database Syst Rev 2:CD005397

Hillman TA, Chen DA, Arriaga MA (2004) Vestibular nerve section versus intratympanic gentamicin for Menière's disease. Laryngoscope 114(2):216–222

Hoffmann SO (2008) Psychodynamische Therapie von Angststörungen. Einführung und Manual für die kurz- und mittelfristige Therapie. Schattauer, Stuttgart

Holmberg J, Karlberg M, Harlacher U, Magnusson M (2007) One-year follow-up of cognitive behavioral therapy for phobic postural vertigo. J Neurol 254:1189e92

Huang TS (ed) (1991) Menière's disease: recent advances in basic and clinical aspects. Acta Otolaryngol Suppl 485:7–154

Huon LK, Fang TY, Wang PC (2012) Outcomes of intratympanic gentamicin injection to treat Menière's disease. Otol Neurotol 33:706–714

Jahnke K (1994) Stadiengerechte Therapie der Menièreschen Krankheit. Dtsch Arztebl 91:428–434

James AI, Burton MJ (2011) Betahistine for Menière's disease syndrome. Cochrane Database Syst Rev. https://doi.org/10.1002/14651858.CD001873

Kitahara M (ed) (1990) Menière's disease. Springer, Berlin/Heidelberg/New York

Kocsis JH, Leon AC, Markowitz JC, Manber R, Arnow B, Klein DN, Thase ME (2009) Patient preference as a moderator of outcome for chronic forms of major depressive disorder treated with nefazodone, cognitive behavioral analysis system of psychotherapy, or their combination. J Clin Psychiat 3:354–361. http://psycnet.apa.org/doi/10.4088/JCP.08m04371; https://doi.org/10.4088/JCP.08m04371

Lang J (2003) Anatomie des vestibulären Systems. In: Haid CT (Hrsg). aus interdisziplinärer Sicht. Thieme, Stuttgart, pp 4–16

Lange G (1977) Die intratympanale Behandlung des Morbus Menière mit ototoxischen Antibiotika. Laryngorhinotologie 56:409–411

Lange G (1998) Die Gentamicin-Injektionstechnik: Eine Vereinfachung der transtympanalen Therapie des Morbus Menière. HNO 46:1000–1002

Link R, Berendes J, Zöller F (Hrsg) (1980) Handbuch der HNO-Heilkunde, Bd III, Teil II. Thieme, Stuttgart

Löhle E (1980) Der Einfluss einer sechswöchigen Vitaminmangelernährung auf die Sinneszellen des Innenohrs. Z Ernährungswiss 19:203–214

Magnusson M, Padoan S, Karlberg M, Johansson R (1991) Delayed onset of ototoxic effects of gentamicin in patients with Menière's disease. Acta Otolaryngol Suppl 485:120–122

Martinez D (1972) The effect of Serc (betahistine hydrochloride) on the circulation of the inner ear in experimental animals. Acta Otolaryngol 305:29–47

Moller MN, Caye-Tomasen P, Thomsen JH (2009) Vestibular nerve section in the treatment of morbus Menière. Ugeskr Laeger 171(12):1000–1003

Montandon PB, Häusler RJ, Kimura RS (1985) Treatment of endolymphatic hydrops with cochleosacculotomy. Clinical results and experimental findings. Otolaryngol Head Neck Surg 93:615–621

Morgenstern C (1985) Pathophysiologie, Klinik und konservative Therapie der Menièreschen Erkrankung. Arch Otorhinolaryngol 1:1–66

Morgenstern C (1994) Morbus Menière. In: Naumann HH, Helms J, Herberhold C, Kastenabuer C (Hrsg) Oto-Rhino-Laryngologie in Klinik und Praxis, Bd 1: Ohr. Thieme, Stuttgart, S. 768–775

Naganuma H, Kawahara K, Tokumasu K, Okamoto M (2006) Water may cure patients with Menière disease. Laryngoscope 116(8):1455–1460

Nevoux J, Viengchareun S, Lema I, Lecoq AL, Ferrary E, Lombès M (2015) Glucocorticoids stimulate endolymphatic water reabsorption in inner ear through aquaporin 3 regulation. Pflugers Arch 467(9):1931–1943

Novoa E, Gärtner M, Henzen C (2014) Systemic effects of intratympanic dexamethasone therapy. Endocr Connect 3:127–131

Paparella MM (2006) Endolymphatic sac revision for recurrent intractable Menière's disease. Otolaryngol Clin N Am 4:713–721

Park JJ, Luedeke I, Luecke K, Emmerling O, Westhofen M (2013) Eustachian tube function in patients with inner ear disorders. Eur Arch Otorhinolaryngol 270:1615–1621

Patel M, Agarwal K, Arshad Q, Hariri M, Rea P, Seemungal BM, Golding JF, Harcourt JP, Bronstein AM (2016) Intratympanic methylprednisolone versus gentamicin in patients with unilateral Ménière's disease: a randomised, double-blind, comparative eff ectiveness trial. Lancet 388:2753–2762

Plontke SK (2011) Evaluation of the round window niche before local drug delivery to the inner ear using a new mini-otoscope. Otol Neurotol 32:183–185

Plontke SK, Gürkov R (2015) Morbus Menière. Facharztwissen HNO. LRO 94:530–554

Plontke SK, Mynatt R, Gill RM (2007) Concentration gradient along the scala tympani after local application of gentamicin to the round window membrane. Laryngoscope 117:1191–1198

Popkirov S, Staab JP, Stone J (2018) Persistent postural-perceptual dizziness (PPPD): a common, characteristic and treatable cause of chronic dizziness. Pract Neurol 18:5–13

Postema RJ, Kingma CM, Wit HP (2008) Intratympanic gentamicin therapy for control of vertigo in unilateral Menire's disease: a prospective, double-blind, randomized, placebo-controlled trial. Acta Otolaryngol 128(8):876–880

Pullens B, van Benthem PP (2011) Intratympanic gentamicin for Menière's disease or syndrome Cochrane Database Syst Rev 3:CD008234

Pullens B, Giard JL, Verschuur HP, van Benthem PP. (2021) Surgery for Ménière's disease. Cochrane Database Syst Rev 2010(1):Art. No.:

CD005395. https://doi.org/10.1002/14651858.CD005395.pub2. Accessed 07 February 2021

Quaglieri S, Gatti O, Rebecchi E, Manfrin M, Tinelli C, Mira E, Benazzo M (2014) Intratympanic gentamicin treatment 'as needed' for Meniere's disease. Long-term analysis using the Kaplan-Meier method. Eur Arch Otorhinolaryngol 271:1443–1449

Radeloff A, Hamad M, Baier G, Helms J, Hagen R, Shehata-Dieler W (2009) Die Saccotomie in der Behandlung des M. Menière: Beurteilung der kurz-, mittel- und langfristigen Ergebnisse anhand eines Patientenfragebogens. Laryngorhino otologie 88:653–659

Rah YC, Han JJ, Park J, Choi BY, Koo JW (2014) Management of intractable Menière's disease after intratympanic injection of gentamicin. Laryngoscope 125(4):972–978. https://doi.org/10.1002/lary.v125.4/issuetoc

Rask-Andersen H, Danckwardt-Lilliestrom N, Friberg U (1991) Lymphocyte-macrophage activity in the human endolymphatic sac. Acta Otolaryngol Suppl 485:15–17

Reinecker H (2012) Verhaltenstherapie. In: Senf W, Broda M (Hrsg) Praxis der Psychotherapie. Thieme, Stuttgart, pp 217–219

Saliba I, Gabra N, Alzahrani M et al (2015) Endolymphatic duct blockage: a randomized controlled trial of a novel surgical technique for Menière's disease treatment. Otolaryngol Head Neck Surg 152(1):122–129

Salt AN, Gill RM, Plontke SK (2008) Dependence of hearing changes on the dose of intratympanically applied gentamicin: a meta-analysis using mathematical simulations of clinical drug delivery protocols. Laryngoscope 118:1793–1800

Schaaf H, Holtmann H, Hesse G, Rienhoff U, Brehmer D, Nelting M (2000) Reactive psychogenic dizziness in Menière's disease. In: Sterkers O, Ferrary E, Daumann R, Sauvage JP, Tran Ba Huy R (eds) Menière's disease 1999 – update. Kugler, The Hague, pp 505–511

Schlegel M, Vibert D, Ott SR, Häusler R, Caversaccio MD (2012) Functional results and quality of life after Retrosigmoid vestibular Neurectomy in patients with Ménière's disease. Otol Neurotol 33:1380–1385

Schmid G, Henningsen P, Dieterich M, Sattel H, Lahmann C (2011) Psychotherapy in dizziness: a systematic review. J Neurol Neurosurg Psychiatry 82:601e606. https://doi.org/10.1136/jnnp.2010.237388

Schuknecht HF (1957) Ablation therapy in the management of Menière's disease. Acta Otolaryngol Suppl 132:1–42

Staab J (2012) Chronic subjective dizziness. Continuum 18(5):1118–1141

Stokroos R, Kingma H (2004) Selective vestibular ablation by intratympanic gentamicin in patients with unilateral active Menière's disease: a prospective, double-blind, placebo-controlled, randomized clinical trial. Acta Otolaryngol 124(2):172–175

Thomsen J, Bretlau P, Bretlau P, Tos M, Johnson NJ (1981) Placebo effect in the surgery of Menière's disease: a double blind, placebo-controlled study on endolymphatic sac surgery. Arch Otolaryngol 107:271–277

Trinidade A, Robinson T, Phillips JS (2014) The role of caffeine in otorhinolaryngology: guilty as charged? Eur Arch Otorhinolaryngo 271(8):2097–2102. https://doi.org/10.1007/s00405-013-2648-0

Tschan R, Eckhardt-Henn A, Scheurich V, Best C, Dieterich M, Beutel M (2012) Standfest? Erste Ergebnisse der Entwicklung eines kognitiv-verhaltenstherapeutischen Gruppenschulungsprogramms zur Behandlung des somatoformen Schwindels. Psychother Psychosom Med Psychol 62(3–4):111–119

van Sonsbeek S, Pullens B, van Benthem P (2015) Positive pressure therapy for Menière's disease or syndrome. Cochrane Database Syst Rev 3:Art. No.: CD008419. https://doi.org/10.1002/14651858.CD008419.pub2

Vosteen KH (ed) (1981) Menière's disease. International symposium Düsseldorf. Thieme, Stuttgart

Walther LE (2005) Gestörtes Gleichgewicht: Wiederherstellende Verfahren bei gestörtem Gleichgewicht. Laryngo-Rhino-Otol 84: 70–98 und http://www.thieme-connect.de/ejournals/abstract/lro/doi/10.1055/s-2005-861144)

Wang D, Wang Z (1997) Regeneration and functional restoration of vestibular hair cells in Guinea pigs after gentamicin damage. Zhonghua Er Bi Yan Hou Ke Za Zhi 32:153–156

Weikert S, Rotter A, Scherer H, Hoelzl M (2008) Picrotoxin in der Therapie des Morbus Menière. Laryngorhinootologie 87(12):862–866

Westhofen M (2008) Die operative Therapie des vestibulären Schwindels. Verfahren und Indikationen. HNO 56:1003–1010

Westhofen M (2013) Indikation und Erfolge der operativen Therapie des vestibulären Schwindels. HNO 61:752–761

Wirth W (2000) Psychologische Möglichkeiten bei Schwindel. Tinnitus-Forum 4/2000

Wolpe J (1958) Psychotherapy by reciprocal inhibition. Stanford University Press, Palo Alto

Yardley L, Kirby S (2006) Evaluation of booklet-based self-management of symptoms in Menière disease: a randomized controlled trial. Psychosom Med 68(5):762–769

Bilateral Disease

Contents

8.1 Consequences – 250
8.1.1 For Therapy – 250
8.1.2 In Case of Bilateral Vestibular Loss – 251

8.2 Perspectives – 252

Literature – 253

H. Schaaf, *Ménière's Disease*, https://doi.org/10.1007/978-3-662-63610-7_8

Sometimes a tinnitus in the other ear, but too often a fluctuating hearing in the second (contralateral) ear is interpreted as a sign of bilateral Ménière's disease. In addition to this, hardly an ENT examiner will have had the possibility to distinguish between an organically caused and a (reactively) psychogenic added vertigo or dizziness.

Green et al. (1991) found in a follow-up period of 18 years: The longer the period between the onset of the disease and the examination of the patients, the higher the number of those who are found to have bilateral Ménière's *symptoms*. Thus, at the beginning of their investigation, they found 13% bilaterally affected patients, at the end 45%. This tendency and the percentages in this order of magnitude are confirmed by others, for example by Stahle et al. (in: Huang 1991, pp. 78–83) in 161 Swedish patients who were examined over 9 years, as well as by a Japanese multi-center study (Kitahara in: Huang 1991, pp. 74–77).

A review by House et al. (2006) over 4 decades showed that 11% of patients already had bilateral symptoms at initial diagnosis. A further 12% developed Ménière's symptoms in the other ear over a period of 5 years after initially having symptoms on one side. The average duration until the appearance of a complete Ménière's disease on the opposite ear was about 7.6 years.

More encouraging is a recent study by Perez et al. (2004). The result was "only" 5% bilateral Ménière's disease. This number deviates perhaps also because they had looked more closely and did not classify every endolymphatic fluctuation as a new Ménière's disease. Thus, the authors distinguished the additional low-frequency hearing loss occurring in 16% of unilateral Ménière's patients in the other ear as an additional hearing loss – and did not classify it as "now bilateral" Ménière's disease.

We also assume, without being able to examine it in detail, that Ménière's disease can be present on one side, while on the other side, for whatever reason, endolymphatic fluctuations can be present, which do not necessarily mean bilateral Ménière's disease.

8.1 Consequences

8.1.1 For Therapy

However, if bilateral Ménière's disease is present, it is treated with the same symptom-oriented measures as a unilateral condition. This certainly includes the trial of intratympanal administered cortisone. There are different opinions about the way of gentamycin elimination in the second affected ear.

The advocates of the saccotomy would also perform it bilaterally (Kitahara et al. 2014).

- **Gentamycin Via the Bloodstream**

Lang (2003) would not hesitate to use low doses of gentamycin on both sides. Jahnke (1999), on the other hand, tries to administer gentamycin cautiously via the blood route when conservative therapy is not effective. He assumes that here the line between the destruction of the vestibular organ and the destruction of hearing is wider than with the procedure via the middle ear.

In normal-weight patients, he initially administers 120 mg gentamycin/day twice over an initial period of 1 week, dissolved in 500 ml Ringer's solution over 2–3 hours and over a period of 5–6 days. If necessary, further gentamycin is applied in a second series (Jahnke and Arweiler 1997). With regard to vertigo the success rate was high with a follow-up period of about 5 years: 5 out of 6 patients were symptom-free.

8.1.2 In Case of Bilateral Vestibular Loss

Sometimes bilateral Ménière's disease can progress to the point where both sides show serious loss of function. In this case, the attacks of dizziness and vertigo may stop, but there is also a loss of balance with unsteady gait. Since the vestibulo-ocular reflex (VOR) can no longer be effective, the affected person experiences his surroundings during a head movement as others do through a camera: The image shakes with the movement. When the affected person shakes his head, it looks to him as if the opposite person is jumping or moving.

Uncertainty increases when orientation via the eyes is restricted, for example in the dark, when the toilet has to be visited at night. Uncertainty also increases when the sensitive nerves of the soles of the feet are restricted, then orientation via the standing and walking surface is more difficult.

For example, bilateral sufferers have a hard time when they have to walk in the dark on a surface that is unfamiliar to them, perhaps still irregular or even slippery. Most learn to avoid this, or they use a stick or hold on to someone.

The most important thing in treatment is to improve the ability to compensate. These include:

- Provide for the optimal supply for visual acuity (glasses)
- Avoidance of all things that can impair the vestibular system (especially alcohol, which damages the sensitive

nerve endings, e.g. under the feet, and the structures in the brain, but also sedative drugs).
- Establishment and knowledge of walking routes and their possible obstacles, as far as possible – at least at home and at work.
- Optimal hearing aids or cochlea implants

Balance Training and Fall Prevention

Preventing falls involves avoiding risks that can be avoided, such as standing too close to a platform (before the train stops) or even diving.

Many things can be changed at home to reduce the risk of falls.
- Well-fitting shoes that provide a firm grip, especially in the heel area, are important.
- Tripping hazards such as small rugs, ledges on doorsteps and loose cables should be removed.
- Adequate space can be created between furniture to allow for wide enough walkways.
- The path from the bed to the toilet must be free of tripping hazards and illuminated at night Motion detectors with bright but not blinding lighting can help.
- In case of urge to urinate at night, man can also help himself with a urine bottle, and woman with a toilet chair next to the bed
- Installing handholds, non-slip bath mats in the bathtub or shower
- Handrails or railings on stairs
- Beds need to be high enough so that you don't have to stand up from bending over
- The use of hip protectors has resulted in a significant reduction in fractures after falls. What is needed is proper training in the use of hip protectors.
- And just in case, for people living alone: a functioning simple emergency call system (alarm systems at the bedside).

Always balance training possibly with neurofeedback (Basta and Ernst 2008), can be useful.

8.2 Perspectives

Although the outlook for bilateral disease isn't rosy, an upright gait is possible even after complete loss of both vestibular organs.

■ Cochlea Implant and "Lips Reading" Training

With regard to hearing compensation, the development is becoming more and more hopeful. In the case of hearing loss that can no longer be compensated by hearing aids, "cochlea implants" are now being used. Together with "lips reading" training (although there is nothing "to read" from the lips), the ability to communicate can be restored to a large extent. In most cases, patients can even use the telephone again.

Of course, I myself am also afraid that I could still be facing something in this respect. However, the knowledge of a possible, humane way of dealing with it and, above all, the experiences I had after stopping my vertigo with gentamycin give me hope, that even bilateral Ménière's disease does not mean the end of a life.

■ Signs Accompanying Spoken Languages, Speech Computer

For me, it is sometimes also helpful to deal with the worst possibility, even if the danger of becoming completely deaf is not very likely. I am closely following the development of speech computers and would like to learn more about visual recognition techniques.

Literature

Basta D, Ernst A (2008) Moderne Rehabilitation von Gleichgewichtsstörungen mit Hilfe von Neurofeedback-Trainingsverfahren. HNO 56:990–995

Green D, Blum DJ, Harner SG (1991) Longitudinal follow-up of patients with Menière's disease. Otolaryngol Head Neck Surg 104:783–788

House JW, Doherty JK, Fisher LM, Derebery MJ, Berliner KI (2006) Menière's disease: prevalence of contralateral ear involvement. Otol Neurotol 27:355–361

Huang TS (ed) (1991) Menière's disease: recent advances in basic and clinical aspects. Acta Otolaryngol Suppl 485:7–154

Jahnke K (1999) Interview zu M. Menière. Tinnitus Forum 2:14

Jahnke K, Arweiler D (1997) Die intravenöse Gentamycintherapie bei beidseitigem M. Menière. Laryngorhinootologie 76:519–522

Kitahara T, Horii A, Imai T, Ohta Y, Morihana T, Inohara H, Sakagami M (2014) Does endolymphatic sac decompression surgery prevent bilateral development of unilateral Ménière disease? Laryngoscope 124:1932–1936

Lang J (2003) Anatomie des vestibulären Systems. In: Haid CT (ed) Schwindel aus interdisziplinärer Sicht. Thieme, Stuttgart, pp 4–16

Perez R, Chen JM, Nedzelski JM (2004) The status of the contralateral ear in established unilateral Menière's disease. Laryngoscope 114(8): 1373–1376

What Might Make a Good Therapist?

Contents

9.1 Careful Diagnostics – 257

9.2 Comprehensible Enlightenment – 257

9.3 Therapeutic Measures – 258

9.4 Support and Therapy Between Vertigo Attacks – 259

9.5 Psychological Measures – 259

9.6 What Might Make a Good Patient? – 260

9.6.1 Factors that Can Be Influenced – 260

9.6.2 Compensable Factors – 260

9.6.3 And myself? – 261

Literature – 262

H. Schaaf, *Ménière's Disease*, https://doi.org/10.1007/978-3-662-63610-7_9

The answer therefore remains complex and – as already suspected – in the end somewhat open. This is also due to the fact that there is neither "the *Ménière's disease*" nor "the Ménière's patient".

For example, there are:

- Ménière's sufferers who are quickly back on their feet after the attack and a relatively short period of rest and tick off the attack
- Ménière's disease sufferers who are distressed for a long time afterwards and depressively relive the event
- Quite a few Ménière's sufferers who anxiously await the next attack, so that the psychogenic anxiety and dizziness component becomes the decisive part of Ménière's disease

Even if one wants to know "with certainty" what exactly constitutes Ménière's disease, one encounters definitional and demarcation difficulties up to the view that Ménière's disease does not exist at all, and there is only a syndrome that is named after Prosper Meniere. The only thing that is sure is that it has to be an inner ear disease, that is accompanied by vertigo, hearing loss and tinnitus and can possibly be influenced by many organic and psychosomatic factors.

Unfortunately, it is also still sure that there is no real cure for Ménière's disease. Instead, the number of therapeutic suggestions is as large as it is confusing with regard to success criteria and not infrequently depending on the point of view.

▪ Effects on the Whole Person

It is certain that the symptoms triggered by the inner ear disease – at least with – have effects on the whole person. Thus, the typical spinning attacks are often accompanied by fears of death and destruction. If this event, which is experienced as existentially threatening, occurs more often, the fear of repetition understandably grows. In the process, the fear can become so dominant, that it is itself experienced as insecurity and vertigo, up to and including a feeling of rotary vertigo, and becomes a disease component in its own right.

That's why it would make more sense to ask: who is to recommend for what in the disease? So who can help in time of need?

In principle, Ménière's disease falls within the field of expertise of the ENT physician. Also neurologists can be involved within the scope of their competence in vertigo, but normally general practitioners come in contact first with the patients and remain companions during the disease, if it is shaped well for the patient. Psychosomatics are also (usually the last) to see essential aspects in the development and maintenance of Ménière's disease that cannot be covered by the organists.

It can seem striking how different the opinions are from a more surgical, neurological or psychosomatic point of view. Since in the end, there are realistically many ways to help and alleviate symptoms for Ménière's disease.

- **If Possible, Get a Second Opinion**

Many differences between the various views and specialist groups could be clarified if there were agreement on whether one's proposals are about measures to alleviate symptoms (e.g. attack vertigo or permanent vertigo should be reduced, hearing should be maintained or improved) or whether one assumes that one can really "cure".

It is probable that the Ménière's patient will meet more or less suitable specialists in the various phases of his illness. In principle, it makes sense to get a second opinion, no matter how well-intentioned and well-founded the first one may be, at the price of having to make one's own decision for one's own life afterwards.

9.1 Careful Diagnostics

What is useful at the beginning?

Favorable for Ménière's patients is when medical professionals:

- be able to diagnose the disease, for which knowledge in the field of otorhinolaryngology is indispensable;
- know possible differential diagnoses (especially migraine), which falls predominantly into the specialist area of neurologists.

A good diagnosis is often not so easy, especially in the early stages. Many diseases can show symptoms similar to those of Ménière's disease (▶ Chap. 5). It is helpful to record eye movements during a vertigo attack and to test hearing promptly using modern "mobile technology" (▶ Chap. 6).

9.2 Comprehensible Enlightenment

What should be done if Ménière's disease is correctly diagnosed?

After the exact diagnosis, it helps to provide information that is comprehensible to those affected. This should actually be self-evident, but is nevertheless often difficult to obtain. Often it must be supplemented by the patient's own efforts (research on the Internet, literature that is as helpful as possible and, last but not least, self-help groups).

Perhaps even more than with other diseases with physical and mental components, organic understanding in the sense of understanding and knowledge is necessary with Ménière's disease. The better the disease can be understood and the more practicable ways of dealing with the problems arising from it, such as vertigo and general insecurity, become understandable, the fewer secondary problems arise. This is especially true for the phenomena of psychogenic dizziness and the extension of the anxiety component.

▪ **Sympathetic Approach Important**

What is needed here on the part of the "expert physician" is a Sympathetic approach to the patient's need for knowledge and distress. At the same time, it is also difficult for a physician to endure not being able to be "healing".

> Ménière's disease is not a diagnosis of death or destruction, but refers to a disease of the inner ear, which is benign in all – mostly unilateral – functional deficits and is not a disease of the central nervous system such as a "stroke".

9.3 Therapeutic Measures

In the following, it is important to explore what is still possible, but without pretending a feasibility, which is quickly disappointed.

Even though the disease itself is not curable, nevertheless:

- many effects of Ménière's disease can be compensated in many parts,
- many effects of Ménière's disease can be influenced favorably,
- many unfavorable factors effects can be alleviated.

Favorable for Ménière's patients is when medical professionals:

- carry out or arrange for the acute therapy,
- support the patient in his or her own competence, if possible.

If the diagnosis is confirmed or at least likely, it is probably worth trying intratympanal cortisone. On the one hand, one can do little wrong and on the other hand – at least many – experience an improvement.

If the – inner ear-related! – vertigo occurs more often than 2 times a week and the hearing in the speech area has failed, eliminating measures can be considered. These include the administration of the "ear poisonous" gentamycin directly in front of the inner ear or the severing (neurectomy) of the vestibular nerve, which is always considered last.

9.4 Support and Therapy Between Vertigo Attacks

Also and especially between the attacks, the medical support remains important regarding the questions and needs of the patients. In particular, it is often necessary to clarify what is possible and what is not, if hearing aids are useful and to what extent the dizziness and the fear of dizziness show larger psychological dimensions.

■ An Open Ear for Emotional Concerns

It is favorable for Ménière's patients if medical professionals:

- know about the course and the changeability of the clinical picture;
- consider the fact that a Ménière's patient does not always suffer from Ménière's vertigo and dizziness, but may – more than others – develop benign positional vertigo and often has a (reactive) psychogenic dizziness component or may even suffer from migraine;
- perceive and respect the psychological side and, if necessary, be able to set a professional course, whereby relaxation methods such as progressive muscle relaxation or autogenic training can already initiate a changed way of dealing with the illness.

What usually exceeds the possibilities are the time-consuming intermediate steps and the professional – psychotherapeutic processing of the distress of affected persons. However, this treatment is often necessary and useful.

9.5 Psychological Measures

Psychological measures beyond learning relaxation techniques should be considered if problems with coping with the illness occur and the ability to live, relate and work is at risk. Psychotherapeutic help is particularly necessary if psychogenic dizziness develops. It is important to clarify whether the "vertigo attacks" are attacks from the inner ear or psychogenic vertigo events, which can feel similar or the same for those affected. In our indoor patients we found more frequent reactive psychogenic dizziness, determining the clinical picture,

Much can be gained if psychotherapeutic work can be done to limit vertigo experience to the purely organic attacks.

It is favorable for Ménière's patients if psychologists:

- organically – at least roughly – know or are informed,
- do not interpret every dizziness as psychogenic – that is the wish and the requirement for non-physician psychotherapists.

9.6 What Might Make a Good Patient?

It is favorable for the Ménière's patient if he himself – despite all dizziness and despair – has the own motivation and will to work on the changeable parts and to deal with the unchangeable parts.

9.6.1 Factors that Can Be Influenced

- Psychologically treatable constellations that lead to vertigo and – perhaps also via a tension that does not dissipate – to alterations in the inner ear
- Extension of the vertigo coming from the inner ear to psychogenic dizziness with its – possible – repercussions on the inner ear events
- Mixing with other forms of dizziness (blood pressure, anxiety, visual defects, etc.)

9.6.2 Compensable Factors

- Deafness
- Experience of the disease
- Social impact
- Interpersonal intrusions and challenges

How Do I Deal with Irreversible Suffering?

From my point of view, the most important thing is to get his fate back into his own hands. Unfortunately, this can hardly be found in books and ultimately remains an existential question. It touches on the life question "How do I deal with a suffering that cannot be undone, without waiting – mostly in vain – for redemption from outside or persisting in accusations to whomever?". It is also the question "How can I – in spite of this – work out and use opportunities?"

Less helpful and "meaningful" is the question: "Why did I get sick?" and then of course the question: "Why do I of all people have Ménière's disease?"

We cannot choose the questions that life asks us. But the answers we give to them are, according to Frankl (2019), "testimonies of our very own attitude, as it were fingerprints of our life."

Since I cannot now choose whether I am ill and how severely I have been ill up to now, it makes sense to develop a perspective in the search for what is healthy and what is helpful, in which shaping is possible again. Thus, Ménière's patients show a more favorable processing, who – even in the disease – can experience and recognize positive aspects (Stephens et al. 2007). This includes the perception of the needs of other and of their own needs, which in turn leads to them being able to cope better with the disease.

9.6.3 And myself?

It took me years to see that my Ménière's disease had initiated a turnaround that was now positive for me, even if I would have wished a less dizzying drama. In the meantime, I still live and work, with "one ear" and one vestibular organ and sometime dizziness from migraine.

Probably only through the loss of balance I have learned better to perceive the coordinates of the balance system in its organic and psychological components. So, I would not like to exchange my very different occupation and the handling of my – health any more for my former one.

I am grateful to have had supportive people and good professional help in hard and dizzy times. The fact that I am a doctor myself has often helped me, but it has also made things more difficult when dealing with colleagues. Without the psychotherapeutic support of Irene Wielpütz from Cologne, I do not know whether I would have got through the tight spots of life. I owe her and my – later – psychotherapeutic trainer, Dr. Volker Warnke from Kiel, many life-saving impulses.

Nevertheless, of course I am still afraid of having to go through the dizziness of a Ménière's disease again.

Here, in addition to self-awareness, it is often helpful for me to deal with patients who, in many cases, have much worse hearing – and yet can communicate with me. So in addition to the Ménière's patients whom I can help, there are also always those whom I can only admire in their ability to get up again after a vertigo attack – and learn a lot from them.

Last but not least, my own experience of having already overcome a crisis and the fact that I am looking towards technical aids give me hope that even bilateral Ménière's disease does not mean the end of a life worth living.

But it is easier said than done. And you cannot always get through these times alone. However, experienced and endured suffering also makes one a bit more "clear-sighted", if that is the right word.

As a doctor, I wish you as a reader – not only in the treatment of Ménière's disease – a medicine that can view the human being as a whole and accompany you in your search for new possibilities in a therapeutically professional and humanly supportive way.

Such medicine is exhausting and anything but easy. Nor does it come free of charge for patients: It requires the departure from a consumerist attitude towards personal initiative, patience and occasionally also coping with conditions that seem almost unbearable. In return, the regaining of responsibility and self-responsible possibilities of shaping one's own health with possibly new results of a – certainly not easy – search can be won.

▪ **What Else?**

Ultimately, the point of all therapeutic encounters is to enable people to come into their own in the search for possible solutions, i.e. to find their own way.

You probably would not find a therapist that often combines everything a Ménière's patient needs. Sometimes there is an interrelated, coordinated team in a clinic that regularly work with Ménière's patients. But even though they may be far away, their expertise – unlike 20 years ago – is accessible in various forms.

Literature

Frankl V (2019) Man's search for meaning. Beacon Press, Boston, p 192. ISBN-10: 0807092150

Stephens D, Kentala E, Varpa K, Pyykko I (2007) Positive experiences associated with Menière‘s disorder. Otol Neurotol 14:1531–7129

Short Answers to Frequently Asked Questions

For Readers in a Hurry

Contents

10.1 What Is Ménière's Disease? – 265

10.2 What Causes Ménière's Disease? – 265

10.3 How Common Is Ménière's Disease – 265

10.4 Are Hearing Fluctuations in the Low-Frequency Range with Low Tone Tinnitus a Sign of Ménière's Disease? – 265

10.5 Can Ménière's Disease Be Bilateral? – 266

10.6 Is There a Cure for Ménière's Disease? – 266

10.7 When Can Therapy Be Helpful for Ménière's Disease? – 266

10.8 Is There a Connection Between Migraine and Ménière's Disease? – 267

10.9 Are Ménière's Sufferers Allowed to Drive? – 267

10.10 Are Ménière's Sufferers Allowed to Travel (Fly)? – 268

10.11 Are Ménière's Patients Allowed to Swim and What Do they Need to Be Aware of? – 268

10.12 Are Ménière's Sufferers Allowed to Dive? – 269

H. Schaaf, *Ménière's Disease*, https://doi.org/10.1007/978-3-662-63610-7_10

10.13 Is Ménière's Disease Hereditary? – 269

10.14 Does Ménière's Disease Affect Pregnancy? – 269

10.15 Do Hearing Aids Help with Ménière's Disease? – 269

10.16 Can Anesthesia Influence Ménière's Symptoms? – 270

10.17 And What Other Use Is There? – 270

Literature – 270

10.1 What Is Ménière's Disease?

Ménière's disease affects the inner ear with the balance- and hearing parts. This manifest themselves in typical, unpredictable, attack vertigo as well as in hearing loss and in roaring in the ears (tinnitus). In the case of repeated attacks, the fear of and during vertigo can also develop to reactive psychogenic dizziness. Despite a clear description, many different diseases gather together behind the term Ménière's disease. This also makes the assessment of diagnostic and treatment measures, and not least research, so difficult.

10.2 What Causes Ménière's Disease?

In Ménière's patients, a so-called endolymphatic hydrops is found. For the endolymphatic hydrops, a reduced resorption of endolymphatic fluid in the saccus endolymphaticus is held responsible. It is possible that the endolymphatic sac may be overloaded with immune defense tasks, for which it is arguably also responsible, so that it cannot adequately perform this dual task. In the end, it must be said that the organic "end route" of the disease is known, but it is not known exactly what causes or significantly influences it.

10.3 How Common Is Ménière's Disease

The frequency of Ménière's disease is assumed to be around 1:1000 (0.1%) in industrial nations.

10.4 Are Hearing Fluctuations in the Low-Frequency Range with Low Tone Tinnitus a Sign of Ménière's Disease?

No. A usually buzzing, droning deep tinnitus, which is often associated with repeated hearing fluctuations in the low-frequency range, is a relatively common feature of the inner ear. Although this special form of tinnitus and hearing loss is often misjudged as a precursor to Ménière's disease, it is very likely that it is an independent clinical picture. So-called endolymphatic fluctuations in the "auditory tube" of the cochlea form the organic part of this disease. Although it is true, that a Ménière's disease can begin with endolymphatic fluctuations before the full picture of Ménière's disease develops, it is also true that only very few people with endolymphatic fluctuations develop Ménière's disease.

10.5 Can Ménière's Disease Be Bilateral?

Unfortunately, yes. However, we can only speak of a bilateral Ménière's disease if all three symptoms, hearing loss, ringing in the ears and inner ear-related (!) vertigo (not an additional psychogenic dizziness), are also found on the other side. Above all, the ringing in the ears very often occurs on both sides without a new trouble in the inner ear.

10.6 Is There a Cure for Ménière's Disease?

Up to now, there is no known cure in the classical sense. This already follows from the fact that no exact cause is known. Unfortunately, until now it is only clear how the disease affects the inner ear. However, effective symptomatic measures do exist. For the acute, violent attacks of vertigo, a safe symptom control with drugs against the nausea (antiemetics) is known. Ultimately, inner vertigo can be eliminated if the vertigo attacks occur too often and too violently. However, the hearing part is often affected as well.

10.7 When Can Therapy Be Helpful for Ménière's Disease?

If Ménière's disease develops in its serious form, this entails measures far beyond the medicinal acute therapy. It is helpful to have an understandable, comprehensible, *explanation of the clinical picture*, both with regard to the nature of the clinical picture and with regard to dealing with the resulting possible problems, such as dizziness and uncertainty. It is extremely important to clarify whether the "vertigo attacks" are attacks from the inner ear or whether they are accompanying or reactive psychogenic dizziness and/or depressive crises, which can feel similar or the same in the experience. Here two very different therapies and coping approaches arise.

Patel's (2016) study raises hope that cortisone, if it can be given directly into the middle ear – after appropriate anesthesia of the tympanic membrane – may lead to the reduction of vertigo.

An important role is played by *balance training*, which can compensate for the loss of balance. *Hearing aids* can help decisively with hearing loss, a cochlea implant in deafness.

A *psychological treatment* of the life situation changed by the disease is necessary at the latest when the disease in its organic and psychological part leads to reactive changes with anxiety and depression.

If vertigo dominates life, measures to reduce vertigo should be considered.

The reduction and *elimination of the vestibular function* with gentamycin seems – according to the current state – to be the safest measure.

In inpatient treatment, a medically, psychologically and movement-therapeutically coordinated and interlocking therapy can enable the start of a long-term and fundamental stabilization.

10.8 Is There a Connection Between Migraine and Ménière's Disease?

Both diseases are sometimes confusingly similar in symptoms. In some patients, they are observed simultaneously or at different times. Thus, links between migraine and Ménière's disease are suspected. However, it could also be that this connection is raised so often because ultimately the demarcations are possible in the long term, but difficult in the acute stage.

10.9 Are Ménière's Sufferers Allowed to Drive?

Since Ménière's vertigo attacks usually come on suddenly, it is in your own interest to refrain from driving a motor vehicle. This must apply all the more when Tumarkin attacks (▶ Sect. 4.2) occur. It should always be borne in mind, that not only the patient's own person but also others are put at extreme risk. After definitive elimination of the vertiginous vestibular organ, as after gentamycin therapy and neurectomy, reconsideration can be made. If freedom from vertigo has been achieved over a longer period of time *and* at the same time sufficient compensation has occurred, it should actually be possible to drive a vehicle again during the day (!), but not in darkness. However, this is certainly a case-by-case decision under specialist medical advice.

10.10 Are Ménière's Sufferers Allowed to Travel (Fly)?

In principle, Ménière's patients can travel – even for longer periods. A Ménière's attack cannot – by definition – be provoked by an external event.

If Ménière's disease has led to a partial or complete loss of balance, accelerations can be compensated more poorly via the reflex to the eyes (vestibulo-ocular reflex), which can be experienced as – temporary – dizziness. It is relatively unimportant for the vestibular organ whether the speed changes forward or – as during take-off and landing in an aircraft – diagonally.

Constant speeds also do not trigger any further changes in the vestibular organ. Accordingly, there is nothing to be said against travelling by train or plane. Changing speeds and probably the most frequent changes of direction are most likely to take place in a car.

The question is rather how to behave in a Ménière's attack. It is just as difficult as it is usually not justifiable to bring trains, ships or planes to a halt. This would not change the progress of the attack. Therapy with Antivertiginosa remains the same and is generally also possible on trains and planes.

10.11 Are Ménière's Patients Allowed to Swim and What Do they Need to Be Aware of?

As long as Ménière's attacks can still occur, no Ménière's patient should go swimming alone, since orientation in the water – also for up and down – is lost during an attack.

Even if balance attacks no longer occur, the difference between the healthy and diseased side can cause problems in special situations. For example, dizziness and an associated feeling of anxiety can occur when swimming – especially in cold water.

The reason is a "stimulation" of the vestibular organs by the water in the ear. The effect is the same as with the diagnostic caloric testing, only that the effect is unintentional when swimming. This leads to an asymmetrical and thus vertigo-inducing result, because both ears are no longer equally functional.

Here the solution is relatively simple:

- In case of complete failure of an organ, an earplug in the healthy ear is sufficient!
- In the case of partial loss, one earplug is needed for each ear.

10.12 Are Ménière's Sufferers Allowed to Dive?

For purely physical reasons, there is nothing to be said against "diving" even for Ménière's sufferers, but against "sport-" and performance diving at greater depths. But even when diving in the swimming pool, as long as the possibility of an attack exists, one should not expose oneself to the danger that can then occur under water.

10.13 Is Ménière's Disease Hereditary?

In the meantime, some studies suggest that a certain predisposition or "readiness" to Ménière's disease could also be partly hereditary (Arweiler-Harbeck et al. 2011; Frykholm et al. 2006). The mode of inheritance is presumed to be "autosomal" with incomplete expression, i.e. it is sufficient for one parent to carry the predisposition. However, it is generally true that "only" the probability of contracting a disease is inherited rather than acquired. The severity of the disease and its effects, as well as the chance of getting the disease, probably depend much more on acquired opportunities and coping strategies. Thus, it is certainly more important to develop a livable concept than to lament the – possible – inherited damage.

10.14 Does Ménière's Disease Affect Pregnancy?

There are women whose symptoms improve during pregnancy and others whose symptoms do not change at all. Pregnant women must be careful with any kind of permanent medication; the package inserts are usually of little help here. This also applies to emergency medication in the event of a dizzy spell. Although single doses are certainly less dangerous than continuous doses, there is no absolute safety for any medication. However, the use of drugs containing the active ingredient diazepam, which has been on the market for a very long time and is apparently not known to have any serious side effects, appears to be of least concern in the control of Ménière's attacks (not in long-term treatment).

10.15 Do Hearing Aids Help with Ménière's Disease?

Yes!!! Hearing loss, often an important component of Ménière's disease, can lead to acoustic and social isolation. Thus, hearing aids are also essential for symptomatic help with hearing loss in

Ménière's patients. However, the hearing threshold of Ménière's disease patients often shifts, so the hearing aid must be readjusted from time to time. However, this should not prevent sufferers from using this important communication aid if their hearing is correspondingly impaired – even on one side. In cases of unilateral deafness, a so-called contralateral routing of signals (CROS) device can improve directional hearing. In cases of unilateral deafness, a cochlear implant is also recommended – and at an early stage and in the case of – rare – bilateral deafness, a "cochlear implant" would further enable communication.

10.16 Can Anesthesia Influence Ménière's Symptoms?

With the so-called spinal anesthesia, it *can* (rarely!) happen that with outflow of spinal fluid in some patients, a – usually temporary – low tone tinnitus, usually together with a low tone impairment, is noticed. If a patient already exhibits fluctuating hearing before the operation, as in the context of Ménière's disease, the use of spinal anesthesia should be carefully considered – and in case of doubt, "normal general anesthesia" should be preferred. If low-frequency tinnitus with low-tone hearing loss appears after spinal anesthesia as part of a "post-spinal" syndrome, bed rest should be observed and plenty of fluids should be administered. If this does not help, anesthetists can usually perform a so-called "blood patch" (plug with the patient's own blood), which can close the small gap.

10.17 And What Other Use Is There?

Help in and by self-help groups can be useful.

Literature

Arweiler-Harbeck D, Horsthemke B, Jahnke K, Hennies HC (2011) Genetic aspects of familial Ménière's disease. Otol Neurotol 4:695–700

Frykholm C, Larsen HC, Dahl N (2006) Familial Menière's disease in five generations. Otol Neurotol 27:681–686

Patel M, Agarwal K, Arshad Q, Hariri M, Rea P, Seemungal BM, Golding JF, Harcourt, JP, Bronstein AM (2016) Intratympanic methylprednisolone versus gentamicin in patients with unilateral Ménière's disease: a randomised, double-blind, comparative eff ectiveness trial. Lancet 388:2753–2762

Supplementary Information

Self-help Groups – 272

Glossary – 273

Literature – 279

Index – 295

H. Schaaf, *Ménière's Disease*, https://doi.org/10.1007/978-3-662-63610-7

Self-help Groups

Meniere's Society

Ménière's Society, The Rookery, Surrey Hills Business Park, Wotton, Surrey, RH5 6Q

► https://www.menieres.org.uk/, e-mail: info@menieres.org.uk

K.I.M.M. e. V.: Kommunikation und Information M. Menière

Internet: ► http://www.kimm-ev.de, email: info@kimm-ev.de

Deutsche Tinnitus Liga (DTL): German Tinnitus League e. V.

Am Lohsiepen 18, 42353 Wuppertal, Germany

Internet: ► http://www.tinnitus-liga.de, email: ► dtl@tinnitus-liga.de

Glossary

Aetiology (gr.) This is used in the broadest sense for having the cause in itself.

Allergy Hypersensitivity to certain substances

Aminoglycosides A class of antibiotics to which belong the substances gentamycin and streptomycin.

Anatomy The study of the form and structure of the body

Antiemetic Emesis (gr.): vomiting, anti (gr.): against

Autonomic (also unconscious) nervous system Consists of 2 counterparts: the sympathetic portion and the parasympathetic portion. The sympathetic part contributes, for example, to the blood vessels constricting, the parasympathetic part causes the vessels to dilate.

BERA Brainstem Evoked Response Audiometry, Sound impressions are played on the ear and, as in the case of an EEG, the brain waves generated as a result are derived and evaluated at the head. This is mainly used to exclude a brain tumour along the auditory nerve (acoustic neuroma).

Causal (lat.) Concerning the causes

Cholesteatoma Progressive inflammation in the middle ear that can "eat into the bone" and requires surgery. Often makes itself felt as a "running ear", usually the leaking fluid smells, so that the ear doctor is visited.

Cochlea Anatomical structure in the inner ear; contains the hearing organ

Cognitions Ideas that people form about the world and themselves. Thoughts and feelings influence feelings and actions

Conservative This term is used by physicians to refer to preservative and, in particular, non-surgical interventions. However, this distinction certainly is not always correct, because drugs can also have a destructive effect, e.g. in the case of gentamycin.

Ductus cochlearis Ductus: duct, cochlearis: of the cochlea, cochlea duct; corresponds to the auditory canal.

Ductus endolymphaticus Duct of the membranous labyrinth filled with endolymph.

Dura Med. for meninges

Efferent (lat.) Away from the brain; in contrast to afferent: towards the brain

Electrocochleography Special examination of the inner ear; stimulation currents are measured via a small probe through the middle ear.

Electrolytes Small charged particles, e.g. sodium and potassium

Endolymph Fluid in the membranous portion of the inner ear.

Endolymphatic hydrops Accumulation of the fluid "endolymph" in the auditory canal alone or in the semi-circular canals, too, like in Meniere's disease.

Epithelium (gr.) Cell association

Fibrosis Functional tissue is replaced "by simple" connective tissue; this is, of course, a loss in relation to the function previously exercised

Fracture Med. for (bone) fracture

Helicotrema The **helicotrema** is the part of the cochlear labyrinth where the scala tympani and the scala vestibuli meet. It is the main component of the cochlear apex. The hair cells near this area best detect low frequency sounds

Hertz (Hz) Unit for frequency. It indicates the number of repeating processes per second.

Hydrops (gr.) Accumulation of (body) water: ►endolymphatic hydrops

Idiopathic Explained (only) by itself, without an identifiable cause.

Intratympanal Into the middle ear (the space between the eardrum and the inner ear).

Invasive Intervening; usually refers to surgical procedures.

Ischemia Bloodless

Lamina Thin structure, ledge

Local anaesthetics Local anaesthetics

Medical history Medical and/or psychological history of the disease.

Membrana tectoria (lat.) Membrane belonging to the roof of the Corti Organ

Ménière's disease Textbook term for Ménière's disease;

Modiolus (Lat.) Axis

Morbus (Lat.) Disease

Morphological According to form, according to structure

Morphology (gr.) The sciens of the form of the body, including the shape and structures of the internal organs.

Neurectomy Neur (gr.): nerve, ectomy (gr.): to cut out; the nerve is cut out or completely severed and thus all connections are cut.

Neurotological examination Examination of the specific pathways of the hearing- and vestibular organ

Neurosis Non-optimal attempt to solve an unresolved mental conflict. This does not have to be pathological, but can lead to problems in coping with everyday life. According to Watzlawick, neurosis is the attempt to achieve a goal with "more and more of the same", where a qualitatively different solution would be more promising.

Nystagmus Eye tremor caused by jerky, involuntary eye movements. A fast and a slow phase are observed; after the fast phase, the direction is named

Organ of Corti Sensory organ; named after the first describer Graf A. Corti (1851).

Otoacoustic emissions The outer hair cells in the inner ear can generate sound waves themselves, which can be recorded with the aid of extremely fine microphones in the outer ear and used for special diagnostics.

Otoliths Smallest lime crystals in the equilibrium membrane.

Parasympathetic nervous system Part of the autonomic nervous system

Pathophysiology The study of the pathological processes of life

Perilymph Fluid around the membranous portion of the inner ear, or between the membranous and bony portions.

Physiology (gr.) The science of the normal processes of life

Placebo (lat.) I may please; placebo effects mean that a measure that is assumed (by orthodox medicine) to be ineffective has been taken, but it is suggested that it works. Often improvements occur nevertheless, because the patients assume that they are helped. Certainly, however, with each placebo, highly effective endogenous substances are mobilized, which can contribute "quite objectively" to the healing. Important side effects could be disappointed hopes

Polytraumatic therapy Multifaceted therapy, usually a combination of many forms of treatment in the absence of a safe, well proved form of therapy.

Prognosis Prediction about the course of a disease

Prospective (lat.) study A prospective study; in which experimental and success criteria are considered before the study begins; the opposite of a retrospective (looking back) study. A prospective study is significantly more informative about what it is investigating than a retrospective study.

Psyche (Greek) professional word for soul

Psychopathogenesis A "history of the origin" of the disease of the psyche.

Psychovegetative From the psyche to the autonomic nervous system, consisting of the two interacting antagonists, the sympathetic and parasympathetic nervous systems.

Reissner's membrane Membrane in the inner ear that separates the ear canal from the surrounding fluid. It was named after its first describer Reissner

Retrospective Retrospective, as opposed to prospective.

Saccotomy (Latin) "cutting" at the saccus.

Saccule Small bag; part of the vestibular organ, responsible for the perception of "above and below", not to be confused with the saccus endolymphaticus.

Saccus endolymphaticus (Lat.) Sack in which the endolymph is absorbed and removed (reabsorbed), not to be confused with the saccule.

Scala (Lat.) Staircase; one is near the balance organ (scala vestibuli), the other near the tympanic cavity, the tympanum (scala tympani). The designation is based on the spatiality

Semi-circular canals Anatomical structure of the inner ear with sensory organs for rotational movements.

Spontaneous regression Regression means a mostly unconscious "falling back" on earlier, mostly early childhood attempts to solve mental problems.

Stapes Small bone in the middle ear

Stria vascularis Stria (lat.): stripe, vascularis (lat.): vascular, i.e. blood vessels are found here.

Subarachnoid space Fluid-filled, soft cerebral membrane

Sympathetic nervous system Part oft the autonomic nervous system

Symptoms Clinical signs

Symptomatic treatment A treatment that only combats the symptoms and effects of the disease, but not the cause.

Tinnitus Buzzing in the ears, ringing in the ears; tinnire (lat.): ringing, roaring, buzzing.

Trauma (gr.) Wound; today used in a broader sense, e.g. for a generally unexpected violent impact on the body from outside.

This also includes, for example, an operation. Psychologically it denotes a slight and/or injury when dealing with people.

Trigger (Term from cybernetics): switching element for triggering a switching process; in this case, triggering moment.

Tuba auditiva Eustachian tube

Tympanometry Examination of the middle ear in which the function of the eardrum and the reflexes of the middle ear mucosa to sound stimuli are tested.

Uniform Uniform

Utricle Anatomical structure in the vestibular organ: the vesicle on which the three semi-circular canals are based and which is itself responsible for the perception of "left and right" (horizontal).

Verum Drug with a proven effect in orthodox medicine, counter term to "placebo"

Vestibular Associated with the balance organ

Vestibular evoked myogenic potentials (VEMP) A sound stimulus to the sacculus in the vestibular organ triggers a reflex whose muscular response is measured at the cervical muscle (c-VEMP) or at the ocular muscle (o-VEMP)

Vestibulo-ocular reflex (VOR) The reflex to stabilize gaze during head movement, with eye movement due to activation of the vestibular system. The reflex acts to stabilize images on the retinas of the eye during head movement, holding gaze is held steadily on a location, by producing eye movements in the direction opposite to head movement.

Viscosity Toughness of a liquid

(VOR) → vestibulo-ocular reflex

Zonulae occludentes Zonula (Lat.): small, circumscribed district; occludens (Lat.): occluded.

Literature

Recommended Books for Therapists

M. Meniere

Ruckenstein MJ (2010) Ménière's disease. Evidence and outcomes. Plural publishing, San Diego, Oxford, Brisbane, p S162

Balance System and Dizzines

Bronstein A, Lempert T (2017) Dizziness. A practical approach to diagnosis an mangement. 2nd edn. Cambridge clinical guides. Cambridge University Press, Cambridge, p 200

Goldberg J, Wilson V, Cullen K, Angelaki D, Broussard D, Buttner-Ennever J, Fukushima K, Minor L (2021) The vestibular system: a sixth sense. Oxford University Press, New York

Herdman SJ, Clendaniel R (2014) Vestibular rehabilitation, 4th edn. Contemporary perspectives in rehabilitation. F.A. Davis Company, Philadelphia, p 656

Schaaf H (2016) Psychotherapie bei Schwindelerkrankungen. 4. Aufl. Asanger, Kröning, p 174

Literature Cited

Adrion C, Fischer CS, Wagner J, Gürkov R, Mansmann U, Strupp M (2016) Efficacy and safety of betahistine treatment in patients with Menière's disease: primary results of a long term, multicentre, double blind, randomised, placebo controlled, dose defining trial (BEMED trial). BMJ 352:h6816. https://doi.org/10.1136/bmj.h6816

Ammon HPT (1991) Arzneimittelneben- und -wechselwirkungen. Wissenschaftliche Verlagsgesellschaft, Stuttgart

Anderson JP, Harris JP (2001) Impact of Meniere's disease on quality of life. Otol Neurotol 22:888–894

Andersson G, Hagnebo C, Yardley L (1997) Stress and symptoms of Menière's disease: a time-series analysis. J Psychosom Res 43(6):595–603

Arnold W (2001) Die Qual der Wahl bei der Behandlung des Morbus Menière. HNO 49:163–165

Arroll M, Dancey CP, Attree EA, Smith S, James T (2012) People with symptoms of Meniere's disease: the relationship between illness intrusiveness, illness uncertainty, dizziness handicap, and depression. Otol Neurotol 33(5):816–823

Arweiler DJ, Jahnke K, Grosse-Wilde H (1995) Morbus Menière als autosomal dominant vererbte Erkrankung. Laryngol Rhinol Otol 74:412–415

Arweiler-Harbeck D, Horsthemke B, Jahnke K, Hennies HC (2011) Genetic aspects of familial Ménière's disease. Otol Neurotol 4:695–700

Baier G, Ott I (2008) Die chirurgische Therapie des M. Menière Entwicklung und heutiger Stand. HNO 56:553–566

Balaban CD, Jacob RG, Furman JM (2011) Neurologic bases for comorbidity of balance disorders, anxiety disorders and migraine: neurotherapeutic implications. Expert Rev Neurother 11(3):379–394. https://doi.org/10.1586/ern.11.19

Baloh RW, Jacobson K, Winder T (1990) Drop attacks with Menière's syndrome. Ann Neurol 28:384–387

Basecqz G (1969) Aspects psychodynamiques de la maladie Menière. Laval Med 40:838–843

Basta D, Ernst A (2008) Moderne Rehabilitation von Gleichgewichtsstörungen mit Hilfe von Neurofeedback-Trainingsverfahren. HNO 56:990–995

Basura GJ, Adams ME, Monfared A, Schwartz SR, Antonelli PJ, Burkard R, Bush ML, Bykowski J, Colandrea M, Derebery J, Kelly EA, Kerber KA, Koopman CF, Kuch AA, Marcolini E, McKinnon BJ, Ruckenstein MJ, Valenzuela CV, Vosooney A, Walsh SA, Nnacheta LC, Dhepyasuwan N, Buchanan EM (2020) Clinical practice guideline: Ménière's disease. Executive summary. Otolaryngol Head Neck Surg 162(4):415–434

Beck JS (1997) Praxis der kognitiven Therapie. Weinheim, Beltz PVU

Blodow A, Helbig R, Wichmann N (2013) Der Video-Kopfimpulstest: Erste klinische Erfahrungen. HNO 61:327–334

Blumenbach L (1955) Menière's Originalarbeiten. Musterschmidt, Göttingen

Boenninghaus HG (1990) Hals-Nasen-Ohrenheilkunde. Springer, Berlin, Heidelberg, New York

Boenninghaus HG, Lenarz T (2007) Hals-Nasen-Ohren-Heilkunde, 13. Aufl. Springer, Berlin, Heidelberg, New York, Tokyo

Brandt TH, Dieterich M (1986) Phobischer Attackenschwindel. MMW 128:247–250

Brandt T, Dieterich M, Strupp M (2012) Vertigo. Leitsymptom Schwindel. Steinkopff, Darmstadt

Bronstein AM (1995) Visual vertigo syndrome: clinical an posturography findings. J Neurol Neurosurg Psychiatry 59(5):472–476

Buki B, Platz M, Haslwanter T, Junger H, Avan P (2011) Results of electrocochleography in Menière's disease after successful vertigo control by single intratympanic gentamicin injection. Audiol Neurootol 16(1):49–54

Burgess A, Kundu S (2010) Diuretics for Menière's disease or syndrome. Cochrane Database of Syst Rev (4):CD003599

Calzada AP, Lopez IA, Ishiyama G, Ishiyama A (2012) Otolithic membrane damage in patients with endolymphatic hydrops and drop attacks. Otol Neurotol 33:1593–1598

Carrey J, Nivee A (2006) Evolutionary changes in the cochlea and labyrinth: solving the problem of sound transmission to the balance organs of the inner ear the anatomical record part A. Anat Rec A Discov Mol Cell Evol Biol 288A:482–490

Casani A, Piaggi P, Cerchiai N, Seccia V, Franceschini SS, Dallan I (2012) Intratympanic treatment of intractable unilateral Menière disease. Gentamicin or dexamethasone? A randomized controlled trial. Otolaryngol Head Neck Surg 146(3):430–437

Cawthorne TE, Friedmann G (1969) Head movement exercises in the therapy of disorders of the equilibrium. Schweiz Med Wochenschr 99:156–158

Celestino D, Rosini E, Carucci ML, Marconi PL, Vercillo E (2003) Ménière's disease and anxiety disorders. Acta Otorhinolaryngol Ital 23(6):421–427

Choung YH, Park K, Kim CH, Kim HJ, Kim K (2006) Rare cases of Menière's disease in children. J Laryngol Otol 120(4):343–352

Claes GM, De Valck CF, Van de Heyning P (2012) Does 'Cochlear Meniere's Disease' exist? An ELECTROCOCHLEOGRAPHIC and audiometric study. Audiol Neurotol 18:63–70

Clarke AH, Schönfeld U, Hamann C, Scherer H (2001) Measuring unilateral otolith function via the otolith-ocular response and the subjective visual vertical. Acta Otolaryngol Suppl 545:457–464

Coker NJ, Coker RR, Jenkins HA, Vincent KR (1989) Psychological profile of patients with Menière's disease. Arch Otolaryngol Head Neck Surg 115(11):1355–1357

Colletti V, Carner M, Colletti L (2007) Auditory results after vestibular nerve section and intratympanic gentamicin for Menière's disease. Otol Neurotol 28(2):145–151

Committee on Hearing and Equilibrium (1995) Guidelines for the diagnosis and evaluation of therapy in Menière's disease. Otolaryngol Head Neck Surg 113:181–185

Cooksey FS (1946) Rehabilitation in vestibular injuries. Proc R Soc Med 39:273–278

Costa PT, McCrae RR (1992) Revised NEO Personality Inventory (NEO-PI-R) and NEO Five-Factor Inventory (NEO-FFI) professional manual. Psychological Assessment Resources, Odessa

Crane BT, Minor LB, Della Santina CC, Carey JP (2009) Middle ear exploration in patients with Ménière's disease who have failed outpatient intratympanic gentamicin therapy. Otol Neurotol 30:619–624

Czubalski K, Bochenek W, Zawisza E (1976) Psychological stress and personality in Menière's disorder. J Psychosom Res 20(3):187–191

Dandy W (1933) Treatment of Menière's disease by section of only the vestibular portion of the acoustic nerve. Bull Johns Hopkins Hosp 53:53

De Burlet HM (1934) Zur vergleichenden Anatomie und Physiologie des perilymphatischen Raumes. Acta Otolaryngol 13:153–187

Decot E (2005) Psychosomatische Störungen. Laryngo-Rhino-Otol 84:272–287

Derogatis LR (1992) SCL-90–R, administration, scoring & procedures manual-II for the R(evised) version and other instruments of the Psychopathology Rating Scale Series. Clinical Psychometric Research Inc, Townson

De Valck CF, Wuyts FL, Vanspauwen R, Walravens S, Van de Heyning PH (2007) Conscientiousness in patients with Menière's disease. Otol Neurotol 28(3):365–368

Devantier L, Guldfred FL, Djurhuus BD, Handel MN, Schmidt JH, Hougaard DD, Edemann-Callesen H (2019a) Positive pressure device treatment for Meniere's disease: an overview of the current evidence and a meta-analysis. Eur Arch Otorhinolaryngol 276(5):1263–1273

Devantier L, Schmidt JH, Djurhuus BD, Hougaard DD, Händel MN, Liviu-Adelin Guldfred F, Edemann-Callesen H (2019b) Current state of evidence for endolymphatic sac surgery in Menière's disease: a systematic review. Acta Otolaryngol 139(11):953–958. https://doi.org/10.1080/00016489.2019.1657240

Devantier L, Hougaard D, Händel MN, Liviu-Adelin Guldfred F, Schmidt JH, Djurhuus B, Callesen HE (2020) Using betahistine in the treatment of patients with Menière's disease: a meta-analysis with the current randomized-controlled evidence. Acta Otolaryngol 140(10):845–853. https://doi.org/10.1080/00016489.2020.1777326. Epub 2020 Jun 25. PMID: 32580600

Diamond SG, Markham CH (1983) Ocular counterrolling as an indicator of vestibular otolith function. Neurology 33:1460–1469

Dieterich M, Eckhardt-Henn A (2004) Neurologische und somatoforme Schwindelsyndrome. Nervenarzt 75:281–302

Dix MR, Hallpike CS (1952) The pathology, symptomatology and diagnosis of certain common disorders of the vestibular system. Ann Otol 61:987–1016

Düwel P, Ilgner J, Ilgner J, Westhofen MM (2005a) Differenzierung von Bogengangs- und Otolithenfunktionsstörungen im zeitlichen Verlauf des M. Menière. Laryngorhinootologie 84:589–593

Düwel P, Walther LE, Haasler T, Westhofen M, Lückhoff A (2005b) Neue Konzepte zu einer Pathophysiologie des M. Menière auf zellulärer Ebene. Laryngorhinootologie 84:412–417

Düwel P, Walther LE, Sanders M, Ilgner J, Westhofen M (2005c) Otolithenfunktionstests – Ein differenziertes, qualitätsgesichertes Screeningsystem. Laryngorhinootologie 84:653–659
Eckhardt-Henn A (2013) Dizziness from a psychosomatic perspective. Ophthalmologe 110(1):26–30
Eckhardt-Henn A, Hoffmann SO, Tettenborn B, Thomalske C, Hopf HC (1997) "Phobischer Schwankschwindel"- Eine weitere Differenzierung psychogener Schwindelzustände erscheint erforderlich. Nervenarzt 68:806–812
Eckhardt-Henn A, Tschan R, Best C, Dieterich M (2009) Somatoforme Schwindelsyndrome. Nervenarzt 80:909–917
Ellis A (1977) Grundlagen und Methode der Rational-Emotiven Verhaltenstherapie. Pfeiffer, München, p 256
Epley JM (1992) The canalith repositioning procedure: for treatment of benign paroxysmal positional vertigo. Otolaryngol Head Neck Surg 107:399–404
Ermann M (2004) Psychosomatische Medizin und Psychotherapie. 4. Aufl. Ein Lehrbuch auf psychoanalytischer Grundlage. Kohlhammer, Stuttgart
Ernst A (2011) Perspektiven der Gleichgewichtsdiagnostik und -therapie. Laryngo-Rhino-Otol 90(Supplement 1):S35–S43
Ernst A, Basta D (2012) Gleichgewichtsstörungen. Diagnostik und Therapie beim Leitsymptom Schwindel. Thieme, Stuttgart
Feldenkrais M (1978) Bewußtheit durch Bewegung. Der aufrechte Gang. Suhrkamp, Frankfurt a.M.
Feldenkrais M (1987) Die Entdeckung des Selbstverständlichen. Suhrkamp, Frankfurt a.M.
Feldmann H, Lennarz H, Wedel H von (1998) Tinnitus, 2. Aufl. Thieme, Stuttgart
Fisher LM, Derebery MJ, Friedman RA (2012) Oral steroid treatment for hearing improvement in Ménière's disease and endolymphatic hydrops. Otol Neurotol 33(9):1685–1691. https://doi.org/10.1097/MAO.0b013e31826dba83
Flatz WH, Gürkov R, Ertl-Wagner B, Berghaus A, Reiser M (2010) Visualisierung und Evaluation von Endolymph-Hydrops bei der Menier'schen Erkrankung. LRO. https://doi.org/10.1055/s-0030-1252584
Forge A, Li L, Nevill G (1998) Hair cell recovery in the vestibular sensory epithelia of mature guinea pigs. J Comp Neurol 397:69–88
Foster CA, Breeze RE (2013) Endolymphatic hydrops in Meniere's disease: cause, consequence, or epiphenomenon? Otol Neurotol 34:1210–1214
Fowler EP (1948) Streptomycine treatment of vertigo. Trans Am Acad Ophthalmol Otol 53:293–301
Fowler EP Jr, Zeckel A (1952) Psychosomatic aspects of Menière's disease. JAMA 148:1265–1271
Frankl V (1996) Der Mensch vor der Frage nach dem Sinn. Eine Auswahl aus dem Gesamtwerk, 8. Aufl. Piper, München
Frykholm C, Larsen HC, Dahl N (2006) Familial Menière's disease in five generations. Otol Neurotol 27:681–686
Gabra N, Asmar MH, Berbiche D, Saliba I (2016) Endolymphatic duct blockage: quality of life assessment of a novel surgical technique for Menière disease. Eur Arch. https://doi.org/10.1007/s00405-015-3890-4
Gacek RR (2015) Recovery of hearing in Meniere's disease after antiviral treatment. Am J Otolaryngol 36(3):315–323
Garduno-Anaya MA, Couthino De Toledo H, Hinojosa GR, Pane PC, Rios Castaneda LC (2005) Dexamethasone inner ear perfusion by intratympanic injection in unilateral Menière's disease: a two-year prospective,

placebo-controlled, double-blind, randomized trial. RJ: Otolaryngol Head Neck Surg 133(2):285–294
Gleich O, Strutz J, Schmid K (2008) Endolymph-Homöostase und M. Menière Grundlagen, pathologische Veränderungen, Aminoglykoside. HNO 56:1243–1252
Godemann F, Schuller J, Uhlemann H (2009) Psychodynamic vulnerability factors in the development of panic disordersda prospective trial in patients after vestibular neuritis. Psychopathology 42:99e107
Gottshall KR, Hoffer ME, Moore RJ (2005) The role of vestibular rehabilitation in the treatment of Menière's disease. Otolaryngol Head Neck Surg 133(3):p326–p328
Green D, Blum DJ, Harner SG (1991) Longitudinal follow-up of patients with Menière's disease. Otolaryngol Head Neck Surg 104:783–788
Green JD, Verrall A, Gates GA (2007) Quality of life instruments in Menière's disease. Laryngoscope 117(9):1622–1628
Groen JJ (1983) Psychosomatic aspects of Menière's disease. Acta Otolaryngol 95:407–416
Gstöttner W, Adunka O (2004) Labyrinthanästhesie bei M. Menière. HNO 52:265
Gürkov R, Flatz W, Louza J, Strupp M, Ertl-Wagner B, Krause E (2012a) In-vivo visualized endolymphatic hydrops and inner ear functions in patients with electrocochleographically confirmed Menière's disease. Otol Neurotol 33(6):1040–1045
Gürkov R, Flatz W, Louza J (2012b) Herniation of the membranous labyrinth into the horizontal semicircularcanal is correlated with impaired caloric response in Meniere's disease. Otol Neurotol 33:1375–1379
Gürkov R, Flatz W, Keeser D (2013) Effect of standard-dose Betahistine on endolymphatic hydrops: an MRI pilot study. Eur Arch Otorhinolaryngol 270:1231–1235
Gürkov R, Berman A, Dietrich O (2015) MR volumetric assessment of endolymphatic hydrops. Eur Radiol 25:585–595
Gürkov R, Pyyko I, Zou J, Kentala E (2016) What is Menière's disease? A contemporary re-evaluation of endolymphatic hydrops. J Neurol 263(Suppl 1):71–81
Hallpike CS, Cairns H (1938) Observations on the pathology of Menière's syndrome. J Laryngol Otol 53:625–655
Hamann KF (2002) Fahrtüchtigkeit bei vestibulären Läsionen. HNO 50:1086–1088
Hamann KF, Haarfeld R (2006) Vestibulär evozierte myogene Potenziale. HNO 54:415–428
Hasler F (2012) Neuromythologie. Transcript, Bielefeld
Havia M, Kentala E, Pyykkö I (2005) Prevalence of Menière's disease in general population of Southern Finland. Otolaryngol Head Neck Surg 133:762–768
Helling K (2008) Otolithenfunktionsstörungen und Therapieoptionen. HNO 56:996–1002
Helling K (2011) HNO update. Vestibuläre Störungen. In: Iro H, Werner JA (eds) HNO update 2011 – Handbuch HNO 2011/2012. In: Iro H, Werner JA (eds) HNO-update 2011. med update, Wiesbaden
Helling K (2012) HNO update. Vestibuläre Störungen. In: Iro H, Werner JA (eds) HNO update 2012 – Handbuch HNO 2012/2013. med update, Wiesbaden
Helling K (2013) HNO update. Vestibuläre Störungen. In: Iro H, Werner JA (eds) HNO update 2013 – Handbuch HNO 2013/2014. med update, Wiesbaden

Helling K (2014) HNO update. Vestibuläre Störungen. In: Iro H, Werner JA (eds) HNO update 2014 – Handbuch HNO 2014/2015. med update, Wiesbaden

Helling K (2015) HNO update. Vestibuläre Störungen. In: Iro H, Werner JA (eds) HNO update 2015 – Handbuch HNO 2015/2016. med update, Wiesbaden

Helling K, Halbach A, Schönfeld U, Scherer H, Clarke AH (2004) Funktionsstörungen von Sakkulus und Utrikulus beim Morbus Ménière – Verlaufsmessungen vor und nach Gentamicintherapie. Laryngorhinootologie 83. https://doi.org/10.1055/s-2004-823468

Helms J (1985) Die chirurgische Therapie des Morbus Menière. In: Verhandlungsbericht der Deutschen Gesellschaft für Hals-Nasen-Ohrenheilkunde. Arch Otorhinolaryngol Suppl 1:67–118

Herrmann C, Buss U (1994) Vorstellung und Validierung einer deutschen Version der Hospital Anxiety and Depression Scale (HAD-Skala), ein Fragebogen zur Erfassung des psychischen Befindens bei Patienten mit körperlichen Beschwerden. Diagnostica 40:143–154

Hesse G (2013) HNO update. Innenohrschwerhörigkeit, Tinnitus. In: Iro H, Werner JA (eds) HNO-update 2013. med update, Wiesbaden

Hesse G (Hg) (2015) Tinnitus. 2. Aufl. Thieme, Stuttgart

Hesse G, Schaaf H (2012) Hörtherapie. Ein Manual. Thieme, Stuttgart

Hillier SL, McDonnell M (2011) Vestibular rehabilitation for unilateral peripheral vestibular dysfunction. Cochrane Database Syst Rev (2):CD005397

Hillman TA, Chen DA, Arriaga MA (2004) Vestibular nerve section versus intratympanic gentamicin for Menière's disease. Laryngoscope 114(2):216–222

Hinchcliffe R (1967) Emotions as a precipitating factor in Menière's disease. J Laryngol Otol 81:471–475

Hoffmann SO (2008) Psychodynamische Therapie von Angststörungen. Einführung und Manual für die kurz- und mittelfristige Therapie. Schattauer, Stuttgart

Holmberg J, Karlberg M, Harlacher U, Magnusson M (2007) One-year follow-up of cognitive behavioral therapy for phobic postural vertigo. J Neurol 254:1189e92

Hong SK, Nam SW, Lee HJ (2013) Clinical observation on acute low-frequency hearing loss without vertigo: the role of cochlear hydrops analysis masking procedure as initial prognostic parameter. Ear Hear 34:229–235

House JW, Doherty JK, Fisher LM, Derebery MJ, Berliner KI (2006) Menière's disease: prevalence of contralateral ear involvement. Otol Neurotol 27:355–361

Huang TS (ed) (1991) Menière's disease: recent advances in basic and clinical aspects. Acta Otolaryngol Suppl 485:7–154

Huang CH, Young YH (2012) Ocular and cervical vestibular-evoked myogenic potentials in tumarkin falls. Otol Neurotol 33:1251–1256

Hülse M, Neuhuber W, Wolff HD (Hrsg) (2005) Die obere Halswirbelsäule, Pathophysiologie und Klinik. Springer, Heidelberg

Huon LK, Fang TY, Wang PC (2012) Outcomes of intratympanic gentamicin injection to treat Menière's disease. Otol Neurotol 33:706–714

Jacob RG, Woody SR, Clark DB (1993) Discomfort with space an motion: a possible marker of vestibular dysfunction by the situational characteristics questinoaire. J Psychopathol Behav Assess 15(4):299–325

Jahnke K (1977) Zur Pathogenese der akuten Symptome des Morbus Menière. Laryngorhinootologie 56:402–406

Jahnke K (1994) Stadiengerechte Therapie der Menièreschen Krankheit. Dtsch Arztebl 91:428–434

Jahnke K, Arweiler D (1997) Die intravenöse Gentamycintherapie bei beidseitigem M. Menière. Laryngorhinootologie 76:519–522
James AI, Burton MJ (2011) Betahistine for Menière's disease syndrome. Cochrane Database Syst Rev. https://doi.org/10.1002/14651858.CD001873
Junicho M, Aso S, Fujisaka M (2008) Prognosis of low-tone sudden deafness – does it inevitably progress to Menière's disease? Acta Otolaryngol 128(3):304–308
Kato M, Teranishi M, Katayama N, Sone M, Naganawa S, Nakashima T (2011) Association between endolymphatic hydrops as revealed by magnetic resonance imaging and caloric response. Otol Neurotol 32:1480–1485
Kempf HG, Jahnke K (1989) Lermoyez syndrome. Clinical aspects and follow-up. HNO 37:276–280
Kentala E, Havia M, Pyykko I (2001) Short-lasting drop attacks in Menière's disease. Otolaryngol Head Neck Surg 124:526–530
Kirby SE, Yardley L (2009) Cognitions associated with anxiety in Menière's disease. J Psychosom Res 66(2):111
Kitahara M (ed) (1990) Menière's disease. Springer, Berlin Heidelberg New York
Kitahara T, Horii A, Imai T, Ohta Y, Morihana T, Inohara H, Sakagami M (2014) Does endolymphatic sac decompression surgery prevent bilateral development of unilateral Ménière disease? Laryngoscope 124:1932–1936
Kocsis JH, Leon AC, Markowitz JC, Manber R, Arnow B, Klein DN, Thase ME (2009) Patient preference as a moderator of outcome for chronic forms of major depressive disorder treated with nefazodone, cognitive behavioral analysis system of psychotherapy, or their combination. J Clin Psychiatry (3):354–361. https://doi.org/10.4088/JCP.08m04371
Kraft R (1992) Das Schleifchen. Tinnitus Forum 4:89
Kurre A, van Gool CJ, Bastiaenen CH, Gloor-Juzi T, Straumann D, de Bruin ED (2009) Translation, cross-cultural adaptation and reliability of the German version of the dizziness handicap inventory. Otol Neurotol:1537–4505
Lahmann C, Henningsen P, Brandt T, Strupp M, Jahn K, Dieterich M, Eckhardt-Henn A, Feuerecker R, Dinkel A, Schmid G (2015) Psychiatric comorbidity and psychosocial impairment among patients with vertigo and dizziness. J Neurol Neurosurg Psychiatry. https://doi.org/10.1136/jnnp-2014-307601
Lamparter U (2002) Schwindel. In: Ahrens S, Schneider W (Hrsg) Lehrbuch der Psychotherapie und psychosomatischen Medizin, 2. Aufl. Schattauer, Stuttgart, S. 354–361
Landino A (1985) Zur Psychosomatik des Morbus Menière. Material Psychoanal 11:104–147
Lang J (2003) Anatomie des vestibulären Systems. In: Haid CT (Hrsg). aus interdisziplinärer Sicht. Thieme, Stuttgart, pp 4–16
Lange G (1977) Die intratympanale Behandlung des Morbus Menière mit ototoxischen Antibiotika. Laryngorhinotologie 56:409–411
Lange G (1995) 27 Jahre Erfahrung mit der transtympanalen Aminoglykosid-Behandlung des Morbus Menière. Laryngorhinootologie 74:720–723
Lange G (1998) Die Gentamicin-Injektionstechnik: Eine Vereinfachung der transtympanalen Therapie des Morbus Menière. HNO 46:1000–1002
Lange G, Mann W, Maurer J (2003) Intratympanale Intervalltherapie des Morbus Menière mit Gentamicin unter Erhalt der Cochleafunktion. HNO 51:898–902
Lehnhardt E (1984) Klinik der Innenohrschwerhörigkeiten: Tieftonschwerhörigkeit. Arch Otorhinolaryngol Suppl 1:58–218

Lempert T (1995) Benign positional vertigo: recognition and treatment. BMJ 311:489–491

Lempert T (2005) Schwindelattacken: Differenzialdiagnose und Therapie. Fortschr Neurol Psychiatr 10:605–620

Lempert T (2009) Vestibuläre Migräne. Nervenarzt 80:895–899

Lermoyez M (1919) Le vertige qui fait entendre. Presse Mèd 27:13

Levo H, Stephens D, Poe D (2010) Use of ICF in assessing the effects of Meniere's disorder on life. Ann Otol Rhinol Laryngol 119:583–589

Link R, Berendes J, Zöller F (Hrsg) (1980) Handbuch der HNO-Heilkunde, Bd III, Teil II. Thieme, Stuttgart

Löhle E (1980) Der Einfluss einer sechswöchigen Vitaminmangelernährung auf die Sinneszellen des Innenohrs. Z Ernährungswiss 19:203–214

Lopez-Escamez JA, Carey J, Chung WH, Goebel JA, Magnusson M, Mandalà M, Newman-Toker DE, Strupp M, Suzuki M, Trabalzini F, Bisdorff A (2015) Diagnostic criteria for Menière's disease. J Vestib Res 25(1):1–7. https://doi.org/10.3233/VES-150549

Löwe B, Spitzer RL, Zipfel S, Herzog W (2002) PHQ-D Gesundheitsbogen für Patienten. Manual Komplettversion und Kurzform, 2. Aufl. Pfizer, Karlsruhe

Luers JC, Hüttenbrink KB (2013) Akustische und vestibuläre Effekte bei einer Dehiszenz des oberen Bogengangs. HNO. https://doi.org/10.1007/s00106-013-2747-7

Lukas E (1997) Sehnsucht nach Sinn. Profil, München

Magnusson M, Padoan S, Karlberg M, Johansson R (1991) Delayed onset of ototoxic effects of gentamicin in patients with Menière's disease. Acta Otolaryngol Suppl 485:120–122

Mahoney A, Edelman S, Cremer P (2013) Cognitive behavior therapy for chronic subjective dizziness: longer-term gains and predictors of disability. Am J Otolaryngol 34(2):115–120

Manzari L, Burgess AM, Curthoys IS (2012) Vestibular function in Lermoyez syndrome at attack. Eur Arch Otorhinolaryngol 269:685–691

Marks I (1981) Space "phobia": a pseudo-agoraphobic syndrome: J Neurol Neurosurg Psychiatry. In: Arbeitskreis OPD (Hrsg) Operationalisierte Psychodynamische Diagnostik OPD-2 – Das Manual für Diagnose und Therapieplanung. Huber, Bern, S 44: 387–391

Martinez D (1972) The effect of Serc (betahistine hydrochloride) on the circulation of the inner ear in experimental animals. Acta Otolaryngol 305:29–47

McRackan TR, Best J, Pearce EC, Bennett ML, Dietrich M, Wanna GB, Haynes DS, Labadie RF (2014) Intratympanic dexamethasone as a symptomatic treatment for Ménière's disease. Otol Neurotol 35:1638–1640

Menière P (1861) Mémoire sur les lésions de l'oreille interne donnant lieu à des symptômes de congestion cérébrale apoplectiforme. Gaz Méd Paris Sér 16:597–601

Meyer zum Gottesberge A, Stupp H (1980) Menièresche Krankheit. In: Link R, Berendes J, Zöller F (Hrsg) Handbuch der HNO-Heilkunde, Bd III, Teil II. Kap. 38, S. 16. Thieme, Stuttgart

Michel O (1998) Morbus Menière und verwandte Gleichgewichtsstörungen. Thieme, Stuttgart – nicht mehr lieferbar

Modestin J (1983) Schwindel als psychosomatisches Phänomen. Psychother Psychosom Med Psychol 33:77–86

Moller MN, Caye-Tomasen P, Thomsen JH (2009) Vestibular nerve section in the treatment of morbus Menière. Ugeskr Laeger 171(12):1000–1003

Montandon PB, Häusler RJ, Kimura RS (1985) Treatment of endolymphatic hydrops with cochleosacculotomy. Clinical results and experimental findings. Otolaryngol Head Neck Surg 93:615–621

Morgenstern C (1985) Pathophysiologie, Klinik und konservative Therapie der Menièreschen Erkrankung. Arch Otorhinolaryngol 1:1–66
Morgenstern C (1994) Morbus Menière. In: Naumann HH, Helms J, Herberhold C, Kastenabuer C (Hrsg) Oto-Rhino-Laryngologie in Klinik und Praxis, Bd 1: Ohr. Thieme, Stuttgart, S. 768–775
Morrison AW, Bailey ME, Morrison GA (2009) Familial Menière's disease: clinical and genetic aspects. J Laryngol Otol 123(1):29–37
Mrowinski D, Scholz G, Krompaß S, Nubel K (1996) Diagnosis of endolymphatic hydrops by low-frequency masking. Audiol Neurootol 1:125–134
Nadol JB (ed) (1989) Menière's disease. Pathogenesis, pathophysiology, diagnosis and treatment. Kugler & Ghendi, The Hague
Naganuma H, Kawahara K, Tokumasu K, Okamoto M (2006) Water may cure patients with Menière disease. Laryngoscope 116(8):1455–1460
Neuhauser HK (2009) Epidemiologie von Schwindelerkrankungen. Nervenarzt 80:887–894
Nevoux J, Viengchareun S, Lema I, Lecoq AL, Ferrary E, Lombès M (2015) Glucocorticoids stimulate endolymphatic water reabsorption in inner ear through aquaporin 3 regulation. Pflugers Arch 467(9):1931–1943
Nguyen KD, Minor LB, Della Santina CC, Carey JP (2009) Time course of repeated intratympanic gentamicin for Menière's disease. Laryngoscope 119(4):792–798
Novoa E, Gärtner M, Henzen C (2014) Systemic effects of intratympanic dexamethasone therapy. Endocr Connect 3:127–131
Onuki J, Takahashi M, Odagiri K (2005) Comparative study of the daily lifestyle of patients with Menière's disease and controls. Ann Otol Rhinol Laryngol 114(12):927–933
Paparella MM (1991) Methods of diagnosis and treatment of Menière's disease. In: Huang TS (ed) Menière's disease: recent advances in basic and clinical aspects. Acta Otolaryngol Suppl 485: 108–119
Paparella MM (2006) Endolymphatic sac revision for recurrent intractable Menière's disease. Otolaryngol Clin N Am 4:713–721
Paparella MM, Djalilian HR (2002) Etiology, pathophysiology of symptoms, and pathogenesis of Menière's disease. Otolaryngol Clin N Am 35:529–545
Park JJ, Luedeke I, Luecke K, Emmerling O, Westhofen M (2013) Eustachian tube function in patients with inner ear disorders. Eur Arch Otorhinolaryngol 270:1615–1621
Patel M, Agarwal K, Arshad Q, Hariri M, Rea P, Seemungal BM, Golding JF, Harcourt JP, Bronstein AM (2016) Intratympanic methylprednisolone versus gentamicin in patients with unilateral Ménière's disease: a randomised, double-blind, comparative eff ectiveness trial. Lancet 388:2753–2762
Pawlow IP (1927) Conditioned reflexes. Claredon, London
Perez R, Chen JM, Nedzelski JM (2004) The status of the contralateral ear in established unilateral Menière's disease. Laryngoscope 114(8):1373–1376
Pfaltz CR (ed) (1986) Controversial aspects of Menière's disease. Thieme, Stuttgart
Phillips JS, Westerberg B (2011) Intratympanic steroids for Menière's disease or syndrome. Cochrane Database Syst Rev (7):CD008514
Plester D (1979) Morbus Menière. Therapiewoche 29:1334–1342
Plontke SK (2011) Evaluation of the round window niche before local drug delivery to the inner ear using a new mini-otoscope. Otol Neurotol 32:183–185
Plontke SK, Gürkov R (2015) Morbus Menière. Facharztwissen HNO. LRO 94:530–554

Plontke SK, Mynatt R, Gill RM (2007) Concentration gradient along the scala tympani after local application of gentamicin to the round window membrane. Laryngoscope 117:1191–1198

Popkirov S, Staab JP, Stone J (2018) Persistent postural-perceptual dizziness (PPPD): a common, characteristic and treatable cause of chronic dizziness. Pract Neurol 18:5–13

Portmann G (1927) The saccus endolymphaticus and an operation for draining the same for relief of vertigo. J Laryngol 42:809

Postema RJ, Kingma CM, Wit HP (2008) Intratympanic gentamicin therapy for control of vertigo in unilateral Menire's disease: a prospective, double-blind, randomized, placebo-controlled trial. Acta Otolaryngol 128(8):876–880

Praetorius C (1995) Krankheitserleben und Bewältigungsformen bei Morbus Menière-Patienten. Neuthor, Michelstadt

Preyer S, Bootz F (1995) Tinnitusmodelle zur Verwendung bei der Tinnituscounsellingtherapie des chronischen Tinnitus. HNO 43:338–351

Pullens B, van Benthem PP (2011) Intratympanic gentamicin for Menière's disease or syndrome. Cochrane Database Syst Rev (3):CD008234

Pullens B, Giard JL, Verschuur HP, van Benthem PP (2021) Surgery for Ménière's disease. Cochrane Database Syst Rev 2010 (1):CD005395. https://doi.org/10.1002/14651858.CD005395.pub2. Accessed 07 Feb 2021

Pyykkö I, Manchaiah V, Zou J, Levo H, Kentala E (2019) Association between Syncope and Tumarkin attacks in Ménière's disease. J Int Adv Otol 15(1):135–140

Quaglieri S, Gatti O, Rebecchi E, Manfrin M, Tinelli C, Mira E, Benazzo M (2014) Intratympanic gentamicin treatment 'as needed' for Meniere's disease. Long-term analysis using the Kaplan-Meier method. Eur Arch Otorhinolaryngol 271:1443–1449

Radeloff A, Hamad M, Baier G, Helms J, Hagen R, Shehata-Dieler W (2009) Die Saccotomie in der Behandlung des M. Menière: Beurteilung der kurz-, mittel- und langfristigen Ergebnisse anhand eines Patientenfragebogens. Laryngorhino Otol 88:653–659

Rah YC, Han JJ, Park J, Choi BY, Koo JW (2014) Management of intractable Menière's disease after intratympanic injection of gentamicin. Laryngoscope 125(4):972–978. https://doi.org/10.1002/lary.v125.4/issuetoc

Rask-Andersen H, Danckwardt-Lilliestrom N, Friberg U (1991) Lymphocyte-macrophage activity in the human endolymphatic sac. Acta Otolaryngol Suppl 485:15–17

Redon C, Lopez C, Bernard-Demanze L, Dumitrescu M, Magnan J, Lacour M, Borel L (2010) Betahistine treatment improves the recovery of static symptoms in patients with unilateral vestibular loss. J Clin Pharmacol 51(4):538–548. https://doi.org/10.1177/0091270010369241

Reinecker H (2012) Verhaltenstherapie. In: Senf W, Broda M (Hrsg) Praxis der Psychotherapie. Thieme, Stuttgart, pp 217–219

Reineke M (2002) Morbus Menière – Behandlungsmöglichkeiten aus rehabilitationspädagogischer Sicht. Diplomarbeit am Institut für Rehabilitationswissenschaften an der Humboldt-Universität zu Berlin, 104 S

Reiß M, Reiß G (2015) Gleichgewichtsdiagnostik. Videonystagmographie und neue Untersuchungsmethoden. Springer, Berlin Heidelberg

Ritter K (2003) Die Entwicklungsgeschichte des Innenohrs. In: Haid CT (Hrsg) Schwindel aus interdisziplinärer Sicht. Thieme, Stuttgart, pp 1–3

Ruckenstein M, Staab JP (2009) Chronic subjective dizziness. Otolaryngol Clin N Am 42(1):71–77

Rudack C (1995) Immunologie des Innenohres. Ein Überblick. HNO 43:275–281
Rüster P (1989) Psychosomatik und Psychopathologie von Morbus Menière. Diss. Universität Hamburg
Saliba I, Gabra N, Alzahrani M et al (2015) Endolymphatic duct blockage: a randomized controlled trial of a novel surgical technique for Menière's disease treatment. Otolaryngol Head Neck Surg 152(1):122–129
Salt AN, Plontke SK (2010) Endolymphatic hydrops: pathophysiology and experimental models. Otolaryngol Clin N Am 43(5):971–983
Salt AN, Gill RM, Plontke SK (2008) Dependence of hearing changes on the dose of intratympanically applied gentamicin: a meta-analysis using mathematical simulations of clinical drug delivery protocols. Laryngoscope 118:1793–1800
Sandhu JS, Low RH, Rea PA, Saunders NC (2012) Altered frequency dynamics of cervical and ocular vestibular evoked myogenic potentials in patients with Ménière's disease. Otol Neurotol 33:444–449
Savastano M, Maron MB, Mangialaio M, Longhi P, Rizzardo R (1996) Illness behaviour, personality traits, anxiety, and depression in patients with Menière's disease. J Otolaryngol:329–333
Savastano M, Guerrieri V, Marioni G (2006) Evolution of audiometric pattern in Menière's disease: long-term survey of 380 cases evaluated according to the 1995 guidelines of the American Academy of Otolaryngology-Head and Neck Surgery. J Otolaryngol 35(1):26–29
Savastano M, Marioni G, Aita M (2007) Psychological characteristics of patients with Menière's disease compared with patients with vertigo, tinnitus, or hearing loss. Ear Nose Throat 86(3):148–156
Schaaf H (2011) Psychotherapie bei Schwindelerkrankungen. 3. Aufl. Asanger, Kröning
Schaaf H, Haid C-T (2003) Reaktiver psychogener Schwindel bei M. Menière. Dtsch Arztebl 13:853–857
Schaaf H, Hesse G (2007) Sind rezidivierende Tiefton-Hörverluste – ohne Schwindel – die Vorstufe eines M. Menière? Eine Längsschnittuntersuchung nach 4 und nach 10 Jahren. HNO 55:630–637
Schaaf H, Hesse G (2011) Tinnitus: Leiden und Chance 3. Aufl. Profil, München: 112 S
Schaaf H, Hesse G (2012a) Hörtherapie manual. Thieme, Stuttgart
Schaaf H, Hesse G (2012b) Endolymphschwankungen: Stau im Höranteil – Turbulenten im Gleichgewichtsorgan. DTL, Wuppertal
Schaaf H, Hesse G (2015) Patients with long-lasting dizziness. A follow-up after neurotological and psychotherapeutic inpatient treatment after a period of at least one year. Eur Arch Oto-Rhino-Laryngol Head Neck. https://doi.org/10.1007/s00405-014-3447-y
Schaaf H, Holtmann H, Hesse G, Rienhoff N, Kolbe U et al (2000) Reactive psychogenic dizziness in Menière's disease. In: Sterkers O, Ferrary E, Daumann R, Sauvage JP, Tran Ba Huy R (eds) Menière's disease 1999 – update. Proceedings of the 4th international Symposium of Menière's disease in Paris, Kugler Publikcations, The Hague, pp 505–511
Scherer H (1997) Das Gleichgewicht, 2. akt. Aufl. Springer, Berlin Heidelberg New York
Schilder P (1942) The vestibular apparatus. In: Schilder P (ed) Mind, perception & thought in their constructive aspects. Columbia University Press, New York, pp 83–134
Schlegel M, Vibert D, Ott SR, Häusler R, Caversaccio MD (2012) Functional results and quality of life after retrosigmoid vestibular neurectomy in patients with Ménière's disease. Otol Neurotol 33:1380–1385

Schmerber S, Dumas G, Morel N, Chahine K, Karkas A (2009) Vestibular neurectomy vs. chemical labyrinthectomy in the treatment of disabling Menière's disease: a long-term comparative study. Auris Nasus Larynx 36(4):400–405

Schmid G, Henningsen P, Dieterich M, Sattel H, Lahmann C (2011) Psychotherapy in dizziness: a systematic review. J Neurol Neurosurg Psychiatry 82:601e606. https://doi.org/10.1136/jnnp.2010.237388

Schuknecht HF (1957) Ablation therapy in the management of Menière's disease. Acta Otolaryngol Suppl 132:1–42

Semont A, Freyss G, Vitte E (1988) Curing the BPPV with a liberatory maneuver. Adv Otorhinolaryngol 42:290–293

Shojaku H, Watanabe Y, Yagi T, Takahashi M, Takeda T, Ikezono T, Ito J, Kubo T, Suzuki M, Takumida M, Takeda N, Furuya N, Yamashita H (2009) Changes in the characteristics of definite Menière's disease over time in Japan: a long-term survey by the Peripheral Vestibular Disorder Research Committee of Japan, formerly the Menière's Disease Research Committee of Japan. Acta Otolaryngol 129(2):155–160

Silverstein H, Wazen J, Van Ess MJ (2010) Intratympanic gentamicin treatment of patients with Menière's disease with normal hearing. Otolaryngol Head Neck Surg 142(4):570–575

Soderman AC, Moller J, Bagger-Sjoback D (2004) Stress as a trigger of attacks in Menière's disease. A case-crossover study. Laryngoscope 114(10):1843–1848

Staab J (2006) Assessment and management; of psychological problems in the dizzy patient. Continuum:189–213

Staab J (2012) Chronic subjective dizziness. Continuum 18(5):1118–1141

Staab JP (2020) Persistent Postural-Perceptual Dizziness. Semin Neurol 40(1):130–137. https://doi.org/10.1055/s-0039-3402736

Staab JP, Eckhardt-Henn A, Horii A, Jacob R, Strupp M, Brandt T, Bronstein A (2017) Diagnostic criteria for persistent postural-perceptual dizziness (PPPD): consensus document of the Committee for the Classification of Vestibular Disorders of the Bárány Society. J Vestib Res 27(4):191–208. https://doi.org/10.3233/VES-170622. PMID: 29036855

Stephens D, Kentala E, Varpa K, Pyykko I (2007) Positive experiences associated with Menière's disorder. Otol Neurotol 14:1531–7129

Stokroos R, Kingma H (2004) Selective vestibular ablation by intratympanic gentamicin in patients with unilateral active Menière's disease: a prospective, double-blind, placebo-controlled, randomized clinical trial. Acta Otolaryngol 124(2):172–175

Stoll W, Most E, Tegenthoff M (Hrsg) (2004) Schwindel und Gleichgewichtsstörungen. 4. überarb. Aufl. Thieme, Stuttgart

Strupp M, Zingler VC, Arbusow V, Niklas D, Maag KP, Dieterich M, Bense S, Theil D, Jahn K, Brandt T (2004) Methylprednisolone, valacyclovir, or the combination for vestibular neuritis. N Engl J Med 351:354–361

Strupp M, Hupert D, Frenzel C, Wagner J, Hahn A, Jahn K, Zingler VC, Mansmann U, Brandt T (2008) Long-term prophylactic treatment of attacks of vertigo in Menière's disease-comparison of a high with a low dosage of betahistine in an open trial. Acta Otolaryngol 128(5):520–524

Takahama AJ, Volz-Sidiropoulou E, Ilgner J, Westhofen M (2008) Validierung der deutschsprachigen Version des "Dizziness Handicap Inventory" (DHI) zur Evaluation von Schwindelbeschwerden. http://www.egms.de/en/meetings/hnod2008/08hnod410.shtml

Takahashi M, Ishida K, Iida M, Yamashita H, Sugawara K (2001) Analysis of lifestyle and behavioral characteristics in Meniere's disease patients and a control population. Acta Otolaryngol 121(2):254–256

Taura A, Funabiki K, Ohgita H, Ogino E, Torii H, Matsunaga M, Ito J (2014) One-third of vertiginous episodes during the follow-up period are caused by benign paroxysmal positional vertigo in patients with Meniere's disease. Acta Otolaryngol 134(11):1140–1145. https://doi.org/10.3109/00016489.2014.936624
Teranishi M, Naganawa S, Katayama N (2009) Image evaluation of endolymphatic space in fluctuating hearing loss without vertigo. Eur Arch Otorhinolaryngol 266:1871–1877
Thomsen J, Bretlau P, Bretlau P, Tos M, Johnson NJ (1981) Placebo effect in the surgery of Menière's disease: a double blind, placebo-controlled study on endolymphatic sac surgery. Arch Otolaryngol 107:271–277
Thorp MA, Shehab ZP, Bance ML (2003) The AAO-HNS Committee on Hearing and Equilibrium guidelines for the diagnosis and evaluation of therapy in Menière's disease: have they been applied in the published literature of the last decade? Clin Otolaryngol 28(3):173–176
Trinidade A, Robinson T, Phillips JS (2014) The role of caffeine in otorhinolaryngology: guilty as charged? Eur Arch Otorhinolaryngo 271(8):2097–2102. https://doi.org/10.1007/s00405-013-2648-0
Trune DR (2006) Ion homeostasis and inner ear disease. In: Hamid M, Sismanis A (eds) Medical otology and neurotology: a clinical guide to auditory and vestibular disorders. Thieme Medical Publishers, New York
Tschan R, Best C, Beutel ME, Knebel A, Wiltink J, Dieterich M, Eckhardt-Henn A (2011) Patients' psychological well-being and resilient coping protect from secondary somatoform vertigo and dizziness (SVD) 1 year after vestibular disease. J Neurol 258(1):104–112
Tschan R, Eckhardt-Henn A, Scheurich V, Best C, Dieterich M, Beutel M (2012) Standfest? Erste Ergebnisse der Entwicklung eines kognitiv-verhaltenstherapeutischen Gruppenschulungsprogramms zur Behandlung des somatoformen Schwindels. Psychother Psychosom Med Psychol 62(3–4):111–119
Tullio P (1929) Das Ohr und die Entstehung der Sprache und Schrift. Urban & Schwarzenbeck, Berlin
Tumarkin L (1936) Otolithic catastrophe. A new syndrome. Br Med J 1:175–177
Tyrrell J, White MP, Barrett G, Ronan N, Phoenix C, Whinney DJ, Osborne NJ (2015) Mental health and subjective well-being of individuals with Ménière's: cross-sectional analysis in the UK Biobank. Otol Neurotol 36(5):854–861. https://doi.org/10.1097/MAO.0000000000000732
van Cruijsen N, Wit H, Albers F (2003) Psychological aspects of Menière's disease. Acta Otolaryngol 123(3):340–347
van Cruijsen N, Jaspers JP, van de Wiel HB (2006) Psychological assessment of patients with Menière's disease. Int J Audiol 45(9):496–502
van Esch BF, van Benthem PPG, van der Zaag-Loonen HJ, Bruintjes TD (2016) Two common second causes of dizziness in patients with Menière's disease. Otol Neurotol 37:1620–1624
van Sonsbeek S, Pullens B, van Benthem P (2015) Positive pressure therapy for Menière's disease or syndrome. Cochrane Database Syst Rev (3): CD008419. https://doi.org/10.1002/14651858.CD008419.pub2
Vesterhauge S, Katholm M, Mikines P (eds) (1996) Menière's disease. 16. Danavox Symposium, Kolding
Viana LM, Bahmad F, Rauch SD (2014) Intratympanic gentamicin as a treatment for drop attacks in patientes with meniere's disease. Laryngoscope 124:2151–2154
von Weizsäcker V (1956) Pathosophie. Vandenhoeck & Ruprecht, Göttingen
Vosteen KH (ed) (1981) Menière's disease. International symposium Düsseldorf. Thieme, Stuttgart

Waldfahrer F (2014) Fahreignung bei Schwindel und Gleichgewichtsstörungen. HNO 3:155–157

Walther LE (2005) Gestörtes Gleichgewicht: Wiederherstellende Verfahren bei gestörtem Gleichgewicht. Laryngo-Rhino-Otol 84: 70–98 und http://www.thieme-connect.de/ejournals/abstract/lro/doi/10.1055/s-2005-861144

Walther LE, Cebulla M (2015) Frequenzdynamische Analyse der Otolithenfunktion mittels vestibulär evozierter myogener Potenziale (VEMP). Laryngo-Rhino-Otol 94:153–155

Walther LE, Hörmann K, Pfaar O (2010) Die Ableitung zervikaler und okulärer vestibulär evozierter myogener Potentiale. Teil 1. HNO:1031–1045

Walther LE, Schaaf H, Sommer D, Hörmann K (2011) Luftleitungsinduzierte oculäre VEMP I. Methodik und Untersuchungen bei normalen Probanden. Laryngo-Rhino-Otol 90:410–415

Walther LE, Hörmann K, Blochin M, Blödow A (2012) Rezeptorfunktion der Bogengänge Teil 1: Anatomie, Physiologie, Diagnostik und Normalbefunde. HNO 60:75–88

Wang D, Wang Z (1997) Regeneration and functional restoration of vestibular hair cells in guinea pigs after gentamicin damage. Zhonghua Er Bi Yan Hou Ke Za Zhi 32:153–156

Weikert S, Rotter A, Scherer H, Hoelzl M (2008) Picrotoxin in der Therapie des Morbus Menière. Laryngorhinootologie 87(12):862–866

Westhofen M (2008) Die operative Therapie des vestibulären Schwindels. Verfahren und Indikationen. HNO 56:1003–1010

Westhofen M (2009) M. Menière. Evidenzen und Kontroversen. HNO 57:446–454

Westhofen M (2013) Indikation und Erfolge der operativen Therapie des vestibulären Schwindels. HNO 61:752–761

Wexler M, Crary W (1986) Menière's disease: the psychosomatic hypothesis. Am J Otol 7:93–96

Wilson WR, Byl FM, Laird N (1980) The efficacy of steroids in the treatment of idiopathic sudden hearing loss. Arch Otolaryngol 106:772–776

Wirth W (2000) Psychologische Möglichkeiten bei Schwindel. Tinnitus-Forum 4/2000

Wladislavosky-Wasserman P, Facer GW, Mokri B (1984) Menière's disease: a 30–year epidemiologic and clinical study in Rochester, Mn, 1951–1980. Laryngoscope 94:1098–1102

Wolpe J (1958) Psychotherapy by reciprocal inhibition. Stanford University Press, Palo Alto

Yamakawa K (1938) Über pathologische Veränderungen bei einem Menière Kranken. J Otolaryngol Soc Jpn 4:2310–2312

Yamasoba T, Kikuchi S, Sugaswa M, Yagi M, Harada T (1994) Acute low-tone sensorineural hearing loss without vertigo. Arch Otololaryngol Head Neck Surg 120:532–535

Yardley L, Kirby S (2006) Evaluation of booklet-based self-management of symptoms in Menière disease: a randomized controlled trial. Psychosom Med 68(5):762–769

Yardley L, Beech S, Weinman J (2001) Influence of beliefs about the consequences of dizziness on handicap in people with dizziness, and the effect of therapy on beliefs. J Psychosom Res 50(1):1–6

Yoda S, Cureoglu S, Shimizu S, Morita N, Fukushima H, Sato T, Harada T, Paparella MM (2011) Round window membrane in Ménière's disease: a human temporal bone study. Otol Neurotol 32:147–151

Zenner HP (1989) Pathological motility and depolarisation of outer hair cells. Basic steps in K+ induced attacks of Menière's disease. In: Nadol JB (ed) Menière's disease. Pathogenesis, pathophysiology, diagnosis and treatment. Kugler & Ghendi, Amsterdam, pp 247–252
Zenner HP (1994) Hören. Physiologie, Biochemie, Zell- und Neurobiologie. Thieme, Stuttgart, S. 168

Index

A

Acetylsalicylic acid (ASS) 135
Acoustic neuroma 108, 132, 275
Acupuncture 243
Acute therapy 115, 187–192, 258, 266
Adaptation 14, 56, 64, 77, 111, 124
Afferent 21, 24, 34, 51, 64, 110, 123–125, 205, 276
Alcohol 110, 130, 131, 135, 137, 149, 150, 218, 251
Alternative therapy 242
Aminoglycosides 135, 136, 204, 275
Ampoule of the semicircular canal 190
Anticipatory anxiety 229
Antidepressants 14, 74, 104, 135, 136, 187, 217, 238, 239
Antiemetics 187, 188, 190, 266, 275
Anxiety disorder 13, 14, 61, 64, 74, 121–123, 172, 174
Anxiety with vertigo 19, 128, 267
Auditory nerve 34, 62, 63, 166, 200, 211, 212, 275
– sensitive 62–63
Autogenic training 259
Avoidance behaviour 64, 65, 71, 74, 77, 97, 128, 129, 236

B

Balance diary 185, 195
Balance disorder 105, 123, 129, 134, 137, 213
Balance exercises 66, 97, 110–111, 195, 196, 198
Balance, mental 43, 119
Balance training 13, 109–111, 113, 195, 196, 198, 212, 229, 230, 239, 240, 252, 266
Basilar membrane 30, 33, 57, 58, 62, 166, 167
Beta blocker 104, 135, 136
Betahistine 184, 194, 203, 214–219
Blocking 52, 134
Blood pressure fluctuations 13, 95, 131
Bonding, secure 43
Brainstem Electric Response Audiometry (BERA) 132, 167, 275

C

Caloric testing 101, 103, 108, 152, 176, 268
Carbamazepine 117
Cervical nystagmus 134
Cochlea 26, 29–34, 49, 52, 53, 57, 60, 62, 66, 87, 96, 97, 99, 108, 156, 162, 166, 200, 204, 205, 211, 215, 252, 253, 265, 266, 275
Cochleaimplant 66, 252, 253, 266
Cochleosacculotomy 212, 213
Conditioning, classical 63, 68–70
Cortisone
– intratympanic 187–189, 194, 201, 203
– side effects 189
Counselling 14, 181–187
Cover membrane 61
Cupula 25, 26, 32, 35, 38

D

Deafness 57, 61, 187, 210, 223, 260, 266
Deafness, bilateral 270
Depression 14, 73–76, 94, 103, 119, 121, 122, 172–174, 227, 238, 239, 241, 242
Desensitization 97, 229–237
Diagnostic criteria 4, 5, 64, 127
Diazepam 188, 190, 191, 238, 269
Dimenhydrinate 109, 188, 190–192, 214
Diuretics 135, 136, 168, 194, 218, 219
Dizziness, constant 9
Dizziness, psychogenic 8–10
Doctor–patient relationship 183–187
Driving ability 267
Drug side effect 190
Dysacusis 8, 57–58

E

Efference 122
Electrocochleography 101, 166, 167, 276
Endolymph 5, 25–28, 31, 33, 50–53, 55, 57, 96, 99, 100, 105, 114, 116, 154, 157, 167–169, 188, 205, 218, 219, 221, 222, 225, 276
Endolymphatic congestion 100, 107, 166–169
Endolymphatic sinus 28
Endolymph fluctuations 114
Enlightenment 97, 181–187, 257–258
Exercises, therapeutic 58

F

Failure nystagmus 55, 86, 207, 208
Fall prevention 252
Fear 2, 5, 9, 13, 42–44, 64, 65, 67–73, 77, 79–81, 97, 99, 109, 111, 112, 118, 119, 122–125, 128, 129, 187, 195, 196, 209, 230–232, 234–236, 238, 239, 256, 259, 265
Fear of annihilation 93
Feeling of pressure 6, 8, 62–63, 96, 134
Feldenkrais method 197

Frenzel glasses 78, 152, 153
Frequency of illness 147

G

Gaze direction nystagmus 149
Gentamycin 7, 11, 61, 132, 135–137, 160, 198, 201–210, 212, 213, 224, 251, 253, 259, 267
Gentamycin, intratympanic 87, 187, 201, 202, 204

H

Hair cells
– internal 29, 33, 60, 62
– outer 29, 58, 60, 62, 166, 277
– poisoning 57
Head impulse test 56, 108, 144, 151–152, 154, 162
Hearing aid 8, 66, 165, 199, 240, 269, 270
Hearing centre 29, 30, 167
Hearing impairment 8, 61, 62, 92, 96–98, 107, 112, 136, 148, 164, 206, 210
Hearing loss 2–8, 13, 19, 54, 57, 58, 62, 63, 66, 75, 76, 92–95, 97, 99–102, 104, 106, 112, 113, 117, 135, 136, 143, 145, 162–166, 169, 175, 176, 181, 182, 187, 189, 191, 192, 198–201, 204, 208, 210, 213, 214, 240, 241, 250, 253, 256, 265, 266, 269, 270
Hearing test 78, 100, 115, 144–146, 162–168, 257
Hearing training 199–200
Homeopathy 243
Hydrops, endolymphatic 19–21, 49, 51, 52, 61, 96, 164, 166–169, 189, 211, 212, 215, 221, 222, 265, 276

I

Incapacity for work 172, 210
Infusion therapy 188
Inheritability 50, 269
Inhibition, double 63–66, 124
Inner ear 3, 9, 12–13, 19, 21, 28, 30–32, 44, 49–55, 58, 60, 73, 77, 78, 81, 87, 92, 96, 97, 101, 107, 108, 113, 115, 116, 118, 135, 136, 144, 145, 148, 162–164, 166–169, 182, 188, 189, 192, 198, 200, 203–213, 215, 218, 220–222, 225, 226, 232, 240, 256, 258–260, 265, 266
Inner ear processes 12–13
Irritable nystagmus 80

L

Lability, vegetative 121
Labyrinth anaesthesia 225–226
Labyrinth damage 53
Lermoyez syndrome 86
Lips reading training 253
Loss of balance 7, 53, 65, 66, 97, 107–110, 112, 113, 125, 155, 187, 196, 198, 212, 251, 261, 266, 268
Loss of function 51, 52, 56, 110, 143, 157, 182, 203, 251

M

Macular organs 23
Magnetic resonance imaging 129, 168
Medical history 100, 103, 132, 144–147, 149, 169, 170, 172, 230, 243, 277
Meniere, Prosper 4, 107, 256
Migraine 4, 7, 13, 74, 86, 87, 92, 97, 101–105, 124, 126, 143, 145, 147, 169, 180, 181, 187, 203, 257, 259, 261, 267
Migraine aura 102, 103
Migraine dizziness 102
Multiple sclerosis 129, 130
Mumps infection 50
Muscle relaxation according to Jacobsen 63, 104, 226–227

N

Neurectomy 182, 187, 207, 210–213, 259, 267, 277
Neurofeedback procedures 198
Noise sensitivity 58–59
Nystagmus
– direction 149, 158, 159
– optokinetic 36–37
– vestibulo-okulaer,

O

Organ of Corti 29, 33–34, 58, 277
Ossicles 28, 31
Otitis media 62
Otolith dysfunction 117–118
Otoliths 23, 32, 33, 86, 94, 105, 107, 278
Otosclerosis 164

P

Pentoxifylline 189
Perilymph 25–28, 32–34, 50–53, 55, 113, 202, 205
Perilymph fistula 4, 98, 113–116, 143, 167, 203
Picrotoxin 219
Positional manoeuvre 97
Positional vertigo, benign paroxysmal 7, 92–94, 97, 105–107, 112, 134, 145, 149, 152, 181, 216

Potassium poisoning 55, 57
Pregnancy 190–191, 214, 269
Pressure pulse generator 221
Progressive muscle relaxation according to Jacobsen 63, 100, 101, 188, 226, 232
Psychotherapy 95, 97, 183, 227, 228, 237, 239, 240, 242
Psychotropic drugs 150, 238–239
Pure tone audiogram 162–165, 167

Q

Questionnaires 175, 241
Quinidine 135, 136
Quinine 135, 136

R

Reduction of stimulants 218
Reflex, vestibulo-ocular 34–36, 56, 86, 108, 149–152, 268, 280
Reissner membrane 51, 205
Relationship 9, 77, 183, 184, 186, 187, 205, 219, 228, 237
Reset movements 36
Resilience 125, 236
Romberg test 147, 148
Rotational vertigo 6, 67, 102, 107, 143

S

Saccades 36, 37, 39, 66, 149–153
Saccotomy 194, 222, 223, 225, 251, 279
Saccule 22–24, 31, 32, 34, 39, 86, 116, 117, 155–157, 160, 169, 204, 279
Sacculus 22, 26, 28, 31, 33, 49, 53, 86, 108, 116, 155–158, 160, 204
Saccus endolymphaticus 19, 27–28, 32, 49–50, 52, 222, 225, 265, 279
Security 9, 43, 67, 77, 183, 184, 190, 191, 229
Self-help 12, 183, 186, 187, 202, 257, 270
Semicircular canals 24–27, 31, 32, 34, 35, 38, 39, 41, 42, 53, 64, 94, 98, 105, 107, 108, 113–115, 117, 151–155, 157, 159, 203, 279
Sound conduction disorder 164
Sound sensory disorder,
Speech audiogram 165
Spinning attacks 2, 105, 256
Spontaneous nystagmus 102, 149, 152
Stapedius reflex 58
Stimulus generalization 68, 70

T

Tai Chi 198
Therapist 11, 170, 183, 185, 186, 228, 230–232, 234–237, 256–262
Thiethylperazine,
Tinnitus 2–6, 8, 12, 14, 19, 59–62, 66, 68, 75, 76, 92, 93, 95–102, 106, 113, 117, 135, 136, 143, 165, 166, 189, 199–201, 226, 240, 241, 250, 256, 265, 270, 279
Trigger 10, 52–53, 62, 68–70, 79, 80, 113, 119, 125, 183, 214, 230, 231, 268, 280
Tullio phenomenon 31, 116
Tumarkin drop 86–87, 145
Tympanostomy tube 98, 221, 222

U

Unterberger pedal test 147–148
Utricle 22–24, 26, 28, 31, 32, 34, 39, 49, 51, 53, 86, 94, 105, 107–109, 112, 117, 118, 155, 156, 158–162, 188, 204, 280
Utriculus 22, 32, 49, 53

V

Vehicle use, private 267
Vertigo
– chronic, subjective 241
– psychogenic 2, 4, 13, 67–81, 92, 94, 95, 112, 118, 120, 121, 126, 144, 192, 213, 214, 259
– psychosomatic 12
Vestibular cores 41, 63, 103
Vestibular nerve 25, 34, 51, 63, 108, 116, 117, 155, 156, 187, 188, 207, 210–213, 259
Vestibular neuritis 7, 97, 107–113, 119, 124, 152
Vestibular organ 3, 7, 19, 21–28, 31–33, 35, 36, 39, 42, 51, 53, 54, 56, 64, 66, 73, 79, 86, 94, 96, 105, 107, 108, 110, 111, 113, 116, 120, 124, 133, 134, 136, 147–149, 152–154, 158, 162, 181, 202–204, 207, 208, 210, 211, 214, 238, 239, 251, 252, 261, 267
Vestibular paroxysm 4, 116–117, 143
Video oculography 102, 154, 158, 161
Vitamins 220

W

Work ability 11, 226

FSC
www.fsc.org
MIX
Papier aus verantwortungsvollen Quellen
Paper from responsible sources
FSC® C105338

If you have any concerns about our products,
you can contact us on
ProductSafety@springernature.com

In case Publisher is established outside the EU,
the EU authorized representative is:
Springer Nature Customer Service Center GmbH
Europaplatz 3, 69115 Heidelberg, Germany

Printed by Libri Plureos GmbH
in Hamburg, Germany